Practical Applications for the Occupational Therapy Code of Ethics and Ethics Standards

Practical Applications for the Occupational Therapy Code of Ethics and Ethics Standards

Janie B. Scott, MA, OT/L, FAOTA, and
S. Maggie Reitz, PhD, OTR/L, FAOTA, Editors

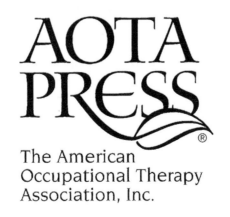

AOTA PRESS

The American
Occupational Therapy
Association, Inc.

AOTA Centennial Vision
We envision that occupational therapy is a powerful, widely recognized, science-driven, and evidence-based profession with a globally connected and diverse workforce meeting society's occupational needs.

Mission Statement
The American Occupational Therapy Association advances the quality, availability, use, and support of occupational therapy through standard-setting, advocacy, education, and research on behalf of its members and the public.

AOTA Staff
Frederick P. Somers, *Executive Director*
Christopher M. Bluhm, *Chief Operating Officer*

Chris Davis, *Director, AOTA Press*
K. Hyde Loomis, *Production Consultant*
Ashley Hofmann, *Development/Production Editor*
Victoria Davis, *Digital/Production Editor*

Beth Ledford, *Director, Marketing*
Amanda F. Fogle, *Marketing Specialist*
Jennifer Folden, *Marketing Specialist*

American Occupational Therapy Association, Inc.
4720 Montgomery Lane
Bethesda, MD 20814
Phone: 301-652-AOTA (2682)
TDD: 800-377-8555
Fax: 301-652-7711
www.aota.org
To order: 1-877-404-AOTA or store.aota.org

Disclaimers
This publication is designed to provide accurate and authoritative information in regard to the subject matter covered. It is sold or distributed with the understanding that the publisher is not engaged in rendering legal, accounting, or other professional service. If legal advice or other expert assistance is required, the services of a competent professional person should be sought.
—*From the Declaration of Principles jointly adopted by the American Bar Association and a Committee of Publishers and Associations*

It is the objective of the American Occupational Therapy Association to be a forum for free expression and interchange of ideas. The opinions expressed by the contributors to this work are their own and not necessarily those of the American Occupational Therapy Association.

ISBN: 978-1-56900-309-1

Library of Congress Control Number: 2012949748

Cover Design by Naylor Design, Inc., Washington, DC
Composition by Manila Typesetting Company, Guadalupe Makati City, Philippines
Printed by Automated Graphic Systems, Inc., White Plains, MD

Contents

Introduction ix
Janie B. Scott, MA, OT/L, FAOTA, and S. Maggie Reitz, PhD, OTR/L, FAOTA

Glossary xix

About the Editors xxv

About the Authors xxvii

Part I. Foundations
Introduction 3
Janie B. Scott, MA, OT/L, FAOTA

Chapter 1. Historical Background of Ethics in Occupational Therapy 5
S. Maggie Reitz, PhD, OTR/L, FAOTA, and Janie B. Scott, MA, OT/L, FAOTA

Chapter 2. Promoting Ethics in Occupational Therapy Practice:
Codes and Consequences 15
Janie B. Scott, MA, OT/L, FAOTA, and S. Maggie Reitz, PhD, OTR/L, FAOTA

Part II. Principles
Introduction 35
Janie B. Scott, MA, OT/L, FAOTA

Chapter 3. Principle 1: Beneficence 37
Janie B. Scott, MA, OT/L, FAOTA, and Dana Burns, MS, OTR/L, CBIS

Chapter 4. Principle 2: Nonmaleficence 45
  S. Maggie Reitz, PhD, OTR/L, FAOTA

Chapter 5. Principle 3: Autonomy and Confidentiality 55
  Janie B. Scott, MA, OT/L, FAOTA

Chapter 6. Principle 4: Social Justice 65
  S. Maggie Reitz, PhD, OTR/L, FAOTA, and Stacey Harcum, MS, OTR/L, CBIS

Chapter 7. Principle 5: Procedural Justice 77
  Janie B. Scott, MA, OT/L, FAOTA

Chapter 8. Principle 6: Veracity 87
  Janie B. Scott, MA, OT/L, FAOTA

Chapter 9. Principle 7: Fidelity 97
  S. Maggie Reitz, PhD, OTR/L, FAOTA

Part III. Models
  Introduction 107
  Janie B. Scott, MA, OT/L, FAOTA

Chapter 10. Solving Ethical Dilemmas 109
  Janie B. Scott, MA, OT/L, FAOTA

Part IV. Applications
  Introduction 121
  Janie B. Scott, MA, OT/L, FAOTA, and S. Maggie Reitz, PhD, OTR/L, FAOTA

Chapter 11. Ethics in Diverse Mental Health Settings 123
  *Susan Haiman, MPS, OTR/L, FAOTA, and Deborah Yarett Slater,
  MS, OT/L, FAOTA*

Chapter 12. Productive Aging 137
  Janie B. Scott, MA, OT/L, FAOTA

**Chapter 13. Children and Youth: Ethics in Service Provision
    Across Contexts** 149
  Susanne Smith Roley, OTD, OTR/L, FAOTA, and Mary Alice Singer, MA, OTR/L

Chapter 14. Ethics in Health Promotion and Wellness 161
  S. Maggie Reitz, PhD, OTR/L, FAOTA

**Chapter 15. Work and Industry: Ethical Considerations in Designing
    an Injury Prevention Program** 169
  Jeff Snodgrass, PhD, MPH, OTR/L

Chapter 16. Participation, Disability, and Rehabilitation 177
Barbara L. Kornblau, JD, OTR, FAOTA

Chapter 17. Administration and Private Practice 189
Tammy Richmond, MS, OTR/L, FAOTA

Chapter 18. Application of Ethics in Higher Education 205
Linda S. Gabriel, PhD, OTR/L

Chapter 19. Ethics in Occupational Therapy Research 215
Elizabeth Larson, PhD, OTR

**Chapter 20. Internal Relationships: Ethical Issues
Within Institutions** 231
S. Maggie Reitz, PhD, OTR/L, FAOTA

**Chapter 21. External Relationships: Ethical Issues in Interactions
Among Institutions** 241
Marian K. Scheinholtz, MS, OT/L, and Janie B. Scott, MA, OT/L, FAOTA

Appendixes
A. *Occupational Therapy Code of Ethics and Ethics Standards (2010)* 255
B. Enforcement Procedures for the *Occupational Therapy Code
    of Ethics and Ethics Standards (2010)* 265
C. Scope of Practice 277
D. *NBCOT® Candidate/Certificant Code of Conduct* 285
E. Procedures for the Enforcement of the *NBCOT® Candidate/Certificant
    Code of Conduct* 287
F. Occupational Therapy Profession—Continuing Competence Requirements 293
G. Ethics Resources 299

Index 301

Introduction

Janie B. Scott, MA, OT/L, FAOTA, and
S. Maggie Reitz, PhD, OTR/L, FAOTA

Practical Applications for the Occupational Therapy Code of Ethics and Ethics Standards was developed to provide occupational therapy practitioners with a resource containing practical case studies to help promote ethical reflection and practice in their increasingly complex and varied professional roles. The following definition of *occupational therapy practice,* developed by the American Occupational Therapy Association (AOTA) to describe occupational therapy to state boards of practice and external entities, clearly highlights the profession's wide-ranging scope and settings:

> The practice of occupational therapy means the therapeutic use of occupations, including everyday life activities with individuals, groups, populations, or organizations to support participation, performance, and function in roles and situations in home, school, workplace, community, and other settings. Occupational therapy services are provided for habilitation, rehabilitation, and the promotion of health and wellness to those who have or are at risk for developing an illness, injury, disease, disorder, condition, impairment, disability, activity limitation, or participation restriction. Occupational therapy addresses the physical, cognitive, psychosocial, sensory–perceptual, and other aspects of performance in a variety of contexts and environments to support engagement in occupations that affect physical and mental health, well-being, and quality of life. (AOTA, 2011, p. S81)

This definition identifies various client groups and settings in which occupational therapy services are delivered. However, the definition does not specifically address the roles of occupational therapy practitioners relative to education, research, advocacy, or volunteerism. The principles articulated in the *Occupational Therapy Code of Ethics and Ethics Standards (2010),* developed by AOTA and most recently revised in 2010 (referred to throughout this book as the "Code and Ethics Standards"), can be used to guide the behaviors and ethical decision making of occupational therapy practitioners in their many roles.

PURPOSES AND GOALS OF THE BOOK

Through this book, occupational therapy practitioners and students have a resource to use in exploring the Code and Ethics Standards to promote ethical reflection and practice in their increasingly complex and varied professional roles. The phrase *occupational therapy practitioner* is used throughout the book to refer to both occupational therapists and occupational therapy assistants. The authors present models and approaches to help readers resolve ethical dilemmas and provide realistic case studies and vignettes to assist practitioners in identifying solutions that range from taking no action or addressing the situation at the local level to involving organizations and agencies to promote ethical practice and protect the public and the profession.

Occupational therapy practitioners fulfill a wide variety of roles, including those of educator, practitioner, consultant, policymaker, advocate, researcher, and volunteer. Ethical dilemmas may arise in any of these roles and across the many contexts in which occupational therapy is practiced. Practitioners can use the principles articulated in the Code and Ethics Standards as a guide for their behaviors and ethical decision making in their many roles and contexts. The overarching goal of this book is to help occupational therapy practitioners and students strive toward the aspirational principles articulated in the Code and Ethics Standards.

CONTENT

This book is divided into four parts. Part I reviews the historical and current foundations for ethical decision making in occupational therapy, Part II discusses the seven principles in the Code and Ethics Standards, Part III describes models for ethical reasoning, and Part IV illustrates applications of ethical reasoning in practice. The first three sections provide the foundation on which to base an understanding of the materials presented in the final section.

Although case studies and vignettes appear primarily in chapters in Part IV (Applications), they also are woven throughout chapters in Part II (Principles). The authors developed their case studies and vignettes on the basis of their experiences as occupational therapy practitioners. They wrote in their own unique voice to help you appreciate the ethical dilemmas that arise in diverse settings and the strategies they have developed to seek good ethical outcomes. In general, the authors describe more complex ethical situations and provide more detail in the case studies than in the vignettes.

Part IV includes chapters on each of the six areas of practice linked to AOTA's *Centennial Vision* (AOTA, 2007). In addition, chapters are included on administration and private practice, education, research, and internal and external institutional relationships. The various case studies and vignettes that appear in this book are listed in Table I.1. From this table, readers can see where specific principles, settings, or populations are addressed.

The chapters emphasize a variety of important themes, including

- Adherence to the Code and Ethics Standards, Accreditation Council for Occupational Therapy Education (2012) standards, and state regulations;
- Support of occupational therapy students' academic education and professional development for ethical practice;
- Fulfillment of state regulatory requirements;
- Promotion of occupational therapy practitioners' ethical reasoning and decision making through continuing education; and
- Compliance with continuing education mandates.

We selected the authors of this book on the basis of their expertise in the subject areas associated with their respective chapters. In Parts II and IV, the authors first introduce a principle or practice area (e.g., research, education) and then discuss the practical application of ethics. The authors approach their assigned ethics topic on the basis of the method best suited to sharing ethical issues in that particular practice area. The authors also include either one central case study or several smaller case studies and vignettes to ensure a common thread of practical application. A glossary, a list of pertinent Web and print resources, and appendixes with ethics-related documents by AOTA and the National Board for Certification in Occupational Therapy also are included. The Code and Ethics Standards are reprinted in Appendix A; consult this and other documents as needed during your progress through this book.

TABLE I.1
Case Studies and Vignettes and the Principles and Populations Covered in Each

CHAPTER	CASE STUDIES AND VIGNETTES	PRINCIPLES COVERED	POPULATIONS AND SETTINGS ADDRESSED
Part II: Principles			
3. Principle 1: Beneficence	Vignette 3.1. Using Expertise to Benefit Clients	1G	Private and community practice
	Case Study 3.1. Developing Competence in Novice Practitioners	1E	Home care
	Case Study 3.2. Using Assessments Appropriately	1B, 1C	Acute care
4. Principle 2: Nonmalefi-cence	Case Study 4.1. Avoiding Exploitation	2A, 2C, 2E, 2G	Hospital Employee relationship
	Vignette 4.1. Preventing Academic Dishonesty	2A, 2C, 2E, 2G	Academia
	Vignette 4.2. Avoiding Potential Harm to Colleagues	2A, 2E, 2G	Skilled nursing
	Vignette 4.3. Analyzing Risks and Benefits in Research	2A, 2L	Community-dwelling older adults Students
	Case Study 4.2. Engaging in Self-Reflection and Mindfulness to Avoid Harm When Making Decisions	2I	Skilled nursing
	Vignette 4.4. Avoiding Conflict of Interest	2I 7E	Professional association
	Vignette 4.5. Avoiding Undue Influences	2E, 2F	Professional conference Distance teaching
	Vignette 4.6. Preventing Conflict of Commitment	2E, 2H	Academia
5. Principle 3: Autonomy and Confidentiality	Vignette 5.1. Maintaining Confidentiality in Testimony	3G, 3H 5C, 5D	Work rehabilitation
	Case Study 5.1. Addressing an Inadvertent Violation of Confidentiality	1M 2A, 2E, 2F 3H, 3J 5D 6E 7B	Public restaurant
	Case Study 5.2. Exploring Health Communication Across Cultures	2K 3I 4F	Community center Hispanic community
	Vignette 5.2. Obtaining Consent for Consultation	3B, 3G	Children and youth Assistive technology
	Vignette 5.3. Balancing Autonomy and Collaboration	3A, 3B	Community practice Older adults

(continued)

TABLE I.1 *(cont.)*

CHAPTER	CASE STUDIES AND VIGNETTES	PRINCIPLES COVERED	POPULATIONS AND SETTINGS ADDRESSED
6. Principle 4: Social Justice	Vignette 6.1. Supporting a Return to Roles and Benefit to the Community	4A, 4B, 4C, 4D, 4E 5A, 5C	Community Leisure Return to work
	Vignette 6.2. Ensuring Respect and Fairness During Intervention	1 2 3 4 5 7	Inpatient, acute care
	Case Study 6.1. Promoting Access to Services	1 4 5 7	Outpatient Older adults
	Vignette 6.3. Extending Services to Underserved Populations	1 2 3I 4	Community nonprofit Asian immigrants
	Vignette 6.4. Promoting Occupational Justice Following a Disaster	4A, 4C, 4E	Community Disaster survivors
	Vignette 6.5. Gaining Competency Before a Disaster	1E, 1G 2 4	Community Disaster survivors
7. Principle 5: Procedural Justice	Case Study 7.1. Addressing a Failure to Maintain Credentials	5E, 5G 6A, 6B	Return to work Older adults
	Vignette 7.1. Fulfilling the Duty to Inform Others	5B, 5G, 5H	Hospital Occupational therapy assistant supervision
	Vignette 7.2. Complying With Institutional Regulations	5A, 5L, 5N 6B, 6C, 6D	Facility Individuals with developmental disabilities
	Vignette 7.3. Addressing Failure to Provide Adequate Supervision	5B, 5G, 5H 7C	Academia Occupational therapy students
	Vignette 7.4. Addressing Failure to Maintain Ethical Principles in Private Practice	1 5H, 5P	Private practice Children and youth Fieldwork students
8. Principle 6: Veracity	Case Study 8.1. Exhibiting Moral Courage to Address a Lack of Veracity	6A, 6B, 6E	Long-term care Subacute Private practice

(continued)

TABLE I.1 *(cont.)*

Chapter	Case Studies and Vignettes	Principles Covered	Populations and Settings Addressed
	Case Study 8.2. Improving Veracity in Client Communication	1H 3A, 3B, 3J	Outpatient hand rehabilitation Adults
	Vignette 8.1. Ensuring Veracity in Multiple Roles	6B, 6D, 6F	Pediatric inpatient rehabilitation People with spinal cord and traumatic head injuries
	Case Study 8.3. Ensuring Veracity in Documentation	1M 5 6D 7C	Not-for-profit teaching hospital
	Vignette 8.2. Failing to Ensure Veracity in Attribution	5K 6B, 6C, 6I	Professional conference
9. Principle 7: Fidelity	Vignette 9.1. Showing Respect	7A, 7B, 7D	Academia
	Vignette 9.2. Promoting a Climate of Civility	2A 4D 7B, 7D	Academia Faculty, students
	Case Study 9.1. Analyzing and Preventing a Potential Ethics Breach	2F, 2G 5 7	Skilled nursing Older adults
	Case Study 9.2. Preventing Conflict by Promoting Transparency	1 2 3 4 5 6F 7A	Community mental health
	Vignette 9.3. Addressing Misuse of Resources	2G 6D 7H	Hospital
Part III. Models 10. Solving Ethical Dilemmas	Case Study 10.1. Addressing the Duty to Report Versus the Right to Privacy	1A 3A, 3H 5A, 5B	Hospital driving program People who experienced a cerebrovascular accident Rural community hospital
	Case Study 10.2. Protecting Professional Boundaries	1H 2C 3G	Occupational therapy assistant
	Case Study 10.3. Taking Responsibility for Ensuring Competence	1L 5A, 5E, 5F, 5H	Outpatient hand clinic

(continued)

TABLE I.1 (*cont.*)

CHAPTER	CASE STUDIES AND VIGNETTES	PRINCIPLES COVERED	POPULATIONS AND SETTINGS ADDRESSED
Part IV. Applications			
11. Ethics in Diverse Mental Health Settings	Case Study 11.1. Addressing a Confidentiality Breach in an Inpatient Facility	2C, 2G 3	Private psychiatric hospital
	Vignette 11.1. Balancing Confidentiality With a Client Orientation in a Partial Hospitalization Program	3G	Partial hospitalization program
	Vignette 11.2. Adhering to Competence Requirements at a Clubhouse	5G, 5H	Community-based club-house Mental health
	Case Study 11.2. Unraveling Ethical Priorities in Private Practice	3A, 3G	Private practice
	Vignette 11.3. Defending the Need for Ethical Practice in a Consumer-Run Organization	2B 4D, 4E	Consumer-run nonprofit
12. Productive Aging	Vignette 12.1. Facilitating a Transition to Retirement With Cultural Competence	3I 4F	Community behavioral health
	Case Study 12.1. Balancing Ethical Obligations to Enable Aging in Place	2E, 2G 7E, 7F, 7H	Community-based senior center Aging-in-place clients
	Case Study 12.2. Addressing Client and Caregiver Needs in Home Care	1 2C 4A, 4E	Home care People who experienced a cerebrovascular accident
	Vignette 12.2. Promoting Client Well-Being in a Skilled Nursing Facility	1A, 1C, 1H 2I 7H	Skilled nursing Older adults
	Vignette 12.3. Advocating for Adequate Discharge Planning	2A 4D, 4E	Inpatient behavioral health Level II fieldwork student
	Vignette 12.4. Addressing a Lack of Vigilance in Hospice	2C, 2G, 2J 5J 6	Hospice
13. Children and Youth: Ethics in Service Provision Across Contexts	Vignette 13.1. Promoting Beneficence in Services to Families	1 2I 3A 5B, 5M, 5P 6F	Early intervention Children with autism

(*continued*)

TABLE I.1 *(cont.)*

Chapter	Case Studies and Vignettes	Principles Covered	Populations and Settings Addressed
	Vignette 13.2. Ensuring the Avoidance of Harm	1I, 1M 2 3I 4D 5B, 5D, 5L 6 7D	Early intervention Children with Down syndrome
	Vignette 13.3. Weighing Confidentiality Against Nonmaleficence	2 3, 3J	School-based practice Children with seizure disorder
	Vignette 13.4. Promoting Access to Services for All	3J 4, 4A, 4E, 4G 5K, 5O	Private practice
	Vignette 13.5. Ensuring Adherence to Legal Obligations	1I 2B 5, 5P 6	Outpatient Children
	Vignette 13.6. Rectifying a Breach of Veracity	1D, 1E, 1F, 1N 6C, 6F	School-based practice Children
	Vignette 13.7. Ensuring Fidelity to Scope of Practice	5L 7D	Rural home health Homebound medically fragile children
14. Ethics in Health Promotion and Wellness	Case Study 14.1. Promoting Competency for Community Practice	1N 2A 5A, 5C	Academia
	Case Study 14.2. Fostering Autonomy in Program Planning	3I, 3J 4C 6I, 6J	Urban hospital Parent program
	Vignette 14.1. Maintaining Fidelity in Program Development	6I, 6J 7D	Community fall prevention
	Vignette 14.2. Observing Fidelity in Assisting Colleagues	3I, 3J 7A	Rural faith-based university
15. Work and Industry: Ethical Considerations in Designing an Injury Prevention Program	Case Study 15.1. Confronting Ethical Dilemmas in a Work Site Program	1 5 6	Work rehabilitation Injured workers

(continued)

TABLE I.1 (*cont.*)

Chapter	Case Studies and Vignettes	Principles Covered	Populations and Settings Addressed
16. Participation, Disability, and Rehabilitation	Case Study 16.1. Advocating for Client Autonomy	1, 1B 3	Subacute care People who experienced a cerebrovascular accident
	Case Study 16.2. Addressing Conflict of Interest and Conflict of Commitment	1A 3 4 7E	Skilled nursing People with spinal cord injury
	Case Study 16.3. Helping or Harming a Recipient of Services	1 2, 2E, 2G 4, 4F 6	Outpatient People with rheumatoid arthritis
	Case Study 16.4. Promoting Confidentiality and Social Justice	3G, 3H 4 6	Manufacturing company Client with traumatic brain injury, amputation
17. Administration and Private Practice	Vignette 17.1. Addressing a Challenge to Personal Morality Case Study 17.1. Addressing a Challenge to Professional Morality	5C 6D, 6F 1 2 4 5	Private practice in development Private practice Family
	Case Study 17.2. Addressing a Challenge to Organizational Morality	2J 4D 5N, 5P 7H	New private practice Hand therapy
18. Application of Ethics in Higher Education	Case Study 18.1. Addressing Academic Dishonesty Among Occupational Therapy Students	1K 2 5 6 7C	Academia Students
	Case Study 18.2. Correcting Unwitting Plagiarism by a Fieldwork Student	6, 6J	Rehabilitation Fieldwork student
	Case Study 18.3. Avoiding the Duty to Report Cheating	1N 5F	Academia
19. Ethics in Occupational Therapy Research	Vignette 19.1. Confronting the Risks of Research for Participants: A Personal Story	1 2 6	Hospital Clinical trial

(*continued*)

TABLE I.1 *(cont.)*

CHAPTER	CASE STUDIES AND VIGNETTES	PRINCIPLES COVERED	POPULATIONS AND SETTINGS ADDRESSED
20. Internal Relationships: Ethical Issues Within Institutions	Vignette 20.1. Rectifying a Conflict of Commitment	2G 7E	County hospital
	Vignette 20.2. Showing Respect for Colleagues	7	University hospital rehabilitation department
	Vignette 20.3. Ensuring Respect for Institutional Rules	1M 2A, 2C 5D, 5H 7D, 7H	Academia
	Case Study 20.1. Combating Discriminatory and Non-inclusive Behavior in a Volunteer Role	2, 2H 7A, 7D	Professional association
	Case Study 20.2. Confronting Bullying in the Workplace	2, 2H 5, 5L 6 7B, 7C, 7D	Large outpatient clinic Relationships among professionals
	Case Study 20.3. Confronting Mobbing in the Workplace	2, 2A, 2C, 2J 4D 5 6, 6B 7, 7D, 7G	Large county hospital
21. External Relationships: Ethical Issues in Interactions Among Institutions	Case Study 21.1. Ensuring Legal Compliance With a Funder's Requirements	3, 3G, 3I, 3J 4, 4D, 4G 5, 5B, 5C, 5L, 5P	Early intervention Infants and toddlers
	Case Study 21.2. Engaging in Due Diligence to Avoid Fraud	1E, 1G, 1I, 1N 2H, 2J, 2G	School system Private practice
	Case Study 21.3. Dealing Ethically With Funding Agencies and Organizations	1L, 1M 2G 5A, 5B 6, 6A, 6B 7D	Academia
	Case Study 21.4. Examining a Duality of Interest	1H 4D 6B, 6D 7, 7E, 7F	Community rehabilitation People with neurological and orthopedic conditions, traumatic brain injury, and pain

(continued)

TABLE I.1 (*cont.*)

CHAPTER	CASE STUDIES AND VIGNETTES	PRINCIPLES COVERED	POPULATIONS AND SETTINGS ADDRESSED
	Case Study 21.5. Assessing an Offer of Gifts	2C, 2K 5J 7F	Nonprofit rehabilitation hospital People with neurological and orthopedic conditions and spinal cord injury
	Case Study 21.6. Promoting Nonmaleficence and Beneficence in a Busy Clinic Vignette 21.1. Weighing Disclosure of Personal Information	1E, 1G 6A 7A 3, 3G	Outpatient rehabilitation Community behavioral health Occupational therapy assistant

CONCLUSION

Ethical dilemmas arise during the academic preparation to become an occupational therapy practitioner and continue throughout all areas of practice. Lifelong ethical education is an important part of becoming and remaining an ethical occupational therapy practitioner. One method to ensure consistently ethical practice is to use tools like this book that provide ethical decision-making models and opportunities to reflect on ethical issues and appropriate responses using the Code and Ethics Standards.

The editors and authors hope this publication will be used in academic settings and in occupational therapy practice to expand the dialogue regarding the ethical practice of occupational therapy. The purpose is to encourage occupational therapy practitioners and students to think of ethics not from a punitive perspective but rather from one that encourages learning, reflection, dialogue, and ethical behavior. Furthermore, we hope this publication will help readers make informed decisions when confronting ethical dilemmas but caution them to consult an attorney or other professional for legal or expert advice.

REFERENCES

Accreditation Council for Occupational Therapy Education. (2012). 2011 Accreditation Council for Occupational Therapy Education (ACOTE®) standards. *American Journal of Occupational Therapy*, 66(6 Suppl.), S6–S74. doi: 10.5014/ajot.2012.66S6

American Occupational Therapy Association. (2007). AOTA's *Centennial Vision* and executive summary. *American Journal of Occupational Therapy*, 61, 613–614. doi: 10.5014/ajot.61.6.613

American Occupational Therapy Association. (2010). Occupational therapy code of ethics and ethics standards (2010). *American Journal of Occupational Therapy*, 64(6 Suppl.), S17–S26. doi: 10.5014/ajot.2010.64S17

American Occupational Therapy Association. (2011). Association Policies: Policy 5.3.1. Definition of occupational therapy practice for state regulation. *American Journal of Occupational Therapy*, 65(6 Suppl.), S81. doi: 10.5014/ajot.2011.65S80

Glossary

The words and phrases in this Glossary are defined through an occupational therapy lens to reflect their application to ethical occupational therapy practice.

accreditation "The process by which an agency or organization evaluates and recognizes a program of study or an institution as meeting certain predetermined qualifications or standards. It applies only to institutions and their programs of study or their services" (American Occupational Therapy Association [AOTA], 2008, p. 36).

altruism "The individual's ability to place the needs of others before their own"; one of the seven occupational therapy core values (AOTA, 2010a, p. S17).

attribution Accurate acknowledgment of the sources of one's ideas, whether taken word for word or adapted from text, an image, or oral communication.

autonomy "(*auto* = self, *nomos* = law) The right of an individual to self-determination" (Slater, 2011, p. 225); "self-rule that is free from both controlling interference by others and from certain limitations ... that prevent meaningful choice" (Beauchamp & Childress, 2009, p. 58).

beneficence "(*bene faceae* = to do well) Doing good for others or bringing about good for them; the duty to confer benefits on others" (Slater, 2011, p. 225).

bioethics "A type of normative ethics involving the application of ethical principles in health care delivery, medical treatment, and research" (Slater, 2011, p. 225).

boundaries (professional) Professional distance that occupational therapy practitioners maintain from the clients they serve and the students they educate to ensure ethical behavior and the avoidance of perceived or real impropriety, overidentification, or transference.

care ethics "An ethical concept found primarily in nursing and feminist literature that states that the attitude of being a moral person is based on the concepts of receptivity, relatedness, and responsiveness by the caregiver to the one being cared for" (Slater, 2011, p. 225).

certification Means of ensuring a desired level of knowledge regarding established occupational therapy standards of practice obtained from the National Board for Certification in Occupational Therapy (NBCOT), AOTA, or other health-related professional organization. Occupational therapists and occupational therapy assistants must successfully complete and pass an assessment such as an examination or a portfolio review to obtain certification and use the associated credentials.

code of ethics Written guidelines for conduct that reflect the values and standards of a group or organization. Occupational therapy professional organizations, state regulatory boards, and agencies have established ethical guidelines with which their members, licensees, or employees are expected to comply.

colleague "A person who provides services in the same or different business (facility or organization) to which a professional relationship exists or may exist" (Slater, 2011, p. 8).

competence Possession of the knowledge and skills essential to protecting the recipients of occupational therapy services and the profession from harm.

complaint An official statement filed by an occupational therapy practitioner or member of the public regarding a breach of ethics or conduct with whomever has jurisdiction over the practitioner (e.g., AOTA, NBCOT, state regulatory board).

confidentiality "Nondisclosure of data or information that should be kept private to prevent harm and to abide by policies, regulations, and laws" (Slater, 2011, p. 225).

conflict of commitment Situation in which a practitioner or student faces overwhelming or opposing obligations from multiple competing roles.

conflict of interest Situation in which a person (or institution) "has personal, financial, professional, or political interests that are likely to undermine his or her ability to meet or fulfill his or her primary professional, ethical, or legal obligations" (Shamoo & Resnick, 2003, p. 139).

consent Written permission from the client or his or her representative to initiate an evaluation or intervention, to include the client as a participant in research, or to make information publicly available; approval from authors to use their intellectual property.

credentials Evidence of legal and ethical authority to use specific designations associated with occupational therapy practice or its

specialty areas. Occupational therapists and occupational therapy assistants must successfully complete and pass an assessment such as an examination or a portfolio review to obtain certification and use the associated credentials.

cultural competence Incorporation of knowledge about clients' primary language, cultural beliefs, values, and traditions into practice whenever possible.

deontology "(*deon* = duty) A classical ethical theory that states that the concept of *duty* is independent of the concept of good or the consequences of the action. People's actions are assessed by their ability to follow such things as religious codes, laws, and professional codes of ethics" (Slater, 2011, p. 225).

dignity Sense of worthiness, promoted in occupational therapy clients by helping them engage in meaningful occupations regardless of level of function; one of the seven occupational therapy core values (AOTA, 2010a).

duty "Actions required of professionals by society or actions that are self-imposed" (Slater, 2011, p. 225).

employee "A person who is hired by a business (facility or organization) to provide occupational therapy services" (Slater, 2011, p. 8).

equality "Fairness in interactions with others"; one of the seven occupational therapy core values (AOTA, 2010a, p. S17).

ethical dilemma A conflict between two divergent moral challenges that one must resolve in deciding on the proper course of action.

ethics "A systematic view of rules of conduct that is grounded in philosophical principles and theory; character and customs of societal values and norms that are assumed in a given cultural, professional, or institutional setting as ways of determining right and wrong" (Slater, 2011, pp. 225–226).

evidence-based practice Use of "the knowledge base of the profession or discipline in one's practice" (AOTA, 2009, p. 790).

fidelity "Faithful fulfillment of vows, promises, and agreements and discharge of fiduciary responsibilities" (Slater, 2011, p. 226).

fiduciary "A person, often in a position of authority, who obligates himself or herself to act on behalf of another (as in managing money or property) and assumes a duty to act in good faith and with care, candor, and loyalty in fulfilling the obligation; one (as an agent) having fiduciary duty to another" (Slater, 2011, p. 226).

fraud Intentional inaccuracy and dishonesty in word or action for the purpose of gaining an advantage that violates expectations articulated in ethical principles and laws.

freedom Exercise of "personal choice," promoted in occupational therapy by allowing "the desires of the client [to] guide our interventions"; one of the seven occupational therapy core values (AOTA, 2010a, p. S17).

guidelines Directions, frameworks, and templates focused on ethical and professional behaviors that support competent practice.

jurisdiction The power and authority AOTA, NBCOT, and state regulatory boards have over their members, certificants, and licensees.

jurisprudence Philosophy and theory of law; body of laws.

jurisprudence exam An exam required by some state regulatory boards for applicants for initial licensure to demonstrate their understanding of the laws and regulations governing occupational therapy practice. This exam is sometimes available to those who are renewing their licenses as recognition of continuing education.

justice "The act of distributing goods and burdens among members of society." Three types include

- **"compensatory justice** The making of reparations for wrongs that have been done."

- **"distributive justice** 'Fair, equitable, and appropriate distribution determined by justified norms that structure the terms of social cooperation. *Distributive justice* refers broadly to the distribution of all rights and responsibilities in society' (Beauchamp & Childress, 2009, p. 226)."

- **"procedural justice** The assurance that processes are organized in a fair manner" (Slater, 2011, p. 226).

Justice is one of the seven occupational therapy core values (AOTA, 2010a, p. S17).

law "A body or system of rules used by an authority to impose control over a system or humans" (Slater, 2011, p. 226).

liability The possibility of financial, professional, or legal repercussions following unethical practice.

licensure Evidence of legal and ethical authority to practice occupational therapy within a specific geographic area regulated by a state or other government agency designed to protect the public and the occupational therapy scope of practice.

moral courage Confidence that one's course of action is correct, particularly when facing and resolving an ethical dilemma.

moral distress "Painful feelings and psychological disequilibrium that result from a moral conflict in which one knows the correct action to take, but constraints prevent implementation of the action" (Jameton, cited in Slater & Brandt, 2011, p. 107).

morality, morals Standards that guide relationships between people to promote a high-quality and ethical life for people or for the community as a whole.

moral treatment An 18th-century social movement for asylum reform promoting humane treatment of people with mental illness, including "a routine of work and recreation, an appeal to reason, and the development of desirable moral traits" (Peloquin, 1989, p. 538).

nonmaleficence "Not harming or causing harm to be done to oneself or others; the duty to ensure that no harm is done" (Slater, 2011, p. 226).

oversight Supervision in one's area of responsibility to ensure careful attention to the needs and behaviors of supervisees to prevent harm or other unethical behaviors.

paternalism "An action taken by one person in the best interests of another without his or her consent."

- **"strong paternalism** Action taken that is exercised against the competent wishes of another."

- **"weak paternalism** Action taken that is presumed to be according to the wishes of the person, usually done because of the individual's age or mental status" (Slater, 2011, p. 226).

plagiarism The reproduction of published and unpublished work of another without credit to the originator. This work may be in written, electronic, or verbal form. Plagiarism violates codes of ethics and copyright laws.

procedural justice Fairness in the formulation and application of laws, regulations, and policies concerning the practice of occupational therapy to ensure fair and equitable treatment.

prudence "Use [of] clinical and ethical reasoning skills, sound judgment, and reflection to make decisions"; one of the seven occupational therapy core values (AOTA, 2010a, p. S18).

public "The community of people at large" (Slater, 2011, p. 8).

regulation Laws governing occupational therapy practice established by individual states, the District of Columbia, and Guam designed to protect the public and the occupational therapy scope of practice.

research participant "A prospective participant or one who has agreed to participate in an approved research project" (Slater, 2011, p. 8).

respect Honor given through actions and words to people, symbols, and objects that hold special meaning for individuals, families, communities, populations, and nations.

rights "Specific legal, moral, and social claims humans possess that require others to act in specific ways toward us. With all rights is the implied obligation or duty on the part of each of us" (Slater, 2011, p. 226).

scope of practice Delineation of "the domain of occupational therapy practice that directs the focus and actions of services provided by occupational therapists and occupational therapy assistants" and that includes "the dynamic process of occupational therapy evaluation and intervention services used to achieve outcomes that support the participation of clients in their everyday life activities" (AOTA, 2010b, p. S70).

social justice Ethical sharing of resources among individuals and groups in a process that is inclusive of all people, recognizing their right to be able to meet basic needs and engage in health-promoting occupations; the responsibility to seek to eliminate inequalities.

stakeholders Key people or groups in any given circumstance, including the client and his or her family members, internal influencers (e.g., supervisor, institution), and external influencers (e.g., third-party payers, state regulatory boards) who have a primary or more distant relationship to the situation.

standards Recognized or agreed-on values, guidelines, and principles promoting ethical and high-quality practice.

state regulatory board (SRB) An agency of a state government that licenses occupational therapy practitioners and oversees their actions for the purpose of protecting the public against injury by incompetent or unqualified practitioners.

stewardship Responsible management of a client's occupational health and well-being, fiscal resources, and the profession's dignity.

student "A person who is enrolled in an accredited occupational therapy education program" (Slater, 2011, p. 8).

trademark A name, symbol, or other mark owned for exclusive use by a professional organization or business. For example, the trademarks *OTR* and *COTA* are owned by NBCOT and may be used only by occupational therapists and occupational therapy assistants who possess these certifications.

truth "Accurate information, both in oral and written form"; one of the seven occupational therapy core values (AOTA, 2010, p. S18).

utilitarianism "An ethical theory that states that right actions are those that maximize utility (the greatest good for the greatest number) and result in the best consequences for all involved" (Slater, 2011, p. 227).

veracity "A duty to tell the truth" (Slater, 2011, p. 227).

REFERENCES

American Occupational Therapy Association. (2008). *The reference manual of the official documents of the American Occupational Therapy Association, Inc.* (13th ed., pp. 35–45). Bethesda, MD: AOTA Press.

American Occupational Therapy Association. (2009). Scholarship in occupational therapy. *American Journal of Occupational Therapy, 63,* 790–793.

American Occupational Therapy Association. (2010a). Occupational therapy code of ethics and ethics standards (2010). *American Journal of Occupational Therapy, 64*(6 Suppl.), S17–S26. doi: 10.5014/ajot2010.64S17

American Occupational Therapy Association. (2010b). Scope of practice. *American Journal of Occupational Therapy, 64*(6 Suppl.), S70–S77. doi: 10.5014/ajot2010.64S70

Beauchamp, T. L., & Childress, J. F. (2009). *Principles of biomedical ethics.* New York: Oxford University Press.

Peloquin, S. M. (1989). Moral treatment: Contexts considered. *American Journal of Occupational Therapy, 43,* 537–544. doi: 10.5014/ajot.43.8.537

Shamoo, A. E., & Resnik, D. B. (2003). *Responsible conduct of research.* New York: Oxford University Press.

Slater, D. Y. (Ed.). (2011). *Reference guide to the Occupational Therapy Code of Ethics and Ethics Standards* (2010 ed.). Bethesda, MD: AOTA Press.

Slater, D. Y., & Brandt, L. C. (2011). Combating moral distress. In D. Y. Slater (Ed.), *Reference guide to the Occupational Therapy Code of Ethics and Ethics Standards* (2010 ed., pp. 107–113). Bethesda, MD: AOTA Press.

About the Editors

Janie B. Scott, MA, OT/L, FAOTA, is an occupational therapy and aging-in-place consultant and adjunct faculty at Towson University, Towson, Maryland. She earned a BS in occupational therapy from Wayne State University and an MA in legal and ethical studies from the University of Baltimore. She has presented nationwide and has published in the area of health care ethics, productive aging, autism, aging in place, consultation, and mental health practice. She has been Ethics Officer, Director of Practice, and Staff Liason to the Special Interest Sections of the American Occupational Therapy Association (AOTA). Her volunteer positions include member of the AOTA Judicial Council and Representative Assembly, trustee and past president for the Maryland Occupational Therapy Association, and president and vice president of the Homes for Life Coalition of Howard County, Maryland.

S. Maggie Reitz, PhD, OTR/L, FAOTA, is chairperson and professor in the Department of Occupational Therapy and Occupational Science at Towson University, Towson, Maryland. She received both her BS and MS degrees in occupational therapy from Towson University and her doctorate in health education from the University of Maryland, College Park. She practiced as an occupational therapist in mental health and physical disabilities in the Anacostia neighborhood of Washington, DC, before beginning her academic career. She has been elected and served as president of the Maryland Occupational Therapy Association and chairperson of AOTA's Ethics Commission. Her areas of interest include occupational therapy theory and philosophy, occupational science, ethics, and health promotion. She has lectured on these topics throughout the United Kingdom, as well as in Australia, Hong Kong, Ireland, Sweden, and the People's Republic of China.

About the Authors

Dana Burns, MS, OTR/L, CBIS, is Occupational Therapist, Kernan Orthopaedics and Rehabilitation, University of Maryland Medical System, Baltimore.

Linda S. Gabriel, PhD, OTR/L, is Assistant Professor and Occupational Therapy Faculty Associate, Center for Health Policy and Ethics, Creighton University, Omaha, NE.

Susan Haiman, MPS, OTR/L, FAOTA, is Associate Professor, Department of Occupational Therapy, College of Science, Health and the Liberal Arts, Philadelphia University, Philadelphia.

Stacey Harcum, MS, OTR/L, CBIS, is Occupational Therapist, Kernan Orthopaedics and Rehabilitation, University of Maryland Medical System, Baltimore.

Barbara L. Kornblau, JD, OTR, FAOTA, is Professor of Occupational Therapy, Florida A&M University, Tallahassee; Founder and Executive Director, Coalition for Disability Health Equity, Arlington, VA; and Executive Director, Society for Participatory Medicine, Arlington, VA.

Elizabeth Larson, PhD, OTR, is Associate Professor, University of Wisconsin–Madison.

Tammy Richmond, MS, OTR/L, FAOTA, is CEO, Go 2 Care, Inc., Los Angeles.

Marian K. Scheinholtz, MS, OT/L, is Public Health Advisor, Substance Abuse and Mental Health Services Administration, Rockville, MD.

Mary Alice Singer, MA, OTR/L, is certified in Ayres Sensory Integration and Owner, Occupational Therapy for Children, Laguna Beach, CA.

Deborah Yarett Slater, MS, OT/L, FAOTA, is Staff Liaison to the Ethics Commission and the Bylaws, Policies, and Procedures Committee, American Occupational Therapy Association, Bethesda, MD.

Susanne Smith Roley, OTD, OTR/L, FAOTA, is Project Director, Sensory Integration Certification Program, Division of Occupational Science and Occupational Therapy, University of Southern California, Los Angeles.

Jeff Snodgrass, PhD, MPH, OTR/L, is Chair and Program Director and Associate Professor, Occupational Therapy Department, Milligan College, Milligan College, TN, and Contributing Faculty, Department of Public Health, School of Health Sciences, Walden University, Minneapolis.

Part I. Foundations

Introduction

Janie B. Scott, MA, OT/L, FAOTA

The historical foundations of ethical thinking that have had the greatest influence on occupational therapy and the *Occupational Therapy Code of Ethics and Ethics Standards (2010)* (referred to as the "Code and Ethics Standards"; American Occupational Therapy Association [AOTA], 2010) are reviewed in Part I. The history of ethics is relevant to the government, philosophy, culture, and beliefs of societies and also to health care delivery in general and occupational therapy theory and practice specifically.

Part I provides glimpses of ethical constructs developed in societies around the world and across time, setting the stage for the remainder of the book by showing readers how ethical thinking in occupational therapy has been influenced by the history of ethics. Readers also will explore how this ethical legacy has been implemented within the profession of occupational therapy, from the roles of certification and state regulation of the profession as a whole to the expectations and enforcement of ethical behavior for individual occupational therapy practitioners. Readers are provided a structure and context for delving into the complex case studies and vignettes involving a variety of practice settings and populations that are presented in the rest of the book.

Chapter 1, "Historical Background of Ethics in Occupational Therapy," outlines the evolution of ethical thinking throughout history, focusing on the ancient world, medieval Europe, and the Age of Enlightenment. Taoist beliefs, the Hippocratic Oath, Socratic tradition, and medieval guilds' behaviors and values are compared with principles in the Code and Ethics Standards. Tables show how AOTA's core values and the principles of the Code and Ethics Standards reflect this history.

The authors of Chapter 2, "Promoting Ethics in Occupational Therapy Practice: Codes and Consequences," discuss the evolution of codes of ethics reflecting the values and standards of occupational therapy groups and organizations and the purpose of these codes in professional life. Readers will review the development of the seven core values on which the ethical practice of occupational therapy practice is based and see how these values were incorporated into the current Code and Ethics Standards. Through a description of AOTA's earlier codes and their parallels with the current Code and Ethics Standards, readers will gain an appreciation of how this document has evolved in response to changes in occupational therapy practice and societal beliefs.

In addition, Chapter 2 describes the entities and mechanisms responsible for ensuring the ethical practice of occupational therapy. Readers will learn when the National Board for Certification in Occupational Therapy (NBCOT) was created and how its policies and procedures and those of state regulatory boards (SRBs) ensure that occupational therapy practitioners engage in ethical practice. The jurisdictions of AOTA, NBCOT, and SRBs are presented and described, as are the disciplinary processes, enforcement procedures, and potential disciplinary actions of each. Within this context, the importance of continuing competence and its relationship to ethical behaviors and regulations is highlighted.

Reference

American Occupational Therapy Association. (2010). Occupational therapy code of ethics and ethics standards (2010). *American Journal of Occupational Therapy, 64*(6 Suppl.), S17–S26. doi: 10.5014/ajot2010.64S17

Historical Background of Ethics in Occupational Therapy

1

*S. Maggie Reitz, PhD, OTR/L, FAOTA, and
Janie B. Scott, MA, OT/L, FAOTA*

History provides a lens through which occupational therapy practitioners can understand the present and a foundation on which we can wisely build the future. As Stattel (1977) noted, "We cannot accurately and professionally comprehend the present or look at the future intelligently until we become acquainted with and study the past" (p. 650). Occupational therapy has a long history—nearly a century in length—that is rich with practice experience, but the ethical principles governing our practice date back millennia. The history of ethics has been shaped by needs and changes within societies over time. An understanding of how this evolution has shaped our society and our profession can help guide our thinking and processes to ensure that our conduct is consistently ethical.

After defining ethics and explaining its function in human society, we provide a snapshot of the ethical contributions of three eras in history—the ancient world, medieval Europe, and the Enlightenment—to the development of the ethics that govern occupational therapy. These time periods are represented in a timeline in Figure 1.1. Chapter 2 focuses on the history of occupational therapy ethics; the development of an occupational therapy code, including an overview of the *Occupational Therapy Code of Ethics and Ethics Standards (2010)* (referred to as the "Code and Ethics Standards"; AOTA,

2010); and the requirements of other occupational therapy regulatory bodies. After reading these two chapters, you will have gained an understanding both of the historical background of the profession's commitment to ethics and of the tools currently available to help you be an ethical practitioner.

Ethics evolved as "a body of moral principles or values" (AOTA, 2011, p. 39). Ethics reflect societal values, morals, and norms as they are applied to the effort of communities, professions, and organizations to determine what is or is not acceptable behavior (Slater, 2011). Codes of professional ethics articulate the duties that members of the discipline have to each other and to society and are based on beliefs and values that a profession supports. Ethics guide behavior, and codes of ethics serve as a guide for individual practitioners and for a profession (Scott, 2007). Professional ethics reflect those morals and values that are endorsed by organizations and serve to guide the behaviors of their members. These beliefs are based on agreements about what is right or wrong in accordance with societal norms. The organization arranges its ethical beliefs into codes that reflect behavioral principles. These principles not only serve as guidelines for the profession but also inform the public of the behavioral expectations of the profession, organization, or agency (AOTA, 2011; Scott, 2007; Slater, 2011).

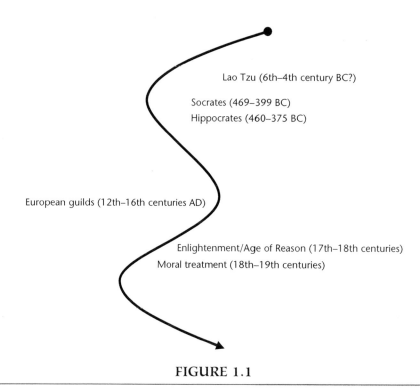

Lao Tzu (6th–4th century BC?)

Socrates (469–399 BC)

Hippocrates (460–375 BC)

European guilds (12th–16th centuries AD)

Enlightenment/Age of Reason (17th–18th centuries)

Moral treatment (18th–19th centuries)

FIGURE 1.1

Milestones in the development of ethical reasoning.

ETHICS THROUGH TIME

Humans are social beings who since their earliest origins have lived in groups for survival and reproductive advantages (Wilcock, 2006). To manage the challenges inherent in living in groups, people have developed increasingly complex systems over time to manage disputes and to promote behavior supportive of the group and larger society. The establishment of norms, values, and rules facilitated the aesthetics, productivity, and survival of the group as a whole and of its individual members. Scientists have proposed that early humans placed a high value on self-help and caring for kin. Once people were able to care for themselves and their kin, they would then display altruism through the sharing of resources with others within their larger social group (Wilcock, 2001b).

Wilcock (2001a) described proto–occupational therapists (i.e., the premodern counterparts of modern occupational therapists) as healers who used occupation as a therapeutic medium, on the basis of their instincts and observations of the results of various actions and inactions, to enhance their health and the health of their social groups.

In addition, they developed "their own methods of justice to create an effective working community to meet the needs of survival" (Wilcock, 2001a, p. 15). Proto–occupational therapists included "medicine men, shamans and priests, along with . . . monks and nuns," among others (Wilcock, 2001a, p. 16). Throughout recorded history, the qualities of ethical healers have included altruism, competency, and caring (Jonsen, 2007).

Modern occupational therapists are also healers; as such, they share the common values and behaviors of those who have healed others through time. Within the fabric of these beliefs, they weave an understanding of the linkages among occupation, natural rhythms, the environment, and health.

Ethics in Society: The Ancient World

Since the earliest societies, religions have provided guidance to followers regarding appropriate behavior. For example, the golden rule—treat others as you wish them to treat you—is a code of conduct embraced by Brahmanism, Buddhism, Christianity, Confucianism, Islam, Judaism, and

Taoism (Kornblau & Burkhardt, 2012). The first documented set of rules guiding the behavior of physicians was the Code of King Hammurabi, found chiseled into stone pillars dating to 2000 BC at the site of ancient Babylon (Wilcock, 2001b). Taoism provides an example of the ethical principles of a society as distant from us in time, geography, and tradition as ancient China. The founder of Taoism, Lao Tzu, lived sometime between the 6th and 4th centuries BC and wrote a code of conduct in Chapter 8 of *Tao Te Ching* (Lao Tzu, 2001) that is summarized in Table 1.1. Six of the seven principles and two of the seven core values from the Code and Ethics Standards can be recognized in Taoist beliefs.

By the time of the ancient Greeks, pragmatic decision making about survival, health, security, and happiness had evolved into organized discussions that would form the basis of Western ethics. Two early Greek philosophers, Hippocrates and Socrates, engaged in such discussions, and their thinking can be seen today in the Code and Ethics Standards. Hippocrates (460–375 BC) and Socrates (469–399 BC) were contemporaries (Wilcock, 2001c). Hippocrates is generally recognized as the father of Western medicine and is credited as the author of the Hippocratic Oath (Hippocrates, 2002), which outlines the behaviors expected of physicians in ancient Greek times. A comparison of the directives appearing in the Hippocratic Oath to the principles in the Code and Ethics Standards is provided in Table 1.2.

The teachings of Socrates on values and their impact on human relationships and behavior, the precursor of the ethics branch of philosophy, were immortalized in his students' writings, those of Plato being the best known (Cavalier, 2002; Wilcock, 2001c). There are no known surviving written works of Socrates. Thus, it is difficult to separate his ideas from those of his students. This has led to disagreement and debate over which ideas were Socrates' and which were those of his pupils. Despite this uncertainty, there is general agreement regarding values and behaviors ascribed to by Socrates (Nails, 2009); a comparison of these values and behaviors to the core values and attitudes and the principles in the Code and Ethics Standards is provided in Table 1.3.

TABLE 1.1
Comparison of Taoist Beliefs to Core Values and Principles of the Code and Ethics Standards

Taoist Belief[a]	Core Values and Principles[b]
In a home it is the site that matters.	Core value—Prudence
	Principle 1—Beneficence
In quality of mind it is the depth that matters.	Principle 1—Beneficence
	Principle 2—Nonmaleficence
	Principle 7—Fidelity (see Principle 7A)
In an ally it is benevolence that matters.	Core value—Altruism
	Principle 1—Beneficence
	Principle 4G—Consideration of pro bono or reduced-fee services
In speech it is good faith that matters.	Principle 7—Fidelity
In government it is order that matters.	Principle 5—Procedural Justice
In affairs it is ability that matters.	Principle 1—Beneficence
In action it is timeliness that matters.	Principle 1—Beneficence (see Principles 1A and 1C)
	Principle 6—Veracity (see Principle 6H)

[a]Lao Tzu (2001).
[b]American Occupational Therapy Association (2010).

TABLE 1.2
Comparison of the Hippocratic Oath to Principles of the Code and Ethics Standards

Hippocratic Oath[a]	Principles[b]
To hold him who taught me this art equally dear to me as my parents, to be a partner in life with him, and to fulfill his needs when required; to look upon his offspring as equals to my own siblings, and to teach them this art, if they shall wish to learn it, without fee or contract; and that by the set rules, lectures, and every other mode of instruction, I will impart a knowledge of the art to my own sons, and those of my teachers, and to students bound by this contract and having sworn this Oath to the law of medicine, but to no others.	Principle 7—Fidelity (see Principle 7A)
I will use those dietary regimens which will benefit my patients according to my greatest ability and judgment, and I will do no harm or injustice to them.	Principle 1—Beneficence
	Principle 2—Nonmaleficence
	Principle 7—Fidelity (see Principle 7A)
I will not give a lethal drug to anyone if I am asked, nor will I advise such a plan; and similarly I will not give a woman a pessary to cause an abortion.	Principle 2—Nonmaleficence
	Principle 5—Procedural Justice
	Principle 7—Fidelity (see Principle 7A)
In purity and according to divine law will I carry out my life and my art.	With the removal of the word *divine:* Principle 1—Beneficence
	Principle 3—Autonomy, Confidentiality
	Principle 5—Procedural Justice
I will not use the knife, even upon those suffering from stones, but I will leave this to those who are trained in this craft.	Principle 2—Nonmaleficence
	Principle 7—Fidelity (see Principle 7A)
Into whatever homes I go, I will enter them for the benefit of the sick, avoiding any voluntary act of impropriety or corruption, including the seduction of women or men, whether they are free men or slaves.	Principle 2—Nonmaleficence (see Principles 2C, 2G, and 2J)
Whatever I see or hear in the lives of my patients, whether in connection with my professional practice or not, which ought not to be spoken of outside, I will keep secret, as considering all such things to be private.	Principle 3—Autonomy, Confidentiality
So long as I maintain this Oath faithfully and without corruption, may it be granted to me to partake of life fully and the practice of my art, gaining the respect of all men for all time. However, should I transgress this Oath and violate it, may the opposite be my fate.	Principle 5—Procedural Justice

[a]Hippocrates (2002).
[b]American Occupational Therapy Association (2010).

TABLE 1.3
Comparison of Socratic Values and Behaviors to Core Values and Principles of the Code and Ethics Standards

Socratic Values and Behaviors	Core Values and Principles[a]
"Postulated a spiritual view of knowledge and conduct . . . and the value of truth, virtue, knowledge and appropriate action and conduct" (Wilcock, 2001c, p. 71)	Core value—Truth
	Principle 3—Veracity
	Principle 7—Fidelity
Declined to accept payment for his work, as he did not see himself as a teacher in the way it was conceptualized in his lifetime; used a conversational probing method of instruction to foster self-analysis that was not valued or accepted at the time	Principle 2—Nonmaleficence (see Principle 2C)
	Principle 3—Autonomy, Confidentiality
	Principle 4—Social Justice (see Principle 4G, consideration of pro bono or reduced-fee services)
Showed greater respect for women than his contemporaries (Nails, 2009)	Core value—Justice
	Principle 4—Social Justice
Believed "the unexamined life is not worth living for a human being" (quoted in Nails, 2009, para. 6)	Core value—Truth
	Principle 3—Autonomy, Confidentiality
Refused to engage in sexual relationships with students, although this was accepted and expected behavior at the time	Principle 2—Nonmaleficence (see Principle 2D)
Refused to escape before his planned execution because he believed that to do so would have broken the law and endangered the city	Core value—Truth
	Principle 2—Nonmaleficence
	Principle 4—Social Justice
	Principle 5—Procedural Justice

[a]American Occupational Therapy Association (2010).

Ethics at Work: Medieval Guilds

During the Middle Ages (1100–1500 AD), people engaged in trades and crafts, including healers, organized themselves into guilds to protect their livelihoods and establish rules about entry into the craft, required training, and standards of work to ensure quality. The guilds held considerable power and enforced their own rules and discipline (Cox, 2007; Naylor, 1921). The standards these guilds established contributed to the later development of professionalism and codes of ethics in medicine (Cox, 2007). Later in the 19th century, social reformers in Europe called, unsuccessfully, for a return to guilds as a way to create social justice (Wilcock, 2001c). A comparison of the activities undertaken by guilds to principles in the Code and Ethics Standards is provided in Table 1.4.

The rules and expectations for behavior set by the guilds are an early example of how people have used values as an aspirational guide for behavior. The Code and Ethics Standards is an aspirational guide in that it provides members of the occupational therapy profession with a description of agreed-on behavior to strive for in order to protect and promote the well-being of both themselves and society.

Ethics in Caring: The Enlightenment

Philosophers and intellectuals identified with the Age of Enlightenment (also called the Age of Reason) in 17th- and 18th-century Europe believed that people could improve the state of humankind by applying reason to solve problems. The goals of humans were thought to be "knowledge, freedom,

TABLE 1.4
Comparison of Medieval Guilds' Activities to Core Values and Principles of the Code and Ethics Standards

Guild Activities[a]	Core Values and Principles[b]
Organized members to protect their livelihood	Core values—Justice, dignity, prudence
	Principle 7—Fidelity
Developed rules governing entry into the guild and necessary training	Core values—Justice, dignity, prudence
	Principle 1—Beneficence (see Principle 1G)
	Principle 5—Procedural Justice
	Principle 6—Veracity (see Principle 6D)
Instituted standards to ensure competency	Core values—Justice, prudence
	Principle 1—Beneficence (see Principle 1E)
	Principle 5—Procedural Justice (see Principles 5F, 5O)
Enforced rules	Core values—Justice, prudence
	Principle 5—Procedural Justice

[a]Cox (2007), Naylor (1921).
[b]American Occupational Therapy Association (2010).

and happiness" (Encyclopedia Britannica, 2011). John Locke, a prominent philosopher of the time, believed that people are born with the capacity to develop through their unique experiences, as opposed to fulfilling a prewritten destiny (Encyclopedia Britannica, 2011). The human capacity to adapt in response to experience is foundational to occupational therapy's belief in the importance of context, doing, and recovery (Christiansen, 1991; Fidler & Fidler, 1978; Mosey, 1981; Wilcock, 2001c). Wilcock (2001b) saw a commonality in Locke's thinking and that of pragmatists who were influential during the time occupational therapy was being developed in the United States (Breines, 1986).

Moral treatment, an 18th-century social movement for asylum reform inspired by the inhumane treatment of people with mental disorders, was heavily influenced by Enlightenment philosophy (Gordon, 2009). Reformers such as Philippe Pinel in France and William Tuke in England realized the need to bring ethical care to people with mental illness. In 1798, Pinel received permission from French Revolution leaders to release people with mental illness from chains, improve their living environments, and provide

some level of autonomy. Pinel's moral treatment included providing liberty and opportunities to engage in individualized, prescribed occupation tailored to the patient's diagnosis (Wilcock, 2001c).

Following the success of moral treatment in France and England, changes were implemented in many U.S. private and state mental hospitals. In 1773 in colonial Williamsburg, the Public Hospital for Persons of Insane and Disordered Minds was opened (Zwelling, 1985), the first public hospital built to care solely for mentally ill patients in British North America (see Figure 1.2). While serving as superintendent of the hospital from 1841 to 1861, John Galt, a physician, implemented an approach consistent with moral treatment (Zwelling, 1985). Eli Todd, a physician associated with the establishment of the Hartford (Connecticut) Retreat for the Insane in 1824, described his view of an asylum as a thoughtful combination of medicine and moral treatment:

It should not be a jail in which for individual and public security the unfortunate are confined, nor should it be merely a hospital where they may have the benefit

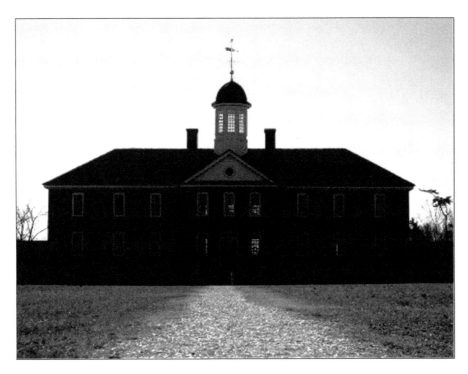

FIGURE 1.2

Public Hospital for Persons of Insane and Disordered Minds, Williamsburg, Virginia.
(Photo courtesy of Jessica Reitz Murphy)

of medical treatment—for without moral management the most judicious course of medication is rarely successful—nor should it be merely a school where the mind is subjected to discipline while the body continues to suffer in consequences of original or symptomatic disease. (quoted in Goodheart, 2003, p. 25)

A variety of factors contributed to the decline and later influence of moral treatment. According to Gordon (2009), the lack of scientific evidence for moral treatment, its use by nonmedical practitioners, and the high regard for the scientific method at the end of the 19th century resulted in moral treatment falling out of favor in the United States. However, Gordon argued that the core beliefs of moral treatment were not lost but became embedded in the foundation of psychiatry. Other forces beyond the preference for the scientific method also may have curtailed moral treatment (Reitz & Scaffa, 2010), including the U.S. Civil War and resulting fiscal constraints (Peloquin, 1989; Zwelling, 1985) and the

push for equal access to care and resultant rapid increase in patient census without the planning and resources needed to cope with this increased volume (Kielhofner, 2004; Peloquin, 1989).

The ideals of moral treatment are ingrained in the values and ethical principles of occupational therapy. Of the seven principles in the Code and Ethics Standards, the values of moral treatment can best be seen in the first four—Beneficence, Nonmaleficence, Autonomy and Confidentiality, and Social Justice. Proponents of moral treatment were motivated by a desire not only to reduce suffering (i.e., Nonmaleficence) but also to bring benefits to patients (i.e., Beneficence) in an atmosphere that provided opportunities for autonomy.

In his 1981 Eleanor Clark Slagle Lecture, Robert K. Bing (1981) explored occupational therapy history. He saw moral treatment both as part of early occupational therapy for people with mental illness and as the foundation of occupational therapy. He also discussed the importance of recognizing and promoting the values of individual clients when delivering occupational therapy services. He encouraged occupational therapy practitioners to recognize and value their past as the profession moves into the future: "The history of occupational therapy is the story of ideals, deeds, hopes, and words of *individuals*" (Bing, 1981, p. 515). Bing's concepts extend beyond the individual practitioner and may be seen as shared values between occupational therapy practitioners and their clients and communities.

CONCLUSION

Codes of ethics establish ideal standards that members of a group strive to achieve. Principles of ethics provide guidelines for today's occupational therapy practitioners to aspire to in their practice. Calling the Code and Ethics Standards an aspirational document underscores the challenge to practice occupational therapy ethically each day. Adhering to ethical principles is not always easy; however, the principles of the Code and Ethics Standards guide practitioners' actions toward ethical behavior and serve as guideposts for examining ethical dilemmas.

Occupational therapy is a profession long concerned with providing caring, competent interventions that benefit clients and society as a whole through altruistic acts and a commitment to an aspirational code of ethics. The profession's concern with supporting ethical occupational therapy practice, as embodied in the evolving Code and Ethics Standards, reflects the long history of ethics and its application to today's societal needs.

REFERENCES

American Occupational Therapy Association. (2010). Occupational therapy code of ethics and ethics standards (2010). *American Journal of Occupational Therapy, 64*(6 Suppl.), S17–S26. doi: 10.5014/ajot2010.64S17.

American Occupational Therapy Association. (2011). Glossary. In *Reference manual of the official documents of the American Occupational Therapy Association* (16th ed., pp. 35–45). Bethesda, MD: AOTA Press.

Bing, R. K. (1981). Occupational therapy revisited: A paraphrastic journey (Eleanor Clarke Slagle Lecture).

American Journal of Occupational Therapy, 35, 499–518. doi: 10.5014/ajot.35.8.499.

Breines, E. (1986). *Origins and adaptations.* Lebanon, NJ: Geri-Rehab.

Cavalier, R. (2002). *Introduction to ethics: Preface—Socrates (469–399 BC).* Retrieved from http://caae.phil.cmu.edu/Cavalier/80130/part1/Preface/PrefaceA.html

Christiansen, C. (1991). Occupational therapy intervention: Intervention for life performance. In C. Christiansen & C. Baum (Eds.), *Occupational therapy: Overcoming human performance deficits* (pp. 1–43). Thorofare, NJ: Slack.

Cox, H. C. (2007). The ethical foundations of professionalism: A sociologic history. *Chest, 131,* 1532–1540.

Encyclopedia Britannica. (2011). *Enlightenment.* Chicago: Author. Retrieved from www.britannica.com/EBchecked/topic/188441/Enlightenment

Fidler, G., & Fidler, J. W. (1978). Doing and becoming: Purposeful action and self-actualization. *American Journal of Occupational Therapy, 32,* 305–310.

Goodheart, L. B. (2003). *Mad Yankees: The Hartford Retreat for the Insane and nineteenth-century psychiatry.* Amherst: University of Massachusetts Press.

Gordon, D. (2009). The history of occupational therapy. In E. B. Crepeau, E. S. Cohn, & B. A. B. Schell (Eds), *Willard and Spackman's occupational therapy* (11th ed., pp. 202–215). Philadelphia: Lippincott Williams & Wilkins.

Hippocrates. (2002). *The Hippocratic oath* (M. North, Trans.). Bethesda, MD: National Library of Medicine. Retrieved from www.nlm.nih.gov/hmd/greek/greek_oath.html

Jonsen, A. (2007). *Bioethics: An introduction to the history, methods, and practice* (2nd ed., pp. 3–16). Boston: Jones & Bartlett.

Kielhofner, G. (2004). The development of occupational therapy knowledge. In *Conceptual foundations of occupational therapy* (3rd ed., pp. 27–63). Philadelphia: F. A. Davis.

Kornblau, B. L., & Burkhardt, A. (2012). Introduction. In *Ethics in rehabilitation* (2nd ed., pp. 3–15). Thorofare, NJ: Slack.

Lao Tzu. (2001). Chapter 8. In *Tao Te Ching* (bilingual ed.; D. C. Lau, Trans.). Hong Kong: Chinese University Press.

Mosey, A. C. (1981). *Occupational therapy: Configuration of a profession.* New York: Raven Press.

Nails, D. (2009). Socrates. In E. N. Zalta (Ed.), *Stanford encyclopedia of philosophy.* Retrieved from http://plato.stanford.edu/archives/spr2010/entries/socrates/

Naylor, E. H. (1921). Historical evolution. In *Trade associations: Their organization and management* (pp. 14–25). New York: Roland Press.

Peloquin, S. M. (1989). Looking back—Moral treatment: Contexts reconsidered. *American Journal of Occupational Therapy, 43,* 537–544. doi: 10.5014/ajot.43.8.537

Reitz, S. M., & Scaffa, M. E. (2010). Public health principles, approaches, and initiatives. In M. E. Scaffa, S. M. Reitz, & M. A. Pizzi (Eds.), *Occupational therapy in the promotion of health and wellness* (pp. 70–95). Philadelphia: F. A. Davis.

Scott, J. B. (2007). Ethical issues in school-based practice and early intervention. In L. Jackson (Ed.), *Occupational therapy practice in education and early childhood settings* (3rd ed., pp. 213–228). Bethesda, MD: AOTA Press.

Slater, D. Y. (2011). Glossary of ethics terms. In D. Y. Slater (Ed.), *Reference guide to the Occupational Therapy Code of Ethics and Ethics Standards* (2010 ed., pp. 225–227). Bethesda, MD: AOTA Press.

Stattel, F. M. (1977). Occupational therapy: Sense of the past—Focus on the present. *American Journal of Occupational Therapy, 31,* 649–650.

Wilcock, A. A. (2001a). A history of occupational therapy. In *Occupation for health* (Vol. 1, pp. 1–19). London: British Association and College of Occupational Therapists.

Wilcock, A. A. (2001b). Nature's regimen in primitive and spiritual times: Evolution, survival and health. In *Occupation for health* (Vol. 1, pp. 20–50). London: British Association and College of Occupational Therapists.

Wilcock, A. A. (2001c). Occupation for health in classical times. In *Occupation for health* (Vol. 1, pp. 52–97). London: British Association and College of Occupational Therapists.

Wilcock, A. A. (2006). An occupational theory of human nature. In *An occupational perspective of health* (2nd ed., pp. 50–74). Thorofare, NJ: Slack.

Zwelling, S. S. (1985). *Quest for a cure: The public hospital in Williamsburg, Virginia, 1773–1885.* Williamsburg, VA: Colonial Williamsburg Foundation.

Promoting Ethics in Occupational Therapy Practice: Codes and Consequences

2

Janie B. Scott, MA, OT/L, FAOTA, and
S. Maggie Reitz, PhD, OTR/L, FAOTA

The historical progression in ethical thought described in Chapter 1 creates a path for the discussion in this chapter of the evolution of codes of ethics reflecting the values and standards of occupational therapy groups and organizations. We compare earlier versions of the occupational therapy codes to the current *Occupational Therapy Code of Ethics and Ethics Standards (2010)* (referred to as the "Code and Ethics Standards"; American Occupational Therapy Association [AOTA], 2010b). The AOTA Ethics Commission (EC) developed the *Enforcement Procedures for the Occupational Therapy Code of Ethics and Ethics Standards* (referred to as the *Enforcement Procedures*) in 1996 (AOTA, 2010a). Possible and actual disciplinary actions from the current *Enforcement Procedures* are presented in this chapter, as are examples of disciplinary actions taken by the National Board for Certification in Occupational Therapy (NBCOT) and state regulatory boards (SRBs).

The focus of this chapter is twofold: (1) to describe the development and structure of the Code and Ethics Standards and (2) to discuss the entities that provide oversight and the mechanisms in place to ensure ethical behavior among occupational therapy practitioners. The case studies and vignettes in future chapters draw on readers' understanding of this material. Figure 2.1 is a timeline showing important milestones in occupational therapy ethics.

ETHICS IN OCCUPATIONAL THERAPY

Two statements of principles predated the first version of the *Occupational Therapy Code of Ethics*, published in 1977. The first statement was penned in 1919 by a physician named William R. Dunton, Jr., who used occupation as a curative and preventive agent. The second statement, the Basic Principles of Occupational Therapy, was developed by a committee of the National Society for the Promotion of Occupational Therapy (the name was changed to AOTA in 1921) that included occupational therapy pioneer Eleanor Clarke Slagle. These principles were published in 1919 and reprinted periodically until 1940 (both statements are reprinted in Reed, 2011). These documents described methods of intervention that modeled behaviors later labeled *Beneficence* and *Nonmaleficence*.

It is not known specifically why the principles were not reprinted after 1940. Initially, one possible reason could have been the disruption in life caused by World War II and the profession's focus on contributions to the war effort and returning soldiers. After World War II, the profession entered a period of great activity. This work included establishing awards such as the Eleanor Clarke Slagle Lectureship, coining definitions of *occupational therapy* and other professional terms, fighting against licensure,

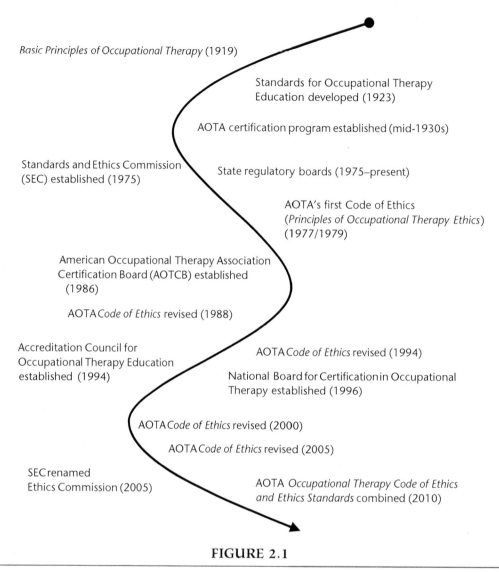

Basic Principles of Occupational Therapy (1919)

Standards for Occupational Therapy
Education developed (1923)

AOTA certification program established (mid-1930s)

Standards and Ethics Commission
(SEC) established (1975)

State regulatory boards (1975–present)

AOTA's first Code of Ethics
(*Principles of Occupational Therapy Ethics*)
(1977/1979)

American Occupational Therapy Association
Certification Board (AOTCB) established
(1986)

AOTA *Code of Ethics* revised (1988)

Accreditation Council for
Occupational Therapy Education
established (1994)

AOTA *Code of Ethics* revised (1994)

National Board for Certification in Occupational
Therapy established (1996)

AOTA *Code of Ethics* revised (2000)

AOTA *Code of Ethics* revised (2005)

SEC renamed
Ethics Commission (2005)

AOTA *Occupational Therapy Code of Ethics
and Ethics Standards* combined (2010)

FIGURE 2.1

Milestones in occupational therapy ethics.
Note. AOTA = American Occupational Therapy Association.

developing a variety of practice areas, and debating entry-level degrees, among other activities (Reed, 2011). Given the dramatic changes in the profession, the original principles may have been viewed as outdated.

The *Occupational Therapy Code of Ethics* (referred to as the "Code") was first adopted in 1977 and has been revised six times: in 1979, 1988, 1994, 2000, 2005, and 2010 (Kyler & Slater, 2011). The revisions to the Code occurred in response to societal changes and AOTA's systematic review process for all of its official documents to ensure that they continue to be relevant and accurate. The current review cycle is every five

years, unless societal changes indicate the need for a sooner revision. Additionally, AOTA member input regarding the relevance and usefulness of the Code and its related documents helps inform the EC's revision of the Code. AOTA members are encouraged to review proposed changes, which are ultimately voted on and approved by the Representative Assembly (RA).

The principles included in the Code have changed over time, as shown in Table 2.1. Beneficence and Autonomy appeared in the first version and in each of the following six revisions, exemplifying the importance to occupational therapy practice of these timeless ethical principles.

TABLE 2.1
Comparison of the 2010 Code and Ethics Standards to Past Codes

PRINCIPLES OF THE 2010 CODE AND ETHICS STANDARDS	PRINCIPLES OF THE PREVIOUS CODES[a]	
	YEAR	WORDING
Principle 1—Beneficence	1977/1979	[Principle I. "Related to the Recipient of Service"]. Occupational therapist demonstrates a beneficent concern for the recipient of services and maintains a goal-directed relationship.
	1988	Principle 1 (Beneficence/Autonomy). Occupational therapy personnel shall demonstrate a concern for the welfare and dignity of the recipient of their services.
	1994	Principle 1. Occupational therapy personnel shall demonstrate a concern for the well-being of the recipients of their services. (Beneficence)
	2000	[Language unchanged]
	2005	Principle 1. Occupational therapy personnel shall demonstrate a concern for the safety and well-being of the recipients of their services. (Beneficence)
	2010	Principle 1. Occupational therapy personnel shall demonstrate a concern for the well-being and safety of the recipients of their services.
Principle 2—Nonmaleficence	1977/1979	[Not addressed]
	1988	[Appears under Principle 1—Beneficence]
	1994	[Appears under Principle 1—Beneficence]
	2000	Principle 2. Occupational therapy personnel shall take reasonable precautions to avoid imposing or inflicting harm upon the recipient of services or to his or her property. (Nonmaleficence)
	2005	Principle 2. Occupational therapy personnel shall take measures to ensure a recipient's safety and avoid imposing or inflicting harm. (Nonmaleficence)
	2010	Occupational therapy personnel shall intentionally refrain from actions that cause harm.
Principle 3—Autonomy, Confidentiality	1977/1979	[Implied under Principle I. "Related to the Recipient of Service"]. The occupational therapist demonstrates a beneficent concern for the recipient of services and maintains a goal-directed relationship. . . . Respect shall be shown for the recipients' rights and the occupational therapist will preserve the confidence of the patient relationship.
	1988	[Autonomy and Confidentiality coupled with Beneficence]

(continued)

TABLE 2.1 (*cont.*)

PRINCIPLES OF THE 2010 CODE AND ETHICS STANDARDS	PRINCIPLES OF THE PREVIOUS CODES[a]	
	YEAR	WORDING
	1994	Principle 2. Occupational therapy personnel shall respect the rights of the recipients of their services. (autonomy, privacy, confidentiality)
	2000	Principle 3. Occupational therapy personnel shall respect the recipient and/or their surrogate(s) as well as the recipient's rights. (autonomy, privacy, confidentiality)
	2005	Principle 3. Occupational therapy personnel shall respect recipients to assure their rights. (Autonomy, Confidentiality)
	2010	Principle 3. Occupational therapy personnel shall respect the right of the individual to self-determination.
Principle 4—Social Justice	1977	[Need to be aware of social issues addressed in Principle 12]
	1979	[Need to be aware of social issues addressed in Principle 13]
	1988	[Not addressed]
	1994	[Not addressed]
	2000	[Not addressed]
	2005	[Not addressed]
	2010	Principle 4. Occupational therapy personnel shall provide services in a fair and equitable manner.
Principle 5—Procedural Justice	1977	[Covered under 6 of the 12 principles]
	1979	[Covered under 7 of the 13 principles]
	1988	Principle 3. Compliance With Laws and Regulations
	1994	Principle 4. Occupational therapy personnel shall comply with laws and Association policies guiding the profession of occupational therapy. (Justice)
	2000	[Language unchanged, now Principle 5]
	2005	[Language unchanged, now referred to as Procedural Justice]
	2010	Principle 5. Occupational therapy personnel shall comply with institutional rules, local, state, federal, and international laws and AOTA documents applicable to the profession of occupational therapy.
Principle 6—Veracity	1977/1979	[Not explicitly stated but implied]
	1988	[Not explicitly stated but implied]

(*continued*)

TABLE 2.1 (*cont.*)

PRINCIPLES OF THE 2010 CODE AND ETHICS STANDARDS	PRINCIPLES OF THE PREVIOUS CODES[a]	
	YEAR	WORDING
	1994	Principle 5. Occupational therapy personnel shall provide accurate information about occupational therapy services. (Veracity)
	2000	[Language unchanged]
	2005	Principle 6. Occupational therapy personnel shall provide accurate information when representing the profession. (Veracity)
	2010	Principle 6. Occupational therapy personnel shall provide comprehensive, accurate, and objective information when representing the profession.
Principle 7—Fidelity	1977	[Covered under 3 of the 12 principles]
	1979	[Covered under 3 of the 13 principles]
	1988	Principle 5 (Professional Relationships). Occupational therapy personnel shall function with discretion and integrity in relations with colleagues and other professionals, and shall be concerned with the quality of their services.
	1994	Principle 6. Occupational therapy personnel shall treat colleagues and other professionals with fairness, discretion, and integrity. (fidelity, veracity)
	2000	[Language unchanged, now Principle 7]
	2005	Principle 7. Occupational therapy personnel shall treat colleagues and other professionals with respect, fairness, discretion, and integrity. (Fidelity)
	2010	[Language unchanged]

[a]Wording not enclosed in brackets is quoted from the source. The full citation for each version of the *Occupational Therapy Code of Ethics* appears in the reference list with American Occupational Therapy Association as the author and the applicable year of publication.

Nonmaleficence first appeared in the 1988 version and has been consistently present since then, although the wording has evolved. The description of Fidelity has remained constant since 1994. Principles related to Procedural Justice were very prominent in the 1977 and 1979 versions (AOTA, 1978, 1983). The changes from the 1977 Code (AOTA, 1978) to the 1979 version (AOTA, 1983), with its emphasis on Procedural Justice, may be a reflection of increased government regulation (e.g., licensure) at that time. The principles and their descriptions in these two versions are identical except for a few wording changes and the addition of a principle regarding advertisement (i.e.,

Principle X. "Related to Advertising") to the 1979 version. Although concern for Social Justice first appeared in the 1977 and 1979 Codes, it was not until the 2010 version that it was included as a separate, distinct principle reflecting the profession's core values and roots in social activism.

DEVELOPMENT OF THE CORE VALUES AND CODE AND ETHICS STANDARDS

Gilfoyle (1984) expressed the need for consistency between our daily practice and our professional values and believed that "values provide unity and become the underlying force in our philosophy" (p. 578). In her 1984 Eleanor Clarke Slagle Lecture, "Transformation of a Profession," Gilfoyle discussed ways occupational therapy could prepare for the future. She encouraged the examination of occupational therapy values, especially the occupation-based belief in "patients' doing" and the commitment "to provide services for severely and chronically disabled" clients (Gilfoyle, 1984, p. 576). This statement resonates with three of what would become occupational therapy's core values: altruism, equality, and justice.

AOTA's formal effort to identify core values for the profession originated with a charge by the RA to the Commission on Practice (COP) and the Commission on Standards and Ethics (SEC) to create a list of knowledge, skills, and attitudes for the profession. The RA is the policymaking body for AOTA and has the authority to direct the work of its commissions and committees. The COP is a commission of the RA responsible for developing and updating the standards and best practices for the profession. The purpose of the SEC (renamed the Ethics Commission [EC] in 2010) is

> to serve the Association members and public through the identification, development, review, interpretation, and education of the AOTA *Occupational Therapy Code of Ethics and Ethics Standards (2010)* and to provide the process whereby the ethics of the Association are enforced. (AOTA, 2011a, p. 24)

AOTA funded the Professional and Technical Role Analysis (PATRA) Study in 1985 "to delineate entry-level practice" for occupational therapists and occupational therapy assistants:

> Knowledge, skills, and attitude statements were to be developed to provide a basis for the role analysis. The PATRA Study completed the knowledge and skills statements. The Executive Board subsequently charged the SEC to develop a statement that would describe the values and attitudes that undergird the profession. (AOTA, 1993, p. 1085)

The PATRA Study yielded a list of terms for the SEC to use in creating the core values document.

The document that resulted from these directives, *Core Values and Attitudes of Occupational Therapy Practice* (AOTA, 1993), was intended to provide the profession with a set of values flexible enough to change over time and yet consistent enough to serve as the core beliefs. *Core Values and Attitudes of Occupational Therapy Practice* includes seven core values—altruism, equality, freedom, justice, dignity, truth, and prudence—that guide occupational therapy practitioners' behaviors (AOTA, 1993, 2010b; see the Glossary for definitions of each core value). In 1993, the SEC believed that these values and beliefs of the profession were reflected in many AOTA official documents and in the occupational therapy literature. The SEC asserted that these values and beliefs should be consistent throughout the professional lives of occupational therapy students and professionals and that our professional behaviors should be based on them (AOTA, 1993). The core values document provides users with a resource to support daily professional ethical behavior and to aid in the resolution of conflicting professional values. Actions that demonstrate the core values are detailed in Table 2.2.

The Code and Ethics Standards were built on the foundation of the seven core values articulated by the SEC in 1993. The Core Values document was never revised and was rescinded in 2010 when it was incorporated into the Code and Ethics Standards (AOTA, 2010c). The SEC originally believed that the document might evolve to reflect the changing values of the profession over time (AOTA, 1993); however, its grounding in professional and societal values has stood the test of time. The most current Code and Ethics Standards continue to refer to the core values—for example, altruism appears in Principle 1, equality in Principle 4, justice in Principles 4 and 5, and truth in Principle 6.

The EC considered input from AOTA members who reported that the existence of three separate documents—the *Occupational Therapy Code of Ethics,* the *Core Values and Attitudes of Occupational Therapy Practice,* and the *Guidelines to the Occupational Therapy Code of Ethics* (AOTA, 2006)—was confusing (D. Slater, personal communication, June 13, 2012). The *Guidelines* document referred to the professional behaviors of honesty, communication, ensuring the common good, competence, confidentiality and protected information,

TABLE 2.2
Behaviors That Exemplify Occupational Therapy Core Values

VALUE	DESCRIPTION
Altruism	Demonstrates "unselfish concern for the welfare of others" (AOTA, 1993, p. 1085) Places the needs of others first (AOTA, 2010b)
Equality	Perceives and acts on belief that all people "have the same fundamental human rights and opportunities" (AOTA, 1993, p. 1085; AOTA, 2010b)
Freedom	Promotes choice for individuals, families, and communities Helps recipients of services "find a balance between autonomy and societal membership that is reflected in the choice of various patterns of interdependence with" people and the environment (AOTA, 1993, p. 1085)
Justice	Provides "occupational therapy services for all individuals who are in need of these services" (AOTA, 1993, p. 1086) Respects "the legal rights of individuals receiving occupational therapy services" (AOTA, 1993, p. 1086) Abides by the local, state, and federal laws governing practice (AOTA, 1993)
Dignity	Demonstrates "an attitude of empathy and respect for self and others" (AOTA, 1993, p. 1086)
Truth	Is "faithful to facts and reality . . . [and] accountable, honest, forthright, accurate, and authentic in . . . attitudes and actions" (AOTA, 1993, p. 1086)
Prudence	Exercises "judiciousness, discretion, vigilance, moderation, care, and circumspection in the management of one's affairs" (AOTA, 1993, p. 1086)

conflict of interest, impaired practitioners, payment for services and other financial arrangements, and resolution of ethical issues with principles from the Code (AOTA, 2006). In 2010, the RA rescinded the *Core Values* and *Guidelines* documents and incorporated the constructs and some of the language into the 2010 Code and Ethics Standards (AOTA, 2010c). Thus, the reference to "ethics standards" in the title of the Code and Ethics Standards reflects the incorporation of the *Core Values* and *Guidelines* documents into a single ethics document (D. Slater, personal communication, July 8, 2012). The new document details the ethical expectations of occupational therapy students and practitioners relative to ethical reasoning throughout occupational therapy practice.

STRUCTURE OF THE CODE AND ETHICS STANDARDS

The Code and Ethics Standards begin with a Preamble that discusses the scope and the objectives of the document. According to the Preamble, the

Code and Ethics Standards have the following purposes:

- Identify and describe the principles supported by the occupational therapy profession.
- Educate the general public and members regarding established principles to which occupational therapy personnel are accountable.
- Socialize occupational therapy personnel to expected standards of conduct.
- Assist occupational therapy personnel in recognition and resolution of ethical dilemmas. (AOTA, 2010b, p. S18)

Thus, preventive education is the primary desired outcome of the Code and Ethics Standards. Through time, this document has also become a tool with which the occupational therapy profession communicates its values and standards to the public, including regulatory bodies and recipients of services.

The body of the Code and Ethics Standards consists of descriptions of each of seven principles and lists of related subprinciples. The principles are described at length in Part II of this book, as follows:

- Principle 1—Beneficence: Chapter 3
- Principle 2—Nonmaleficence: Chapter 4
- Principle 3—Autonomy, Confidentiality: Chapter 5
- Principle 4—Social Justice: Chapter 6
- Principle 5—Procedural Justice: Chapter 7
- Principle 6—Veracity: Chapter 8
- Principle 7—Fidelity: Chapter 9.

The Code and Ethics Standards are reviewed regularly by the EC and AOTA members and the language updated to reflect current values and beliefs, ensuring that this document remains relevant to the practice of occupational therapy and a valuable tool for practitioners and the public as they attempt to solve the ethical dilemmas they may encounter.

OVERSIGHT OF ETHICAL PRACTICE IN OCCUPATIONAL THERAPY

To oversee occupational therapy practitioners' adherence to their respective codes of ethics and conduct, AOTA and other organizations charged with ensuring the ethical practice of occupational therapy have established enforcement procedures. When occupational therapy practitioners become licensed or certified or join a professional organization, they agree to adhere to the code of ethics or conduct of the appropriate body and to abide by its enforcement procedures. Enforcement procedures help ensure that practitioners under a specific jurisdiction (i.e., under an entity's authority to take disciplinary action) who do not adhere to the appropriate code of ethics or guidelines for professional behavior become subject to a process of complaint and investigation that will result in disciplinary action if the complaint is determined to have merit.

If someone (e.g., client, fellow professional) believes that an occupational therapy practitioner has engaged in unethical behavior, enforcement procedures outline the requirements for filing a formal complaint and the investigatory steps that will follow. Typically, a special committee examines the testimonies of the complainant, the respondent,

and any witnesses and considers facts and supporting evidence. The nature of the complaint and the surrounding facts determine whether the committee dismisses the complaint or assesses a fine, takes disciplinary action, or both. The organizations concerned with ethical occupational therapy practice and their enforcement procedures are briefly described in the sections that follow.

American Occupational Therapy Association

The most recent version of AOTA's *Enforcement Procedures* (AOTA, 2010a) was published in 2010, when the new Code and Ethics Standards were adopted (see Appendix B). Jurisdiction, potential disciplinary actions, complaint timeline and processes, and the appeal process are specified in the *Enforcement Procedures*.

A consumer, another occupational therapy practitioner, or any member of the public may file a complaint against an occupational therapy practitioner who is an AOTA member or was a member at the time of the alleged incident. The EC reviews each complaint according to a specified process and, when warranted, issues a disciplinary action against the member. Four of the five disciplinary actions are public and one is private (i.e., between the EC and the people involved). The disciplinary actions are defined in Table 2.3. A summary of AOTA's public disciplinary actions for a recent 1-year period appears in Table 2.4. In addition to disciplinary actions, the EC may write an educative letter, which is private. An educative letter is used when available evidence is insufficient to determine that an ethics violation has occurred but sufficient to indicate a failure to engage in best practice (AOTA, 2010a).

The EC reviews the behaviors that result in disciplinary actions and may develop advisory opinions to help occupational therapy practitioners avoid similar outcomes by understanding the ethical implications of challenging situations. The primary purposes of advisory opinions are to inform and educate occupational therapy practitioners regarding strategies to address ethical issues that arise in everyday practice. These opinions also may be developed in response to themes identified in other communications with AOTA's EC.

TABLE 2.3
Possible Disciplinary Actions in the AOTA Enforcement Procedures

ACTION	DESCRIPTION
Reprimand	"A formal expression of disapproval of conduct communicated privately by letter from the EC Chairperson that is nondisclosable and noncommunicative to other bodies (e.g., state regulatory boards [SRBs], National Board for Certification in Occupational Therapy® [NBCOT®])." (AOTA, 2010a, p. S5)
Censure	"A formal expression of disapproval that is public." (AOTA, 2010a, p. S5)
Probation of membership subject to terms	"Failure to meet terms will subject an AOTA member to any of the disciplinary actions or sanctions." (AOTA, 2010a, p. S5)
Suspension	"Removal of AOTA membership for a specified period of time." (AOTA, 2010a, p. S5)
Revocation	"Permanent denial of AOTA membership." (AOTA, 2010a, p. S5)

Note. AOTA = American Occupational Therapy Association; EC = AOTA's Ethics Commission.

Advisory opinions are made available to AOTA members via the Web site and through AOTA educational products.

National Board for Certification in Occupational Therapy

In the mid-1930s, AOTA established a certification program for occupational therapists; in the 1960s, a similar program was instituted for occupational therapy assistants. *Certification* is a process that agencies use to determine that a professional may "use a certain title if that person has attained entry-level competence" (Willmarth, 2011, p. 455). In 1986, AOTA transferred responsibility for certification of occupational therapy practitioners to a newly formed independent organization, the American Occupational Therapy Certification Board, which was renamed NBCOT in 1998 (Willmarth, 2011). NBCOT has less legal authority over certificants than the SRBs that license occupational therapy practitioners. Since 2006, AOTA has also made available board and specialty certifications in certain practice areas. These certifications are awarded once the practitioner submits an application and fee and their submitted evidence is reviewed and recognized as having met specified qualifications and standards (M. L. Louch, personal communication, June 14, 2012).

NBCOT administers certification exams to graduates of accredited occupational therapy programs who have passed all education and fieldwork components. Candidates who pass an exam and meet other NBCOT requirements are entitled to use the Occupational Therapist Registered (OTR®) or Certified Occupational Therapy Assistant (COTA®) designation. In some states, the OTR or COTA credential is necessary to seek a license or other credential needed to practice in the United States as an occupational therapist or occupational therapy assistant; other states require an alternative examination (AOTA, 2011b). In addition to administering the certification examinations, NBCOT offers a voluntary recertification program that requires practitioners to attest to having earned the minimum number of professional development units to maintain currency in their practice area (NBCOT, 2012). Most SRBs do not require occupational therapy practitioners to renew their NBCOT certification (Moyers, 2009; Willmarth, 2011).

NBCOT has its own code, called the *NBCOT Candidate/Certificant Code of Conduct* (NBCOT, 2010a; see Appendix D). Exam candidates, occupational therapy practitioners who hold initial certification, and those who renew their certification agree to abide by this code. The *NBCOT Candidate/Certificant Code of Conduct* comprises seven principles:

- Principle 1 requires accuracy and truthfulness in information submitted to NBCOT (consistent with Principle 6, Veracity, of the Code and Ethics Standards).

TABLE 2.4
Examples of AOTA Disciplinary Actions in a 1-Year Period

PRINCIPLES VIOLATED IN EACH CASE	DISCIPLINARY ACTION
Principle 2A—Avoid exploiting the recipient of services Principle 4A—Hold appropriate credentials Principle 4F—Duties must match credentials, qualifications, experience, and scope of practice Principle 5—Procedural Justice	Censure
Principle 4A—Hold appropriate credentials Principle 5A—Abide by institutional rules, Association policies, and laws Principle 6A—Represent credentials, qualifications, education, experience, training, and competence accurately	Censure
Principle 4G—Provide appropriate supervision Principle 5—Procedural Justice	Censure
Principle 1G—Ensure competence and weigh potential for harm in emerging technology or practice Principle 4G—Provide appropriate supervision Principle 1E—Provide services within level of competence and scope of practice	Censure
Principle 5A—Abide by institutional rules, Association policies, and laws Principle 5B—Be familiar with revisions in laws and policies and inform others of those changes Principle 6A—Represent credentials, qualifications, education, experience, training, and competence accurately	Censure
Principle 6—Veracity Principle 6B—Refrain from false statements or claims	Censure
Principle 1—Beneficence Principle 4F—Duties must match credentials, qualifications, experience, and scope of practice Principle 4G—Provide appropriate supervision Principle 5A—Abide by institutional rules, Association policies, and laws Principle 7—Fidelity	Suspension of membership for 1 year
Principle 2A—Avoid exploiting the recipient of services Principle 4A—Hold appropriate credentials Principle 4F—Duties must match credentials, qualifications, experience, and scope of practice Principle 5—Procedural Justice	Revocation of membership
Principle 5—Procedural Justice Principle 6—Veracity	Revocation of membership
Principle 6E—Accept responsibility for professional actions that reduce the public's trust in occupational therapy	Revocation of membership

(continued)

TABLE 2.4 (*cont.*)

Principles Violated in Each Case	Disciplinary Action
Principle 5K—Use funds for intended purposes Principle 6B—Refrain from false statements or claims Principle 6E—Accept responsibility for professional actions that reduce the public's trust in occupational therapy Principle 6J—Do not plagiarize Principle 7H—Be diligent stewards of human, financial, and material resources of their employers	Revocation of membership
Principle 3G—Ensure confidentiality and right to privacy Principle 3H—Maintain the confidentiality of all verbal, written, electronic, augmentative, and nonverbal communications Principle 7—Fidelity	Revocation of membership

Note. AOTA = American Occupational Therapy Association.
Source. AOTA (2010d).

- Principle 2 requires cooperation with the NBCOT's investigation process in case of a complaint (consistent with Principle 5, Procedural Justice, of the Code and Ethics Standards).
- Principle 3 requires accuracy and truthfulness in all professional communications (consistent with Principle 6, Veracity, of the Code and Ethics Standards).
- Principle 4 requires compliance with the legal requirements of occupational therapy practice (consistent with Principle 5, Procedural Justice, of the Code and Ethics Standards).
- Principle 5 disqualifies from certification those convicted of crimes related to the practice of occupational therapy (consistent with Principle 5, Procedural Justice, of the Code and Ethics Standards).
- Principle 6 forbids practitioners from threatening the health, well-being, or safety of recipients of occupational therapy services (consistent with Principle 2, Nonmaleficence, of the Code and Ethics Standards).
- Principle 7 prohibits the practice of occupational therapy while the practitioner's ability to practice is impaired because of legal or illegal drug or alcohol use (consistent with Principle 2, Nonmaleficence, of the Code and Ethics Standards).

The *NBCOT Candidate/Certificant Code of Conduct* and the *Procedures for the Enforcement of the NBCOT Candidate/Certificant Code of Conduct* (NBCOT, 2011; see Appendix E) are available on the NBCOT Web site (www.nbcot.org). Breaches of the *NBCOT Candidate/Certificant Code of Conduct* may result in sanctions. Each specific situation is reviewed, and if a violation is found, the candidate or certificant may receive one or more sanctions, including ineligibility for certification, reprimand, censure, probation, suspension, and revocation (NBCOT, 2011). These sanctions mirror AOTA's except that AOTA's disciplinary actions relate to the person's membership in AOTA and include the option of reprimand through an educative letter. NBCOT disciplinary actions for a recent 1-year period are displayed in Table 2.5. A brief comparison of the disciplinary sanctions that might be applied by AOTA, NBCOT, and SRBs appears in Table 2.6.

State Regulatory Boards

SRBs have the legislative authority to license occupational therapy practitioners when they meet specific conditions. The purpose of licensure is to regulate occupational therapy practice and protect the public from injury by incompetent or unqualified practitioners. Licensees are recognized as having met the requirements established by a government agency for a profession (Willmarth, 2011). Occupational therapists were first licensed in 1975 in two states—Florida and New York. By 2011, all 50 states, the District of Columbia,

TABLE 2.5
Summary of NBCOT Principle Violations in a 1-Year Period

NUMBER OF CASES	PRINCIPLE VIOLATED
1	Principle 1. Certificants shall provide accurate and truthful representations to NBCOT concerning all information related to aspects of the Certification Program.
1	Principle 3. Certificants shall be accurate, truthful, and complete in any and all communications relating to their education, professional work, research, and contributions to the field of occupational therapy. Principle 4. Certificants shall comply with laws, regulations, and statutes governing the practice of occupational therapy.
10	Principle 4. Certificants shall comply with laws, regulations, and statutes governing the practice of occupational therapy.

Note. NBCOT = National Board for Certification in Occupational Therapy.

Source. Data courtesy of NBCOT (2010b); wording of principles is from the *NBCOT Candidate/Certificant Code of Conduct* (NBCOT, 2010a).

Guam, and Puerto Rico had some sort of regulation for occupational therapists in place, and all but Hawaii and Colorado had some form of regulation for occupational therapy assistants (Willmarth, 2011). Many SRBs have adopted part or all of AOTA's Code and Ethics Standards and require licensees to adhere to these tenets (Willmarth, 2011).

In addition to regulating the practice of occupational therapy, SRBs publish standards to inform licensees and the public about what constitutes acceptable practice. SRBs also inform the public about what to do in case of a complaint and, in many instances, publish summaries of disciplinary actions taken. Many states also require licensees to meet competence standards (see Appendix F). SRBs have the authority to discipline occupational therapy practitioners under their jurisdiction or fine licensees, or both, for violations of laws

TABLE 2.6
Disciplinary Sanctions by AOTA, NBCOT, and SRBs

AOTA	NBCOT	SRBs
Educative letter	Ineligibility for certification	Civil penalty/disciplinary costs
Reprimand	Reprimand	Probation[a]
Censure	Censure	Suspension of license[a]
Probation of membership subject to terms	Probation	Suspension with probation
Suspension of membership	Suspension of certification	Revocation of license
Revocation of membership	Revocation of certification	Permanent surrender of license

Note. AOTA = American Occupational Therapy Association; NBCOT = National Board for Certification in Occupational Therapy; SRBs = state regulatory boards.

[a]Conditions may apply (e.g., seek psychiatric or substance abuse treatment, attend additional continuing education, receive supervision through a mentor, perform community service).

Sources. American Occupational Therapy Association (2010a); National Board for Certification of Occupational Therapy (2011); Maryland Department of Health and Mental Hygiene, Board of Occupational Therapy Practice (2010); and North Carolina Board of Occupational Therapy (2010).

and regulations. Occupational therapy practitioner behaviors that warranted disciplinary action by two different SRBs in a 1-year period are presented in Table 2.7. Some SRBs publish additional details regarding disciplinary cases on their Web sites.

Jurisdiction

Because AOTA, NBCOT, and SRBs are all concerned with the ethical practice of occupational therapy, confusion can arise regarding the jurisdiction of each organization (i.e., its authority to take disciplinary action) for a specific complaint. As shown in Figure 2.2, jurisdiction depends on the degree of authority that the organization or agency has over the certificant applicant, occupational therapy practitioner, or AOTA member.

The consequences of ethical and legal misconduct vary across jurisdictions. Stakeholders (e.g., AOTA members, NBCOT certificants, consumers, professionals) may report unethical practice to any of the three entities; however, the complaint would move forward for review only if it fell under the jurisdiction of the entity. If the board or organization reviewing the complaint determines that the complaint is not within its jurisdiction, the complainant is notified in writing.

Some actions subject to disciplinary action by one organization also are within the jurisdiction of another; for example, an SRB action may also result in discipline through NBCOT or AOTA if the practitioner is under its jurisdiction. In addition, situations in which client harm occurred may result in legal action against the practitioner and a claim to a liability insurance company.

TABLE 2.7
Summary of SRB Disciplinary Actions in Two States in a 1-Year Period

PRACTITIONER VIOLATION	DISCIPLINARY ACTION
Multiple occurrences of failure to notify the SRB of address change Inadequate or unacceptable continuing education	Probation for 3 years Civil penalty
Failure to submit documentation to contracting agency Violation of HIPAA regulations by keeping medical records and files at home	Probation for 3 years Civil penalty and disciplinary costs Additional continuing competence activity points required for license renewal
Patient fall as a result of negligent transfer	Probation for 2 years Civil penalty and disciplinary costs Additional continuing competence activity points required for 2 renewal years
Failure to comply with continuing competence activity audit	Suspension of license Civil penalty and disciplinary costs
Practice without a valid license Misrepresentation Filing of false reports Negligence Improper use of devices Incompetence	Suspension with probation Discontinuation of unapproved device use Community service Requirement to take ethics and billing courses Requirement to practice under supervision
Reported erratic behavior from patients and employer Positive test for alcohol and cocaine use Negligence	Revocation

(continued)

TABLE 2.7 (*cont.*)

PRACTITIONER VIOLATION	DISCIPLINARY ACTION
Sexual misconduct Exploitation of a client	Surrender of license
Misrepresentation on license application Omission of information about disciplinary actions taken by another state licensing board	Permanent surrender of license
Falsification of patient records	Surrender of license
Forgery of patient and supervisor names Fraudulent billing Filing of false reports Violation of state regulations Breach of code of ethics Misconduct	Suspension and probation Supervision through mentor Requirement to see a psychiatrist
Failure to disclose disciplinary action in license application Fraud in application Failure to possess good moral character	Probation
Practice under the influence (alcohol) and gross misconduct	Suspension (stayed), probation Participation in substance abuse treatment and random drug testing with supervisor notification

Note. HIPAA = Health Insurance Portability and Accountability Act of 1996; SRB = state regulatory board.

Sources. Maryland Department of Health and Mental Hygiene, Board of Occupational Therapy Practice (2010); North Carolina Board of Occupational Therapy (2010).

Reporting on Disciplinary Actions

Systems are in place to gather and report data on occupational therapy practitioners who are found to be in violation of ethics and competence requirements. Publishing the results of disciplinary actions is intended to notify and protect the public by identifying practitioners who have violated laws, regulations, or best practices. Ultimately, these initiatives also protect the occupational therapy profession by identifying these practitioners and preventing their actions that might harm the public and the image of occupational therapy. In addition, public notification serves to remind current practitioners about the importance of legal, ethical, and competent practice.

NBCOT gathers and makes publicly available the outcomes of its disciplinary review processes and those of SRBs on the Disciplinary Action Information Exchange Network (DAIEN), which is available on its Web site. SRBs are encouraged to contribute information about their disciplinary actions to the DAIEN; however, NBCOT has no legal authority to require their compliance with this request (NBCOT, 2009).

AOTA, NBCOT, and SRBs have a legal mandate under Title IV of the Health Care Quality Improvement Act of 1986 to monitor complaints; to gather data regarding disciplinary actions; and to communicate the outcomes of their disciplinary actions publicly on their Web sites, in official publications, or both:

> The intent of Title IV of Public Law 99–660 is to improve the quality of health care by encouraging State licensing boards, hospitals and other health care entities, and professional societies to identify and discipline those who engage in unprofessional behavior; and to restrict the ability of incompetent physicians, dentists, and

QUESTION	JURISDICTION		
	NBCOT	SRB	AOTA
1. Who should I call if I have questions about the following?			
a. Ethical violations that could cause harm or have potential to cause harm to a consumer or the public	X	X	X
b. Violations that do not cause harm or have a limited potential for causing harm to a consumer or the public			X
c. Violations of professional values that do not relate directly to potential harm to the public			X
2. Where did the alleged violation occur, and who was involved in the alleged incident?			
a. Took place in a state with rules, regulations, and disciplinary procedures in place	X	X	X
b. Took place in an unregulated state	X		X
c. Was committed by an AOTA member	X	X	X
d. Was committed by a person who is not an AOTA member	X	X	
3. What is the disciplinary action that you wish as a consequence of filing a complaint?			
a. Restrict or revoke licensure		X	
b. Restrict or revoke certification	X		
c. Restrict or prohibit membership in AOTA			X

Note. AOTA = American Occupational Therapy Association; NBCOT = National Board for Certification in Occupational Therapy; SRB = state regulatory board.

Source. From "Disciplinary Action: Whose Responsibility?" by R. A. Hansen, in *Reference Guide to the Occupational Therapy Code of Ethics and Ethics Standards* (2010 ed., p. 38), edited by D. Y. Slater, 2011, Bethesda, MD: AOTA Press. Copyright © 2011, by the American Occupational Therapy Association. Reprinted with permission.

FIGURE 2.2

Disciplinary jurisdiction.

other health care practitioners to move from State to State without disclosure or discovery of previous medical malpractice payment and adverse action history. (U.S. Department of Health and Human Services [DHHS], 2001, p. A-2)

AOTA, NBCOT, and SRBs also may report disciplinary actions to government-sponsored data collection agencies. For example, the National Practitioner Data Bank (NPDB), a quality assurance division within DHHS, is a database with information about all licensure actions taken against all health care practitioners and health care entities, as well as any negative actions or findings against health care practitioners or organizations by peer review organizations and private accreditation organizations. The NPDB is a confidential clearinghouse responsible for collecting and releasing information about, for example, medical malpractice payments, adverse licensure actions, adverse professional society membership actions, and negative actions by state licensing or certification authorities (DHHS, n.d.). Its legal authority is greater than that of NBCOT and AOTA because its mandates are driven by state or federal regulations, and some of the regulations may affect an individual's ability to practice occupational therapy. Notice of health care provider violations are available to states under specific conditions and may further affect a practitioner's ability to practice.

The number of disciplinary actions taken by AOTA, NBCOT, and the SRBs in a 1-year period is typically larger than that reported in the NPDB. This discrepancy is attributable to several possible reasons; for example, a person reported in more than one state would appear only once in the NPDB, entities incur no legal consequences for not reporting to the NPDB and may not take the time to do so, budget cuts may prevent some states from reporting, and some SRBs report their disciplinary actions to the DAIEN rather than to the NPBD.

CONCLUSION

The profession of occupational therapy protects both the public and its practitioners by developing and enforcing its core values through the Code and Ethics Standards. As the needs of society evolve, new interventions, grounded in evidence, are developed that respond to these changing needs; the core values of the profession, however, remain constant as they have since the inception of the profession (AOTA, 2010b). These core values will continue to inform revisions of the Code and Ethics Standards as principles are modified to provide occupational therapy practitioners with the guidance they need to practice with pride and ethical behavior.

REFERENCES

American Occupational Therapy Association. (1978). Principles of occupational therapy ethics. In H. L. Hopkins & H. D. Smith (Eds.), *Willard and Spackman's occupational therapy* (5th ed., pp. 709–710). Philadelphia: Lippincott.

American Occupational Therapy Association. (1983). Principles of occupational therapy ethics (1979 version). In *Reference manual of the official documents of the American Occupational Therapy Association* (pp. 127–134). Rockville, MD: Author.

American Occupational Therapy Association. (1988). Occupational therapy code of ethics. *American Journal of Occupational Therapy, 42,* 795–796. doi:10.5014/ajot.42.12.795

American Occupational Therapy Association. (1993). Core values and attitudes of occupational therapy practice. *American Journal of Occupational Therapy, 47,* 1085–1086. doi: 10.5014/ajot.47.12.1085

American Occupational Therapy Association. (1994). Occupational therapy code of ethics. *American Journal of Occupational Therapy, 48,* 1037–1038. doi: 10.5014/ajot.48.11.1037

American Occupational Therapy Association. (2000). Occupational therapy code of ethics. *American Journal of Occupational Therapy, 54,* 614–616. doi: 10.5014/ajot.54.6.614

American Occupational Therapy Association. (2005). Occupational therapy code of ethics (2005). *American Journal of Occupational Therapy, 59,* 639–642. doi: 10.5014/ajot.59.6.639

American Occupational Therapy Association. (2006). Guidelines to the occupational therapy code of ethics. *American Journal of Occupational Therapy, 60,* 652–658. doi: 10.5014/ajot.60.6.652

American Occupational Therapy Association. (2010a). Enforcement procedures for the *Occupational Therapy Code of Ethics and Ethics Standards. American Journal of Occupational Therapy, 64*(6 Suppl.), S4–S16. doi: 10.5014/ajot.2010.64S4

American Occupational Therapy Association. (2010b). Occupational therapy code of ethics and ethics standards (2010). *American Journal of Occupational Therapy, 64*(6 Suppl.), S17–S26. doi: 10.5014/ajot2010.64S17

American Occupational Therapy Association. (2010c, April 29). Rescind OT code of ethics (2005), core values and guidelines to ethics. In *Draft minutes of the American Occupational Therapy Association, Inc., Representative Assembly.* Retrieved from www.aota.org/Governance/RA/PastMeetings/Minutes/April-2010.aspx?FT=.pdf

American Occupational Therapy Association. (2010d). *Resources: Disciplinary action.* Retrieved from www.aota.org/Practitioners/Ethics/Enforce.aspx

American Occupational Therapy Association. (2011a). Incorporation papers and bylaws. In *The reference manual of the official documents of the American Occupational Therapy Association* (16th ed., p. 24). Bethesda, MD: AOTA Press.

American Occupational Therapy Association. (2011b). *Jurisdictions regulating occupational therapy assistants (OTAs).* Retrieved from www.aota.org/Practitioners/Licensure/stateRegs/OTRegs/36457.aspx

Gilfoyle, E. M. (1984). Transformation of a profession (Eleanor Clarke Slagle Lecture). *American Journal of Occupational Therapy, 38,* 575–584. doi: 10.5014/ajot.38.9.575

Hansen, R. A. (2011). Disciplinary action: Whose responsibility?" In D. Y. Slater (Ed.), *Reference guide to the Occupational Therapy Code of Ethics and Ethics Standards* (2010 ed., pp. 37–38). Bethesda, MD: AOTA Press.

Health Care Quality Improvement Act of 1986, Pub. L. 99–660, 42 U.S.C. §§ 11101–11152.

Health Insurance Portability and Accountability Act of 1996, Pub. L. 104–191 110 Stat. 1936.

Kyler, P., & Slater, D. Y. (2011). Reference guide to the *Occupational Therapy Code of Ethics and Ethics Standards.* In D. Y. Slater (Ed.), *Reference guide to the Occupational Therapy Code of Ethics and Ethics Standards* (2010 ed., pp. 3–5). Bethesda, MD: AOTA Press.

Maryland Department of Health and Mental Hygiene, Board of Occupational Therapy Practice. (2010, October). *Disciplinary actions.* Retrieved from www.dhmh.state.md.us/botp/SitePages/discipline.aspx

Moyers, P. (2009). Occupational therapy practitioners: Competence and professional development. In E. B. Crepeau, E. S. Cohn, & B. A. B. Schell (Eds.), *Willard and Spackman's occupational therapy* (11th ed., pp. 240–251). Philadelphia: Lippincott Williams & Wilkins.

National Board for Certification in Occupational Therapy. (2009). *The Disciplinary Action Information Exchange Network (DAIEN).* Retrieved from www.nbcot.org/index.php?option=com_content&view=article&id=129:disciplinary-action-information-exchange-network-daien&catid=6:community&Itemid=60

National Board for Certification in Occupational Therapy. (2010a). *NBCOT candidate/certificant code of conduct.* Retrieved from www.nbcot.org/pdf/Candidate-Certificant-Code-of-Conduct.pdf

National Board for Certification in Occupational Therapy. (2010b, Spring/Summer). NBCOT disciplinary actions. *Certification Matters.* Retrieved from www.nbcot.org/pdf/Cert-Matters_Spring-Summer_2010.pdf

National Board for Certification in Occupational Therapy. (2011). *Procedures for the enforcement of the NBCOT Candidate/Certificant Code of Conduct.* Retrieved August 4, 2012, from www.nbcot.org/pdf/Enforcement_Procedures.pdf

National Board for Certification in Occupational Therapy. (2012). *2012 certification renewal application.* Retrieved from www.nbcot.org/pdf/Certification-Renewal-Application.pdf?phpMyAdmin=3710605fd34365e380b9ab41a5078545

North Carolina Board of Occupational Therapy. (2010, September). *Disciplinary actions.* Retrieved from www.ncbot.org/OTpages/disciplinary_actions.html

Reed, K. L. (2011). Occupational therapy values and beliefs: The formative years, 1904–1929. In D. Y. Slater (Ed.), *Reference guide to the Occupational Therapy Code of Ethics and Ethics Standards* (2010 ed., pp. 57–72). Bethesda, MD: AOTA Press.

U.S. Department of Health and Human Services. (2001). *National Practitioner Data Bank guidebook.* Rockville, MD: Health Resources and Services Data Bank. Retrieved from www.npdb-hipdb.hrsa.gov/resources/NPDBGuidebook.pdf

U.S. Department of Health and Human Services. (n.d.). *About us.* Rockville, MD: Health Resources and Services Administration Data Bank. Retrieved from www.npdb-hipdb.hrsa.gov/topNavigation/aboutUs.jsp

Willmarth, C. (2011). State regulation of occupational therapists and occupational therapy assistants. In K. Jacobs & G. L. McCormack (Eds.), *The occupational therapy manager* (5th ed., pp. 455–467). Bethesda, MD: AOTA Press.

Part II. Principles

Introduction

Janie B. Scott, MA, OT/L, FAOTA

Now that a groundwork has been laid for understanding the history of the American Occupational Therapy Association's (AOTA's) *Occupational Therapy Code of Ethics and Ethics Standards (2010)* (referred to as the "Code and Ethics Standards"; AOTA, 2010), Part II proceeds to an examination of its principles. Readers will gain an in-depth understanding of the elements of each ethical principle and its relationship to occupational therapy practice. Through case studies and vignettes, readers will explore the practical applications of each principle, including analytical processes to use in resolving ethical dilemmas, in the context of current occupational therapy practice.

The seven principles reviewed in Part II are as follows:

- *Principle 1: Beneficence.* The ethical principle of Beneficence requires occupational therapy practitioners to work for the well-being and safety of the recipients of their services. Chapter 3 highlights the importance of continuing competence in occupational therapy practices that benefit consumers and promote evidence-based practice. The expectation of continuing competence for occupational therapy practitioners has been articulated by the AOTA in its standards of practice, by the National Board for Certifica-

tion in Occupational Therapy, and by state regulatory boards.
- *Principle 2: Nonmaleficence.* The principle of Nonmaleficence reinforces the obligation of occupational therapy practitioners to avoid exploitation of and prevent harm to recipients of services. Chapter 4 also focuses on the importance of practitioners' own self-care, including vigilance against conflicts of commitment or of interest.
- *Principle 3: Autonomy and Confidentiality.* Occupational therapy practitioners' legal and ethical responsibility to respect the client's right to privacy is the focus of Chapter 5. Practitioners are encouraged to become culturally sensitive in order to support service recipients' autonomy and to focus on supporting client self-determination by engaging in client-centered practice.
- *Principle 4: Social Justice.* The principle of Social Justice is compatible with occupational therapy's roots in social activism. Chapter 6 details the consistency between this principle and its counterparts in the codes of ethics of seven other health-related national organizations. This principle is examined at the institutional and individual levels, reinforcing that social justice is germane to all occupational therapy roles, including those of educator, researcher, volunteer, and practitioner.

- *Principle 5: Procedural Justice.* The principle of Procedural Justice includes occupational therapy practitioners' obligation to adhere to laws, policies, and institutional rules, as well as standards established by AOTA, in all contexts in which occupational therapy is practiced. Chapter 7 discusses these topics, as well as requirements for credentialing and documentation and the importance of informing supervisees, colleagues, and administrators about occupational therapists' ethical and regulatory responsibilities.
- *Principle 6: Veracity.* The principle of Veracity emphasizes truth, honesty, and respect in communication with others (e.g., clients, colleagues, the public). As discussed in Chapter 8, these expectations extend to oral communication and written documentation and include providing proper attributions to the works of others.

- *Principle 7: Fidelity.* The principle of Fidelity involves the constructs of respect, fairness, and integrity as defined from the occupational therapy practitioner's perspective. Chapter 9 discusses the importance of balancing obligations to stakeholders (e.g., clients, colleagues, and other professionals) and provides strategies for preventing breaches of this principle.

Reference

American Occupational Therapy Association. (2010). Occupational therapy code of ethics and ethics standards (2010). *American Journal of Occupational Therapy, 64*(6 Suppl.), S17–S26. doi: 10.5014/ajot2010.64S17

Principle 1: Beneficence

3

Janie B. Scott, MA, OT/L, FAOTA, and
Dana Burns, MS, OTR/L, CBIS

BENEFICENCE

Principle 1. Occupational therapy personnel shall demonstrate a concern for the well-being and safety of the recipients of their services.

Beneficence includes all forms of action intended to benefit other persons. The term *beneficence* connotes acts of mercy, kindness, and charity (Beauchamp & Childress, 2009). Forms of beneficence typically include altruism, love, and humanity. Beneficence requires taking action by helping others, in other words, by promoting good, by preventing harm, and by removing harm. Examples of beneficence include protecting and defending the rights of others, preventing harm from occurring to others, removing conditions that will cause harm to others, helping persons with disabilities, and rescuing persons in danger (Beauchamp & Childress, 2009).

OCCUPATIONAL THERAPY PERSONNEL SHALL

   A. Respond to requests for occupational therapy services (e.g., a referral) in a timely manner as determined by law, regulation, or policy.
   B. Provide appropriate evaluation and a plan of intervention for all recipients of occupational therapy services specific to their needs.
   C. Reevaluate and reassess recipients of service in a timely manner to determine if goals are being achieved and whether intervention plans should be revised.
   D. Avoid the inappropriate use of outdated or obsolete tests/assessments or data obtained from such tests in making intervention decisions or recommendations.
   E. Provide occupational therapy services that are within each practitioner's level of competence and scope of practice (e.g., qualifications, experience, the law).
   F. Use, to the extent possible, evaluation, planning, intervention techniques, and therapeutic equipment that are evidence-based and within the recognized scope of occupational therapy practice.

G. Take responsible steps (e.g., continuing education, research, supervision, training) and use careful judgment to ensure their own competence and weigh potential for client harm when generally recognized standards do not exist in emerging technology or areas of practice.

H. Terminate occupational therapy services in collaboration with the service recipient or responsible party when the needs and goals of the recipient have been met or when services no longer produce a measurable change or outcome.

I. Refer to other health care specialists solely on the basis of the needs of the client.

J. Provide occupational therapy education, continuing education, instruction, and training that are within the instructor's subject area of expertise and level of competence.

K. Provide students and employees with information about the Code and Ethics Standards, opportunities to discuss ethical conflicts, and procedures for reporting unresolved ethical conflicts.

L. Ensure that occupational therapy research is conducted in accordance with currently accepted ethical guidelines and standards for the protection of research participants and the dissemination of results.

M. Report to appropriate authorities any acts in practice, education, and research that appear unethical or illegal.

N. Take responsibility for promoting and practicing occupational therapy on the basis of current knowledge and research and for further developing the profession's body of knowledge.

Source. From the *Occupational Therapy Code of Ethics and Ethics Standards (2010)* (American Occupational Therapy Association, 2010a, pp. S18–S19).

The concept of Beneficence, the first principle of the *Occupational Therapy Code of Ethics and Ethics Standards (2010)* (referred to as the "Code and Ethics Standards"; American Occupational Therapy Association [AOTA], 2010a), has been explored by religious leaders, philosophers, and ethicists, as well as by occupational therapy practitioners. Although the exact wording of their definitions varies, the focus on being helpful to others is consistent. For example, Veatch and Flack (1997) described beneficence in the allied health professions as "the state of doing or producing good . . . [and] the moral principle that actions are right insofar as they produce good" (p. 277).

Beneficence in occupational therapy has similarly been defined as "doing good for others or bringing about good for them; the duty to confer benefits on others" (Slater, 2011, p. 225). Occupational therapy practitioners promote positive outcomes and prevent harm when they adhere to the behavioral expectations described in Principle 1 of the Code and Ethics Standards. This chapter focuses on two such expectations: (1) maintaining competence and (2) engaging in evidence-based practice.

BENEFICENCE THROUGH COMPETENCE

Competence is possession of the knowledge base, skill level, and clinical reasoning ability to deliver occupational therapy services in a safe and consistent manner (Wilson, 1977). State regulatory boards, AOTA, the National Board for Certification in Occupational Therapy (NBCOT), and other organizations and agencies external to occupational therapy each define specific requirements for competence in occupational therapy practitioners (e.g., AOTA, 2010b; see also Appendix F and Chapter 2, this volume). Reed, Ashe, and Slater (2009) reviewed cases considered by the AOTA Ethics Commission, including those that focused on breaches of ethics related to competence. They identified the following components of competence related to Principle 1 that practitioners need to support the ideal of beneficence:

- Qualifications and experience
- Evidence base
- Self-assessment
- Expert education
- Current knowledge

To maintain the ethical obligation of Beneficence, occupational therapy practitioners have a duty to continually maintain their competence by building their knowledge and skills and applying these to clinical, academic, and research practice. The expectation of competence, articulated by AOTA, NBCOT, and state regulatory boards, emphasizes the importance of occupational therapy practitioners developing and maintaining the requisite skills needed to serve clients safely. Competence is thus a value and a standard that encourages high levels of skills and abilities throughout the profession. Continuing education, research, independent reading, attendance at workshops and conferences, and many other vehicles are available to expand the occupational therapy practitioner's knowledge base. Vignette 3.1 describes an example of beneficent practice by a practitioner who has maintained and improved his competence over time.

VIGNETTE 3.1. USING EXPERTISE TO BENEFIT CLIENTS

Darius, an occupational therapist, had worked in the construction industry before entering occupational therapy school. He wanted to integrate his construction experience with occupational therapy and establish his own business once he developed competence in providing occupational therapy rehabilitation services to people recovering from traumatic injuries and neurological and orthopedic conditions. He maintained his entrepreneurial vision through school and during his first 4 years of practice. While gaining his occupational therapy expertise, he continued working part-time on a construction job. He realized that when he began his private practice, his referral base would potentially be greater if he obtained his AOTA Specialty Certification in Environmental Modifications.

After Darius had been in private practice 2 years, he was awarded a consultant contract to assess the internal and external environments of a community center to identify potential hazards that could harm the people with disabilities who attended programs in the center. As part of his contract, Darius also provided recommendations and evidence-based practice guidelines to address the deficiencies he identified. Darius's high level of competence in environmental

assessment and redesign strengthened his ability to provide beneficent occupational therapy services by advocating to reduce potential harm to people with disabilities. The resources and continuing education that he took advantage of through AOTA and other vendors helped him ensure his competence in both practice areas.

Competence is important to clients, to the profession, and to individual occupational therapy practitioners. Most important, high-quality and competent occupational therapy services benefit the recipients, be they individuals or communities (McConnell, 2001). According to the Preamble of the Code and Ethics Standards, "Occupational therapy personnel have an ethical responsibility primarily to recipients of service and secondarily to society" (AOTA, 2010a, p. S17). Moyers (2002) pointed out that unsatisfactory competence can manifest in several ways, including increased expenditures of time and resources. Additionally, practitioner incompetence may worsen clients' condition or cause additional, secondary conditions, which may in turn lead to discontent with or poor quality of life (Moyers, 2002). By maintaining competence, occupational therapy practitioners are better able to prevent the consequences of incompetent practice.

The occupational therapy profession benefits from practitioner competence when practitioners deliver the highest quality services to clients. As stated in the *Centennial Vision* (Baum, 2006), the occupational therapy profession is striving to become "a powerful, widely recognized, science-driven, and evidence-based profession with a globally connected and diverse workforce meeting society's occupational needs" (p. 610). This vision of the profession is dependent on recognition by consumers, providers, and payers that occupational therapy practitioners deliver valuable services with a high level of competence.

Finally, professional competence benefits the practitioner. Continuing education can add meaning to one's professional career; as Bush, Powell, and Herzberg (1993) stated, "therapists must independently navigate their career paths in directions that are personally satisfying and productive" (p. 932). By engaging in continuing education pertaining to one's current position or even to new topics of interest, practitioners are able to direct their professional growth in a meaningful direction. Personal reflection, including that gained through continuing education, can assist occupational therapy practitioners in developing a meaningful and gratifying career, thus ensuring benefits to themselves and their clients (Crist, Wilcox, & McCarron, 1998). According to Wilcox (2005), "Continuing professional development is the means to keep you up to date, safe and competent as a practitioner. It can keep you interested and satisfied in your work, and it can certainly keep you in employment" (p. 44) by opening career opportunities. In Case Study 3.1, novice occupational therapists advocate for the resources they need to increase their competence.

CASE STUDY 3.1. DEVELOPING COMPETENCE IN NOVICE PRACTITIONERS

Azure, an occupational therapist with 10 years of experience, provided physical rehabilitation to clients in hospital settings and in their homes. Azure had worked in home care for the past 5 years and enjoyed the independence, flexibility, and personal client care this setting offered. She had no administrative or supervisory responsibilities for the home care agency.

Three novice occupational therapists working for the same home care agency approached Azure to ask for her assistance in negotiating home care as a practice environment and learning intervention strategies that promote good client care. Although Azure's official role did not include supervision, the novice practitioners sought her assistance to reduce potential harm and optimize care (i.e., promote beneficent practice). Azure stated that her schedule was too busy and her caseload too high to permit her to provide this kind of supervision and support.

The novice occupational therapists wondered if this refusal constituted a breach of Principle 1, Beneficence. They wondered whether Azure's refusal to provide them with the remediation they needed and share the responsibility for their clients' safety conflicted with the duty of providing beneficent care.

Azure, for her part, was concerned about the novice practitioners' lack of knowledge and experi-

ence in a practice area that demands independence and highly competent practice. She consulted the Code and Ethics Standards and found Principle 1E, provide services within the practitioner's level of competence, to be relevant to her concerns. Additionally, Azure reviewed her contract and the *Reference Guide to the Occupational Therapy Code of Ethics and Ethics Standards* (Slater, 2011) for strategies she could use to clarify expectations, roles, and responsibilities for her and the novice practitioners in a way that would promote client care and safety and well-being. In the *Reference Guide,* she found "Combating Moral Distress" (Slater & Brandt, 2011) and "Is It Possible to Be Ethical?" (Morris, 2011) to be particularly helpful. She determined that the most effective approach would be to encourage the occupational therapists to review Principle 1 of the Code and Ethics Standards to understand their responsibilities for continuing competence. She also recommended they contact the home care company's account manager and ask the company to provide either leave time for continuing education or paid supervision until their level of competence improved to a level at which clients would be more likely to benefit from and less likely to be harmed by their services.

On the basis of Azure's recommendations, the novice occupational therapists set up a meeting with the company's representative to discuss their concerns. They thanked Azure for her patience and guidance and for her ability to serve as a good advocate for both clients and colleagues.

BENEFICENCE THROUGH EVIDENCE-BASED PRACTICE

Understanding the evidence base provided by occupational therapy research and incorporating it into practice lead to effective and beneficent practice. Principle 1F urges occupational therapy practitioners to "use, to the extent possible, evaluation, planning, intervention techniques, and therapeutic equipment that are evidence-based and within the recognized scope of occupational therapy practice" (AOTA, 2010a, p. S19). Occupational therapy practitioners must keep abreast of current research outcomes relevant to their practice areas to increase the beneficence of their practice. Craik and Rappolt (2006) suggested that occupational therapy practitioners invest in professional development to ensure they obtain the skills necessary to understand and use research findings.

One important area of evidence-based practice is the use of assessments in occupational therapy evaluation and intervention. Occupational therapy practitioners use assessment results to assist in making decisions for intervention planning (Portney & Watkins, 2009), and they are ethically obligated to use assessments in ways that are supported by the evidence base. Practitioners' responsibility is to respond to an evaluation request in a timely manner (Principle 1A), use current evaluation tools (Principle 1D) that are within their competence (Principle 1E), and use the scoring outcomes to develop an appropriate intervention plan (Principle 1B). The practitioner's obligation to use standardized assessments according to administration and scoring standards exists regardless of setting. As Law and Baum (2005) noted,

> measurement is used to improve our decisions regarding specific clients or programs. As professionals, occupational therapists have an obligation to measure the need for service, design interventions based on knowledge gained from measurement, and evaluate the results of interventions. (p. 15)

Occupational therapy practitioners' obligation in appropriately using assessments to measure client capacities and limitations begins with being knowledgeable about each assessment instrument used. Practitioners must locate the appropriate assessment, master the correct administration procedures, and be sure never to offer test items for practice (Asher, 2007). Using assessments as intended provides valid data regarding clients that can be used to document the value of occupational therapy services. As Law and Baum (2005) affirmed, "as occupational therapists develop evidence-based practice, a valid measurement process is essential in providing evidence of the effectiveness and efficiency of our services" (p. 16). Practitioners must also "review the validity features of the measure to be sure that the test

is designed to offer the kind of information the professional desires" (Dunn, 2005, p. 23).

If assessments are not used according to the developers' instructions and the evidence regarding their use, the client may not receive the full benefit of occupational therapy services because intervention has been planned and implemented on the basis of incomplete, inaccurate, or missing data about important limitations or potential capabilities (Reed, 2011). Reitz, Pizzi, and Scaffa (2010) stated, "Working expediently can be a positive attribute, but it can also lead to unethical behavior if sufficient care is not taken to select the best available assessment, to properly administer the assessment, and to properly report results" (p. 167). Any deficiencies in the application of the test or assessment instrument should be noted in the assessment summary and allowances made for inaccurate interpretation (Reed, 2011), and the client's performance should not be compared with standard scores. Case Study 3.2 describes an occupational therapist's efforts to ensure that assessments are used correctly in her setting.

CASE STUDY 3.2. USING ASSESSMENTS APPROPRIATELY

Julie had practiced as an occupational therapist for 1 year in an urban hospital. She provided care to clients with a variety of physical and cognitive disabilities in both acute care and acute rehabilitation services. She believed she was competent in evaluating clients, planning interventions, and discharging clients appropriately.

Julie attended a session at an occupational therapy conference on the appropriate and ethical use of assessments. Julie remembered studying and learning current administration procedures during her recent academic preparation; however, her coworkers and mentors at her current institution used practices that conflicted with what Julie had learned in academic study and at the conference session. She weighed what she was taught in school and what she learned through continuing education activities against the guidance she received from her coworkers.

For example, it was common practice among Julie's coworkers to use portions of a standardized assessment, rather than the entire assessment, and to ignore scoring guidelines. When Julie questioned a coworker about this type of assessment use, the coworker responded, "I don't record that I am using the assessment. I am just basing my evaluation on how they do on those portions of the assessment. It's not like I am saying they are performing at this level, based on this assessment." In addition, Julie observed several occupational therapists using assessments as an intervention. When Julie asked her coworkers about this practice, one responded, "No one uses the assessments anyway, so why does it matter?"

Julie confirmed that competent assessment administration means documenting when standardized assessments are used. She also concluded that the use of assessments as interventions potentially reduces the validity of the standardization if, in the future, another practitioner were to administer the tool with the same client. Julie determined that administering and using such assessments violated Principles 1B and 1C of the Code and Ethics Standards. She decided to discuss the matter with her immediate supervisor during a private meeting.

Julie and her supervisor agreed that Julie would provide an educational in-service to her peers regarding appropriate and current assessment administration and scoring. After the in-service was held, facility leadership created mandatory competencies for occupational therapy practitioners to ensure their competence in the administration of assessments. Julie felt her presentation was well received by her superiors and peers.

CONCLUSION

The emphasis on continuing competence and evidence-based practice reflects the commitment of the occupational therapy profession to the principle of Beneficence. Maintaining professional competence is a lifelong obligation for all occupational therapy practitioners. A prescribed path for pursuing professional competence does not exist; it is up to each practitioner to identify his or her strengths and needs and create a plan for professional development. As Law and Baum (2005) noted, "What is best practice today

evolves into standard practice in the future. This is how knowledge advances in our discipline. The standard practices of today were best practices of the past that have influenced practice" (pp. 9–10). Therefore, occupational therapy practitioners must constantly critique best practices and incorporate those worthy into their practice. State regulations, the Code and Ethics Standards, and other official documents help guide us to occupational therapy practice that is ethical, beneficent, competent, and evidence based.

REFERENCES

American Occupational Therapy Association. (2010a). Occupational therapy code of ethics and ethics standards (2010). *American Journal of Occupational Therapy, 64*(6 Suppl.), S17–S26. doi: 10.5014/ajot.2010.64S17

American Occupational Therapy Association. (2010b). *Occupational therapy profession—Continuing competence requirements.* Bethesda, MD: Author. Retrieved January 3, 2012, from www.aota.org/Practitioners/Licensure/StateRegs/ContComp/OT-CC-Reqs-August-2010.aspx?FT=.pdf

Asher, I. E. (Ed.). (2007). *Occupational therapy assessment tools: An annotated index* (3rd ed.). Bethesda, MD: AOTA Press.

Baum, M. C. (2006). Presidential Address—Centennial challenges, millennium opportunities. *American Journal of Occupational Therapy, 60,* 609–616. doi: 10.5014/ajot.60.6.609

Beauchamp, T. L., & Childress, J. F. (2009). *Principles of biomedical ethics* (6th ed.). New York: Oxford University Press.

Bush, J. V., Powell, N. J., & Herzberg, G. (1993). Career self-efficacy in occupational therapy practice. *American Journal of Occupational Therapy, 47,* 927–933. doi: 10.5014/ajot.47.10.927

Craik, J., & Rappolt, S. (2006). Enhancing research utilization capacity through multifaceted professional development. *American Journal of Occupational Therapy, 60,* 155–164. doi: 10.5014/ajot.60.2.155

Crist, P., Wilcox, B. L., & McCarron, K. (1998). Transitional portfolios: Orchestrating our professional competence. *American Journal of Occupational Therapy, 52,* 729–736. doi: 10.5014/ajot.52.9.729

Dunn, W. (2005). Measurement issues and practices. In M. Law, C. Baum, & W. Dunn (Eds.), *Measuring occupational performance: Supporting best practice in occupational therapy* (2nd ed., pp. 21–32). Thorofare, NJ: Slack.

Law, M., & Baum, C. (2005). Measurement in occupational therapy. In M. Law, C. Baum, & W. Dunn (Eds.), *Measuring occupational performance: Supporting best practice in occupational therapy* (2nd ed., pp. 3–20). Thorofare, NJ: Slack.

McConnell, E. A. (2001). Competence vs. competency. *Nursing Management, 32*(5), 14.

Morris, J. F. (2011). Is it possible to be ethical? In D. Y. Slater (Ed.), *Reference guide to the Occupational Therapy Code of Ethics and Ethics Standards* (2010 ed., pp. 73–80). Bethesda, MD: AOTA Press.

Moyers, P. A. (2002, September). Continuing competence and competency: What you need to know. *OT Practice, 7*(9), 18–22. Retrieved March 25, 2010, from www1.aota.org/pdt/MoyersOTArticle.htm

Portney, L. G., & Watkins, M. P. (2009). Principles of measurement. In *Foundations of clinical research: Applications to practice* (3rd ed., pp. 63–75). Upper Saddle River, NJ: Pearson Education.

Reed, K. L. (2011). Outdated and obsolete tests and assessment instruments. In D. Y. Slater (Ed.), *Reference guide to the Occupational Therapy Code of Ethics and Ethics Standards* (2010 ed., pp. 193–197). Bethesda, MD: AOTA Press.

Reed, K. L., Ashe, A. M., & Slater, D. Y. (2009, April). *Everyday ethics: Ethical challenges in emerging practice.* Slide show presented at the AOTA Annual Conference & Expo, Houston.

Reitz, S. M., Pizzi, M. A., & Scaffa, M. E. (2010). Evaluation principles in health promotion practice. In M. E. Scaffa, S. M. Reitz, & M. A. Pizzi (Eds.), *Occupational therapy in the promotion of health and wellness* (pp. 157–172). Philadelphia: F. A. Davis.

Slater, D. Y. (Ed.). (2011). *Reference guide to the Occupational Therapy Code of Ethics and Ethics Standards* (2010 ed.). Bethesda, MD: AOTA Press.

Slater, D. Y., & Brandt, L. C. (2011). Combating moral distress. In D. Y. Slater (Ed.), *Reference guide to the Occupational Therapy Code of Ethics and Ethics Standards* (2010 ed., pp. 107–113). Bethesda, MD: AOTA Press.

Veatch, R. M., & Flack, H. E. (1997). *Case studies in allied health ethics.* Upper Saddle River, NJ: Prentice Hall.

Wilcox, A. (2005). How to succeed as a lifelong learner. *Primary Health Care, 15*(10), 43–49.

Wilson, M. A. (1977). A competency assurance program. *American Journal of Occupational Therapy, 31,* 573–579.

Principle 2: Nonmaleficence

4

S. Maggie Reitz, PhD, OTR/L, FAOTA

NONMALEFICENCE

Principle 2. Occupational therapy personnel shall intentionally refrain from actions that cause harm.

Nonmaleficence imparts an obligation to refrain from harming others (Beauchamp & Childress, 2009). The principle of nonmaleficence is grounded in the practitioner's responsibility to refrain from causing harm, inflicting injury, or wronging others. While beneficence requires action to incur benefit, nonmaleficence requires non-action to avoid harm (Beauchamp & Childress, 2009). Nonmaleficence also includes an obligation to not impose risks of harm even if the potential risk is without malicious or harmful intent. This principle often is examined under the context of *due care*. If the standard of due care outweighs the benefit of treatment, then refraining from treatment provision would be ethically indicated (Beauchamp & Childress, 2009).

OCCUPATIONAL THERAPY PERSONNEL SHALL

   A. Avoid inflicting harm or injury to recipients of occupational therapy services, students, research participants, or employees.

   B. Make every effort to ensure continuity of services or options for transition to appropriate services to avoid abandoning the service recipient if the current provider is unavailable due to medical or other absence or loss of employment.

   C. Avoid relationships that exploit the recipient of services, students, research participants, or employees physically, emotionally, psychologically, financially, socially, or in any other manner that conflicts or interferes with professional judgment and objectivity.

   D. Avoid engaging in any sexual relationship or activity, whether consensual or nonconsensual, with any recipient of service, including family or significant other, student, research participant, or employee, while a relationship exists as an occupational therapy practitioner, educator, researcher, supervisor, or employer.

   E. Recognize and take appropriate action to remedy personal problems and limitations that might cause harm to recipients of service, colleagues, students, research participants, or others.

   F. Avoid any undue influences, such as alcohol or drugs, that may compromise the provision of occupational therapy services, education, or research.

G. Avoid situations in which a practitioner, educator, researcher, or employer is unable to maintain clear professional boundaries or objectivity to ensure the safety and well-being of recipients of service, students, research participants, and employees.

H. Maintain awareness of and adherence to the Code and Ethics Standards when participating in volunteer roles.

I. Avoid compromising client rights or well-being based on arbitrary administrative directives by exercising professional judgment and critical analysis.

J. Avoid exploiting any relationship established as an occupational therapist or occupational therapy assistant to further one's own physical, emotional, financial, political, or business interests at the expense of the best interests of recipients of services, students, research participants, employees, or colleagues.

K. Avoid participating in bartering for services because of the potential for exploitation and conflict of interest unless there are clearly no contraindications or bartering is a culturally appropriate custom.

L. Determine the proportion of risk to benefit for participants in research prior to implementing a study.

Source. From the *Occupational Therapy Code of Ethics and Ethics Standards (2010)* (American Occupational Therapy Association, 2010, pp. S19–S20).

Nonmaleficence, Principle 2 of the *Occupational Therapy Code of Ethics and Ethics Standards* (referred to as the "Code and Ethics Standards"; American Occupational Therapy Association [AOTA], 2010), is closely linked to the principle of Beneficence, discussed in Chapter 3 of this volume. The difference is subtle but important; according to Beauchamp and Childress (2009), "while beneficence requires action to incur benefit, nonmaleficence requires non-action to prevent harm" (quoted in AOTA, 2010, p. S19). Nonmaleficence first appeared as a separate principle in the 2000 version of the *Occupational Therapy Code of Ethics* (AOTA, 2000).

Four categories of behaviors are addressed by the principle of Nonmaleficence: (1) avoidance of exploitation, (2) prevention of harm, (3) self-reflection and mindfulness to avoid harm, and (4) self-care (i.e., the protection of one's own health). Although these categories are not mutually exclusive, they constitute a framework for further exploring the complexity of the principle of Nonmaleficence.

AVOIDANCE OF EXPLOITATION

Five of the 12 subprinciples in Principle 2 address the need to refrain from exploitation, and of them

four relate to exploitation in relationships—Principles 2C, 2D, 2G, and 2J; the remaining subprinciple, Principle 2K, refers to exploitation in business. The ability to develop and engage in therapeutic relationships is an essential quality of competent occupational therapy service provision; when these relationships are not in place, intentional and unintentional harm can result. Engaging in bartering that exploits businesses, vendors, or others in the organization can damage the reputation of the profession as well as the employer or institution.

The profession has long paid attention to the importance of relationships within occupational therapy practice. Taylor (2008) described the evolution of thought regarding the optimal use of relationships in occupational therapy practice, including the principles of therapeutic use of self proposed by Frank in 1958 and conscious use of self encouraged by Mosey in 1981. After a review of contemporary literature, Taylor identified two themes in regard to the therapeutic use of relationships in occupational therapy practice: (1) collaboration and client centeredness and (2) caring and empathy. In addition, Taylor discussed the use of narrative and clinical reasoning as valued intervention approaches to develop therapeutic relationships.

Case Study 4.1 shows that exploitation can involve employees, not only clients and students, and exemplifies three important considerations in ethical resolution:

1. Validating perceptions before assuming a violation has occurred,
2. Addressing ethical concerns and perceptions as soon as possible, and
3. Handling concerns locally whenever possible.

CASE STUDY 4.1. AVOIDING EXPLOITATION

Christina, an occupational therapist, was looking forward to being assigned her first new employee to supervise and mentor. She wanted both to share her expertise in evidence-based practice and to help educate the next generation of occupational therapy practitioners. **Serge**, the employee assigned to Christina, was similarly looking forward to starting his first job as an occupational therapist. Christina took Serge to lunch in the hospital cafeteria on his first day to get to know him better and to review the policy manual with him. After reviewing the manual, Christina switched the conversation to more personal topics. During this portion of the conversation, Christina found out that Serge was single and lived with his mother, who ran a house-cleaning service; Serge worked for her on Saturdays. She responded to this news by saying, "I've been looking forever for someone to clean my house but can't find an affordable person. Can your mom give me a deal?"

Serge did not know what to do. He felt bad for his supervisor because he knew that hospital employees had been furloughed because of state budget cutbacks. He also felt guilty that Christina had bought him lunch. However, Serge did not want to undermine the livelihood of the four women who worked for his mother by offering discounted service. He went home and told his mother, **Olga**, about the conversation he had had with Christina. Olga, a first-generation U.S. resident, was anxious for her son to do well. She offered to discount the rate, provided he did the cleaning on a twice-a-month schedule. Olga contacted Christina, and they scheduled the first cleaning. Christina was overjoyed at the deeply discounted rate she had been provided.

As soon as Serge entered Christina's townhouse the following Saturday, he felt uneasy; this feeling intensified over the coming weeks. Christina's large-screen, high-definition television and upscale furnishings contrasted with his assumption that she was financially vulnerable. When he arrived for the second scheduled cleaning session, Christina was just getting out of the shower. He left immediately and waited in his car, reviewing his textbooks in preparation to evaluate a client the following Monday. When Christina left, he reentered the townhouse to complete the cleaning job. He shrugged off her behavior, knowing how easy it was to lose track of time. However, 2 weeks later, when he next went to clean, Christina had left negligees around the townhouse. Serge cleaned around the clothes, being careful not to touch any of them. Although he was feeling increasingly uncomfortable, he did not share his feelings with Christina or anyone else.

Two weeks later, when Serge arrived to clean, Christina had set the table for lunch and was provocatively dressed. She apologized, saying that she had forgotten Serge was scheduled to clean that day. Serge left, but 2 hours later she called and asked if he could return, as her lunch date had unexpectedly been cancelled. When he arrived, she was still dressed for her date and asked him to stay for lunch after he had finished cleaning. He politely said he could not because he was scheduled to clean other homes that afternoon. Hearing this, she then asked him if he was available for dinner. At this point Serge, feeling truly troubled, told Christina that he needed to leave. He called his mother and asked her to schedule one of the other women for future cleanings, stating that he would pay her the money that the cleaner would lose because of the discounted rate.

Serge was worried that Christina would seek revenge for his rejection of the dinner invitation when she completed his probation report, which was due the following month. After a 2-mile run to clear his head, he remembered that in one of his occupational therapy classes, they had reviewed frameworks that could be used when facing an ethical challenge. He found the course material and reviewed the Code and Ethics Standards. From this review, he determined that Christina had possibly violated Principles 2A, 2C, 2E, and 2G. Serge realized, on reflection, that he did not know for certain whether Christina was flirting with him and attempting to engage in a sexual relationship or not, so at this time he did not believe Principle 2D had been violated. However, it became clear to him that the request for discounted cleaning services was inappropriate and that he should not have agreed to ask Olga's cleaning company to work for Christina.

When Serge returned to work on Monday, he asked if he could meet with Christina. At the start of the meeting, he told her that he had become uncomfortable with the house-cleaning arrangement and that he would no longer be able to clean her house. He also shared his concerns that by offering her the discounted cleaning rate, he unwittingly had put her in possible violation of Principles 2A, 2C, 2E, and 2G. At first, Christina became defensive, saying, "I am an extremely competent occupational therapist. The Code of Ethics is to protect clients. I have never harmed a client!" Serge remained calm and responded that she was one of the most competent occupational therapists he had ever had the honor to work with and that he had learned a great deal from watching her work. He then showed her a copy of the Code and Ethics Standards. As Christina read Principle 2, she became visibly more upset. She apologized, saying she had not been aware that her actions were in violation of the Code and Ethics Standards.

Serge then shared that he felt uncomfortable with her invitations for lunch and dinner. At this, Christina started to laugh. Serge became tense. Christina, seeing his anxiety, stopped laughing and explained that although Serge was an attractive young man, she was in a committed relationship. In fact, she said she had been preparing a wardrobe for her wedding and honeymoon and apologized for leaving the garments around the townhouse. She further explained that she had offered him the invitation to lunch and dinner because she did not wish to waste the food she had prepared for her fiancé. She shared that although she was now financially comfortable, she had grown up in a family who needed to use food stamps, and she was always very conscious of wasting food.

Serge believed that he could continue to learn a great deal from Christina. He also was proud that they had worked through a challenging ethical situation together in a positive way. Therefore, he decided he would prefer to continue their current professional relationship but end the house-cleaning arrangement. Christina agreed, saying this decision also would make her most comfortable, and she encouraged Serge to continue to be forthright with her as he had done

that day. Other possible actions that Serge could have considered for addressing this ethical issue are detailed in Table 4.1.

Serge, by following the last option in Table 4.1, addressed all three considerations in ethical resolution. His approach to the first two, validating perceptions and addressing concerns as soon as possible, is readily apparent. The third consideration, handling issues locally, was demonstrated by Serge's speaking directly to Christina rather than reporting her behavior to the department head. Handling issues locally does not preclude using resources such as the staff liaison to AOTA's Ethics Commission or a professional mentor to discuss strategies for approaching the situation, as long as confidentiality is maintained.

PREVENTION OF HARM

Benjamin Franklin is credited with the statement "an ounce of prevention is worth a pound of cure" (Independence Hall Association, 2010, para. 1). The truth of this saying is as evident in ethics as it is in other areas of life. Preventing harm involves being vigilant to avoid circumstances with the potential to evolve into situations in which harm occurs. Principles 2A, 2B, and 2L directly involve the prevention of harm. Vignettes 4.1 and 4.2 both directly relate to Principle 2A, in which occupational therapy practitioners are guided to avoid inflicting harm; these vignettes also show how behaviors associated with the prevention of harm also can be related to the avoidance of exploitation.

VIGNETTE 4.1. PREVENTING ACADEMIC DISHONESTY

Heather and **Lynn** were best friends in different sections of the same graduate course. They were assigned to complete presentations on the same topic. In the week before the presentation, when Lynn had planned on preparing her presentation, her boyfriend broke their engagement and moved to London for a job opportunity. The same day, Lynn lost her wallet, and the next day she was laid off from her job. Overwhelmed, Lynn asked Heather to send her a copy of her draft PowerPoint slides so

TABLE 4.1
Decision Table for Case Study 4.1

POSSIBLE ACTION	POSITIVE OUTCOMES	NEGATIVE CONSEQUENCES
No action	Serge avoids conflict and maintains a comfortable relationship with his supervisor.	Serge allows for possible exploitation of self or others.
Explain, when first asked for the discounted services, that to enter into such a business relationship could be viewed as a conflict of interest and open up the possible or perceived exploitation of each party; refer Christina to another reputable cleaning company; and suggest that Christina read the book *Nickel and Dimed: On (Not) Getting By in America* (Ehrenreich, 2001) so she understands the economic and social justice issues of her looking for deeply discounted services	Serge avoids possible exploitation of self or others. Serge promotes Principle 4: Social Justice.	This action could result in possible conflict and an uncomfortable relationship with his supervisor.
Share his discomfort over the lunch invitation with Christina and clarify their expectations of their relationship	Serge promotes transparency and honest communication earlier in the scenario, preventing further miscommunication. Serge avoids possible exploitation of self.	This action could result in possible conflict and an uncomfortable relationship with his supervisor.
Ask the department head to reassign Serge to another supervisor and mentor while Christina continues to be a customer of Olga's cleaning service, paying the full cost of services	Serge avoids possible exploitation of Olga and Olga's employees.	Principle 1, Beneficence, could be a factor if the new mentor is not a good match for Serge's professional growth.
Continue their current professional relationship and seek a referral from Olga for another reputable cleaning company for Christina	Serge supports Principle 2, Nonmaleficence; Principle 4, Social Justice; and Principle 6, Fidelity.	None foreseen.

that she could make a few changes and submit them as her own work.

Heather knew that such an action would put both herself and Lynn in violation of the Code and Ethics Standards. Although Lynn did not put Heather in danger of physical injury, she jeopardized both her own and Heather's status as occupational therapy students and their future professional careers. In-

stead of agreeing to Lynn's request, Heather suggested that Lynn talk to her professor and adviser about getting an extension on the assignment, seek help from the university counseling center to deal with her personal turmoil, and accept help from a group of volunteers Heather organized to walk Lynn's dog and bring dinner over so that Lynn could catch up on her schoolwork.

Which ethical principles did Heather exhibit? Which ethical principles did Lynne exhibit in accepting Heather's course of action?

VIGNETTE 4.2. AVOIDING POTENTIAL HARM TO COLLEAGUES

The patient census in a skilled nursing facility was low. **Ginger**, an occupational therapist at the facility, decided it was an opportune time to reorganize her office to improve her efficiency and comfort. She went to find **Cliff**, an occupational therapy assistant, and **Sarah**, an occupational therapy student, to help her move some of her office furniture. She was unable to locate either. **Sandy**, another occupational therapist, asked Ginger why she needed Cliff and Sarah. When Ginger explained her plan, Sandy suggested to Ginger that she should get the plan approved by their supervisor, **Bob**. Ginger rolled her eyes and yelled, "Is this really necessary? It's making a mountain out of a molehill!" Trying to lighten the mood, Sandy said, "I don't know anything about moles, only hedgehogs, but you really should talk to Bob." This reply got a smile from Ginger, who went to find Bob.

Bob commended Ginger for using the low patient census time to enhance her work environment to increase productivity and comfort. However, he communicated to Ginger that it was inappropriate to ask a coworker and student to perform tasks that were not within their job descriptions and that put them at risk for incurring injury. Ginger continued to protest until he asked her if it would be appropriate for him to ask her to make him a cup of coffee. She responded, "Certainly not!" She then smiled and said, "OK; whose job is this?" Bob and Ginger talked and were able to schedule the appropriate staff to assist her in her office reorganization project the next day.

Two other principles, Principles 2B and 2L, are related to the prevention of harm. Principle 2B relates to client abandonment. An AOTA Ethics Commission Advisory Opinion provides assistance in upholding this particular principle (Morris, 2011). Principle 2L, in which we are directed to "determine the proportion of risk to benefit for participants in research prior to im-

plementing a study" (AOTA, 2010, p. S20), is the topic of Vignette 4.3 (see also Chapter 19, this volume).

VIGNETTE 4.3. ANALYZING RISKS AND BENEFITS IN RESEARCH

Brianna was an occupational therapy educator working with a group of occupational therapy master's-degree students on examining the link between sports engagement and successful aging among community-dwelling older adults. The research team decided to conduct a focus group with older adults to determine the meaning sports had played in their lives and their current level of engagement in sports. Several students were concerned that if a potential participant was no longer able to engage in favorite sports, their research might provoke sadness and depression.

The concerns of these students led to a lively and reflective discussion. The group decided to take extra care to be explicit in both the marketing and the informed consent materials to ensure that potential participants knew the topic of the research and could make their own decision as to whether to attend the focus group or not. Originally, the students had planned to conduct the focus groups in pairs, with one student asking the questions and the other being responsible for the informed consent form process and taking hand notes during the group. They decided to adjust their plans and have an additional student available in an adjoining room to talk with anyone who became upset during the focus group. The students also reviewed Principle 2L; they believed that the potential risk to participants was low in comparison to the more likely positive social benefits gained from their project. After taking these actions, and knowing that their project would be reviewed by the university's institutional review board, the students felt more comfortable proceeding with their research.

SELF-REFLECTION AND MINDFULNESS TO AVOID HARM

Principles 2H and 2I involve self-reflection and mindfulness to avoid harm. Occupational therapy practitioners are adept in using these behaviors in direct client care, but the need to use them in the course of administrative responsibilities and volunteer roles may be less evident. Case Study 4.2 and Vignette 4.4 address the need to exercise self-reflection and mindfulness when carrying out these roles and responsibilities.

CASE STUDY 4.2. ENGAGING IN SELF-REFLECTION AND MINDFULNESS TO AVOID HARM WHEN MAKING DECISIONS

Juan, an occupational therapy assistant in a skilled nursing facility, was approached by **Mildred** and **Bernice**, residents of the facility who shared a room. Mildred and Bernice were receiving similar occupational therapy for hip fractures from **Ann**, their occupational therapist. Mildred and Bernice wanted to switch their afternoon occupational therapy times. Mildred was currently scheduled at 1 p.m., when her daughter was available to bring Mildred's dog to visit during her lunch hour each day. Bernice was scheduled at 4 p.m., when her favorite television show aired.

Juan thought this was a logical request and approached Ann, the occupational therapist, to ask permission to make the schedule switch. Ann was having a challenging day because one of the other occupational therapists had called in sick. She responded in an agitated voice that she didn't have the time to deal with this change and was concerned that even if she did, it would "open the floodgates" for other similar requests. She then said she needed Juan to return another client to his room right away, effectively ending the conversation.

After Ann's long day ended, she went home and reflected on the day's events. She realized she had made an arbitrary decision because of the stresses of that particular day. The next day, she directed Juan to change Mildred's and Bernice's schedules. In addition, she asked if he was aware of any other clients who were dissatisfied with their current schedule. Juan said he was not but offered to ask each client for the next month and log the time needed to inquire and modify the schedule. Ann commended Juan for his logic and initiative.

One month later, Ann remarked to Juan that the head of Rehabilitation Services had been pleased with the increase in client satisfaction scores with occupational therapy services. She further commented that she believed this increase was attributable, in large part, to Juan's client advocacy efforts and the department's willingness to reconsider previous administrative procedures. Juan had found that only a few clients desired therapy schedule changes. Thus, Ann's concern about needing to spend additional time rearranging schedules was unfounded. In addition, the department realized actual benefits (i.e., an increase in client satisfaction scores) with relatively little effort.

Pleased by the results, Ann asked Juan if he would like to submit a joint proposal for a presentation to the state occupational therapy conference. Juan was excited about this opportunity and readily agreed. Ann thought it would be good to cite the Code and Ethics Standards in their presentation. While reviewing the Code and Ethics Standards for wording about respecting client autonomy, she found Principle 2I, which guides practitioners to "avoid compromising client rights or well-being based on arbitrary administrative directives by exercising professional judgment and critical analysis" (AOTA, 2010, p. S20). After an initial reaction of "Oh, my!" whispered to herself, she smiled and was proud that through self-reflection and Juan's efforts, her actions avoided a potential violation of the Code and Ethics Standards and resulted in several positive outcomes.

VIGNETTE 4.4. AVOIDING CONFLICT OF INTEREST

After relocating to a new state, **Joan** joined the state's occupational therapy conference committee to meet other occupational therapy practitioners. She was excited about the new friendships she made and wanted to be a contributing member of the committee. The conference planning went well, and the committee was ready to print the conference brochure. Joan's uncle, **Jim**, lived in the area and owned a printing business. His business had been losing money, so Joan hoped that she could guide the committee to use his services. She volunteered to find a printer without disclosing that she had a relationship with one of the potential vendors.

After arriving home from the meeting, she called Jim to see if he would like the business. Jim asked her who else was bidding on the opportunity.

She said, "No one else—it's yours for the taking." There was a period of silence on the phone, after which Jim asked whether Joan was aware of the term *conflict of interest*. Joan responded, "Not really." Jim then described what conflict of interest is and told Joan that although he greatly appreciated her efforts, she should get bids from at least two other printers. If the committee deemed his company to provide the best value (i.e., quality for cost) of the three, he would be happy to perform the work. He also asked if the occupational therapy profession had ethical guidelines for situations such as this.

Joan went online and located the Code and Ethics Standards on the AOTA Web page. She saw Principles 2I and 7E, which both pertain to ethical behavior in volunteer roles, with Principle 7E being directly related to conflict of interest. Joan completed the bid process, provided the information to the conference committee, and recused herself from the vendor selection process after disclosing her relationship to one of the bidders, without indicating which business. The conference committee was impressed with her ethical behavior and thanked her for her efforts.

SELF-CARE

Gilfoyle (1986) urged occupational therapists to take care of themselves. She believed that "our future depends on our ability to take care of ourselves both personally and professionally. Taking care of ourselves is the positive force that promotes the ability to seize opportunities for the future" (Gilfoyle, 1986, p. 387). Principles 2E and 2F both involve taking care of ourselves. Vignette 4.5 features an occupational therapy practitioner with a potential alcohol problem and thus relates to both of these principles.

VIGNETTE 4.5. AVOIDING UNDUE INFLUENCES

Stella was attending her state conference many miles away from the university where she taught. After one of the afternoon workshops, a group of local occupational therapy practitioners organized a happy hour outing, suggesting several places with two-for-one drink specials. Not knowing anyone

else at the conference, Stella at first decided to go along with the group. She set her phone alarm to be sure she would get back to the hotel room in time to teach her synchronous online class at 6 p.m. As Stella reflected on her plan, she became concerned that she might be tempted to take advantage of the drink specials and as a result not be in her best form for class that evening. She therefore chose to have an early dinner by herself and skip happy hour. Realizing that she did not trust herself in this situation, she pledged to discuss this self-reflection and her current drinking habits with her physician to determine if she needed to take further action to protect her health.

Stella's actions were consistent with the behavior required by Principles 2E and 2F. At a minimum, she avoided the potential embarrassment of a poor performance while conducting class. She also eliminated the students' potential need to report her performance if it became evident that she was under the influence while conducting class. Her actions also show that she was actively reflecting on her behavior and planned to seek assistance to determine if she needed to further examine her drinking habits to ensure they did not affect either her health or her professional performance.

Vignette 4.6 describes a potential conflict of commitment situation that needs to be avoided to uphold the spirit of Principle 2E: the need to "recognize and take appropriate action to remedy personal problems and limitations that might cause harm to recipients of service, colleagues, students, research participants, or others" (AOTA, 2010, p. S20). *Conflict of commitment* "arises when outside activities substantially interfere with the person's obligation to students, colleagues, or the institution" (University System of Maryland, 2003, para. 5). Conflict of commitment can be thought of broadly as accepting too many professional responsibilities for the available energy and time (AOTA Ethics Commission, 2007).

VIGNETTE 4.6. PREVENTING CONFLICT OF COMMITMENT

After receiving her doctoral degree, **Sally** was excited to be hired as a new tenure-track faculty member at the university from which she had graduated the previous month. She took on with gusto all the responsibilities associated with this new role. Knowing that she had to perform in the areas of teaching, advising, scholarship, and service to obtain tenure, she volunteered to advise the new entering class of occupational therapy students and to revise the course on clinical reasoning. **Jennifer**, the program director, greeted Sally's contributions with relief and appreciation, as they had been short staffed for several years.

Later that fall, Jennifer was surprised to hear that Sally was running for president of the state occupational therapy association, given all of her university commitments and the stresses of a first-year teaching appointment. Jennifer did not voice any concerns, however, until Sally asked Jennifer to nominate her for a leadership position in AOTA. Jennifer, out of concern for Sally's ability to meet her increasing workload, declined to nominate Sally for the opportunity.

Sally was at first offended. Jennifer explained her action, stating that this particular AOTA committee required a great deal of work. She also shared that she was concerned about Sally's potential conflict of commitment and the potential impact on her health and professional success. Jennifer offered to meet with Sally the following week to lay out a 4-year strategy to gradually increase service contributions, both within and outside the university, as Sally became more experienced in teaching and disseminating her scholarly work.

CONCLUSION

Early action, deescalation, and collaboration are all strategies occupational therapy practitioners can use to ensure they do not engage in unethical actions. Good people can make bad decisions. The Code and Ethics Standards are not punitive but rather aspirational, intended to help occupational therapy practitioners as a collective be responsible for protecting the people they treat.

Occupational therapy practitioners are able problem solvers. Coupled with our expertise in communication, we have the necessary prerequisite knowledge and skills to work through challenging ethical situations together and avoid actions that may result in harm.

REFERENCES

American Occupational Therapy Association. (2000). Occupational therapy code of ethics (2000). *American Journal of Occupational Therapy, 54,* 614–616. doi: 10.5014/ajot.54.6.617

American Occupational Therapy Association. (2010). Occupational therapy code of ethics and ethics standards (2010). *American Journal of Occupational Therapy,* 64(6 Suppl.), S17–S26. doi: 10:5014/ajot2010.62S17

American Occupational Therapy Association Ethics Commission. (2007). *Everyday ethics: Core knowledge for occupational therapy practitioners and educators* [Continuing education CD]. Bethesda, MD: Author.

Beauchamp, T. L., & Childress, J. F. (2009). *Principles of biomedical ethics* (6th ed.). New York: Oxford University Press.

Ehrenreich, B. (2001). *Nickel and dimed: On (not) getting by in America.* New York: Metropolitan Books.

Frank, J. D. (1958). Therapeutic use of self. *American Journal of Occupational Therapy, 8,* 215–225.

Gilfoyle, E. M. (1986). Nationally Speaking—Taking care of ourselves as health care providers. *American Journal of Occupational Therapy, 40,* 387–389. doi: 10.5014/ajot.40.6.387

Independence Hall Association. (2010). *The electric Ben Franklin: The quotable Franklin.* Retrieved March 13, 2011, from www.ushistory.org/franklin/quotable/quote67.htm

Morris, J. F. (2011). Patient abandonment. In D. Y. Slater (Ed.), *Reference guide to the Occupational Therapy Code of Ethics and Ethics Standards* (2010 ed., pp. 199–204). Bethesda, MD: AOTA Press.

Mosey, A. C. (1981). *Occupational therapy: Configuration of a profession.* New York: Raven Press.

Taylor, R. R. (2008). Changing landscape of therapeutic use of self. In *The intentional relationship: Occupational therapy and use of self* (pp. 3–18). Philadelphia: F. A. Davis.

University System of Maryland. (2003). *II-3.10—Policy on professional commitment of faculty.* Retrieved March 13, 2011, from www.usmd.edu/regents/bylaws/SectionII/II310.html

Principle 3: Autonomy and Confidentiality

5

Janie B. Scott, MA, OT/L, FAOTA

AUTONOMY, CONFIDENTIALITY

Principle 3. Occupational therapy personnel shall respect the right of the individual to self-determination.

   The principle of autonomy and confidentiality expresses the concept that practitioners have a duty to treat the client according to the client's desires, within the bounds of accepted standards of care and to protect the client's confidential information. Often *autonomy* is referred to as the *self-determination* principle. However, respect for autonomy goes beyond acknowledging an individual as a mere agent and also acknowledges a "person's right to hold views, to make choices, and to take actions based on personal values and beliefs" (Beauchamp & Childress, 2009, p. 103). Autonomy has become a prominent principle in health care ethics; the right to make a determination regarding care decisions that directly impact the life of the service recipient should reside with that individual. The principle of autonomy and confidentiality also applies to students in an educational program, to participants in research studies, and to the public who seek information about occupational therapy services.

OCCUPATIONAL THERAPY PERSONNEL SHALL

   A. Establish a collaborative relationship with recipients of service, including families, significant others, and caregivers, in setting goals and priorities throughout the intervention process. This includes full disclosure of the benefits, risks, and potential outcomes of any intervention; the personnel who will be providing the intervention(s); and/or any reasonable alternatives to the proposed intervention.
   B. Obtain consent before administering any occupational therapy service, including evaluation, and ensure that recipients of service (or their legal representatives) are kept informed of the progress in meeting goals specified in the plan of intervention/care. If the service recipient cannot give consent, the practitioner must be sure that consent has been obtained from the person who is legally responsible for that recipient.

C. Respect the recipient of service's right to refuse occupational therapy services temporarily or permanently without negative consequences.

D. Provide students with access to accurate information regarding educational requirements and academic policies and procedures relative to the occupational therapy program/educational institution.

E. Obtain informed consent from participants involved in research activities, and ensure that they understand the benefits, risks, and potential outcomes as a result of their participation as research subjects.

F. Respect research participants' right to withdraw from a research study without consequences.

G. Ensure that confidentiality and the right to privacy are respected and maintained regarding all information obtained about recipients of service, students, research participants, colleagues, or employees. The only exceptions are when a practitioner or staff member believes that an individual is in serious foreseeable or imminent harm. Laws and regulations may require disclosure to appropriate authorities without consent.

H. Maintain the confidentiality of all verbal, written, electronic, augmentative, and non-verbal communications, including compliance with [Health Insurance Portability and Accountability Act] regulations.

I. Take appropriate steps to facilitate meaningful communication and comprehension in cases in which the recipient of service, student, or research participant has limited ability to communicate (e.g., aphasia or differences in language, literacy, culture).

J. Make every effort to facilitate open and collaborative dialogue with clients and/or responsible parties to facilitate comprehension of services and their potential risks/benefits.

Source. From the *Occupational Therapy Code of Ethics and Ethics Standards (2010)* (American Occupational Therapy Association, 2010, pp. S20–S21).

Principle 3 of the *Occupational Therapy Code of Ethics and Ethics Standards (2010)* (referred to as the "Code and Ethics Standards"; American Occupational Therapy Association [AOTA], 2010) addresses the values of autonomy and confidentiality. In this chapter, Autonomy and Confidentiality are defined to provide a foundation for the exploration of three related ethical issues that support Principle 3: (1) communication, (2) consent, and (3) collaboration.

According to Fremgen (2012), "The principle of *autonomy* means that people have the right to make decisions about their own life" (p. 21). To make such decisions, clients or their representatives need to understand both what is involved in the intervention and its risks and potential benefits. In their roles as service providers, researchers, educators, and students, occupational therapy practitioners must ensure that this information is delivered in a manner that is clear, unbiased, and culturally and linguistically appropriate.

Occupational therapy practitioners and others who have access to confidential information must strictly comply with the preferences of clients; doing less is a breach of ethics and potentially the law. As defined by Fremgen (2012),

> *Confidentiality* refers to keeping private all information about a person (patient) and not disclosing it to a third party without the patient's written consent. . . . Information such as test results, patient histories, and even the fact that a person is a patient cannot be passed on to another person without the patient's consent. (p. 62)

Occupational therapy practitioners must be aware of the influence of clients' family and cultural traditions relative to autonomy and confidentiality. Some clients want practitioners to share all information about their condition, treatment options, and recovery both with the entire health care team directly involved with the provision of care and with their family and friends. Other clients want information about their current status and projected needs shared with only one or two designated people, whereas others may ask that only information about their rehabilitation process be shared with specified people or with no one at all. Taylor (2008) recommended, "As a general guideline, when talking about a client to any other individual, even a family member, always obtain permission from the client before disclosing any information to anyone" (p. 210). By adhering to the client's needs, beliefs, wishes, customs, and rights regarding confidentiality, practitioners support their autonomy.

When speaking about confidentiality, Taylor (2008) encouraged occupational therapy practitioners to be cautious about what information they document in client, student, research participant, colleague, or employee records. Records should include only information that is relevant, not extraneous, to the situation to ensure adherence to standards of confidentiality. For example, occupational therapy practitioners with significant experience in occupational therapy practice may serve as expert witnesses in cases that are reviewed for compliance with laws or policies. As described in Vignette 5.1, when testifying or submitting requested materials, practitioners must make sure to provide only the information specifically requested; any information outside of the scope of the request must be kept confidential (Fremgen, 2012).

VIGNETTE 5.1. MAINTAINING CONFIDENTIALITY IN TESTIMONY

Jasmine provided occupational therapy services to **Miguel** as part of a work rehabilitation program following a back injury. Jasmine was subpoenaed to testify on behalf of Miguel's employer about his recovery and fitness to return to work. She was careful to ensure compliance with Health Insurance Portability and Accountability Act of 1996 (HIPAA) regulations and Principles 3G, 3H, 5C, and 5D of the Code and Ethics Standards. Principles 3G and 3H specifically address confidentiality and the person's right to privacy and underscore the importance of adhering to laws and regulations. Principles 5C and 5D remind occupational therapy practitioners that privacy and

confidentiality laws and regulations require the practitioner to remain current regarding changes to laws, policies, and procedures governing practice; failure to keep up to date can result in a violation of ethical principles and established laws. Jasmine ensured that confidential information Miguel had shared with her that was unrelated to his care was not a part of the medical record that she provided or discussed.

In addition, practitioners must ensure that client records are not left in view of unauthorized people and that confidential information cannot be overheard in conversation. Such carelessness constitutes a violation of Principle 3 and of government regulations, including HIPAA (1996) and the Patient Protection and Affordable Care Act (2010); as in other areas, the law and ethical mandates are in agreement when it comes to confidentiality. Case Study 5.1 describes the consequences of a practitioner's failure to safeguard confidentiality.

CASE STUDY 5.1. ADDRESSING AN INADVERTENT VIOLATION OF CONFIDENTIALITY

Natasha, a licensed occupational therapist, worked in a behavioral health hospital. She had 15 years of experience and was passionate about her work and occupational therapy's role in mental health. Natasha and her friend **Claudia** went out to dinner at a local restaurant after a particularly long and stressful day for Natasha. As she and Claudia unwound over a predinner drink, Natasha began describing her day to Claudia. She talked about the repeated absence of one of the occupational therapists and having to cover his caseload as well as her own and to offer supervision to a student, **Erin**, in her third week of Level II fieldwork. Natasha shared that she had had to attend two case conferences, run three groups by herself that were usually co-led with the absent therapist, complete an evaluation on a new client, and meet with Erin to discuss some behavioral issues she had observed on the unit and in group that day.

Natasha was feeling better when her second drink and dinner arrived. They returned to casual conversation during dinner, and while Claudia was having dessert, Natasha was having her third drink.

Toward the end of dessert, Natasha began to discuss work again. She was a good storyteller, and Claudia found her reports of work events to be entertaining. Natasha told her about a client, **Latoya**, whom she had evaluated after being admitted following a suicide attempt. Latoya had some standing in the community as a volunteer and advocate. Natasha relayed the efforts that were taken to keep the client safe on the unit and in the hospital. She also told Claudia in some detail what Latoya had reported to her were the stressors that prompted her admission.

Unknown to Natasha, the parents of the fieldwork student, Erin, were sitting behind Natasha and Claudia and overheard the entire conversation. When Erin's parents returned home, they repeated the conversation to Erin. Erin was distressed to learn that her supervisor had breached hospital policies, HIPAA, and Principle 3 of the Code and Ethics Standards by discussing confidential client information in a public place. She wondered what course of action she should take. Should she do nothing? This situation involved her supervisor, who had significant influence over her future as an occupational therapy practitioner. Should she present the information she had learned directly to her supervisor or to the department director? Finally, should she report Natasha's alcohol use? Erin had previously noted on a few occasions that Natasha had returned from lunch smelling of alcohol. Table 5.1 reviews some of the courses of action available to Natasha and their consequences.

Erin's review of the Code and Ethics Standards identified several ethical standards that might have been breached or were at risk of being breached through Natasha's behaviors. In addition to Principles 3G and 3H, she realized, her actions also depended on her and Natasha's obligations under Principle 1M (report acts that appear unethical or illegal), Principle 2A (avoid inflicting harm on clients), Principle 2E (take action to remedy personal problems that might cause harm), Principle 2F (avoid undue influences), Principle 6E (accept responsibility for any action that reduces the public's trust in occupational therapy), and Principle 7C (report breaches of the Code and Ethics Standards). In addition, Erin reflected on the potential impacts of her action or inaction. She identified two principles—5D (follow procedures for handling ethics complaints) and 7B (respect private information about colleagues)—that specifically related to her decision making.

Erin decided that keeping this information to herself would potentially do more harm than good. She understood that under optimal circumstances, it is best to discuss ethical dilemmas directly with the person involved. As a student, however, Erin felt she was not on sufficiently equal ground to do this, so she decided to have a confidential conversation with her faculty fieldwork advisor. She hoped that they would present the situation to the department director together and, if the director felt it would be helpful, that both Erin and her faculty advisor would meet with Erin's clinical fieldwork supervisor. Erin was confident that she addressed this sensitive situation in the most ethical way possible.

COMMUNICATION

Client-centered care must be based on the needs and preferences expressed by the client, whether the client is an individual (e.g., patient or student) or community. Principles 3D, 3I, and 3J of the Code and Ethics Standards specifically address the importance of clear communication between the occupational therapy practitioner and others. Principle 3D specifies the occupational therapy practitioner's responsibility to provide clear communication to students regarding the expectations for their academic experiences. Principles 3I and 3J address the need for understandable and open communication between practitioners and students, recipients of services, and others. As noted by the U.S. Department of Health and Human Services (n.d.),

> Effective health communication is as important to health care as clinical skill. To improve individual health and build healthy communities, health care providers need to recognize and address the unique culture, language and health literacy of diverse consumers and communities. (para. 1)

Whether presenting the information verbally, in writing, or electronically, practitioners have an obligation to provide information that is clear and at a level of linguistic clarity that the recipi-

TABLE 5.1
Decision Table for Case Study 5.1

Possible Action	Positive Outcomes	Negative Consequences
Take no action	Erin would avoid dealing with an uncomfortable situation.	Erin's silence would violate Principle 1M. Natasha's behaviors would likely continue and endanger others.
Present information to the academic fieldwork advisor	Natasha's understanding of her obligations under Principles 3G and 3H would increase. Erin would be compliant with the Code and Ethics Standards.	Erin would feel vulnerable. Natasha would be unaware of the concerns about alcohol use and potential harm to patients (Principles 2A and 2F).
Present information to the director	The director has responsibility to patients, the hospital, Natasha, and the profession. The director would fulfill Principle 2E by taking action to confront the situations revealed to her and avoid harm (Principle 2A). The director would review legal and ethical responsibilities with Natasha (Principle 5D).	None. Erin would behave in a professional and ethical way.
Support Natasha's decision to enter treatment to help her control her alcohol use	Erin would fulfill Principle 6E. Natasha would comply with a remediation plan developed in collaboration with the department director, which would help her integrate Principles 7B and 7C.	Erin's inaction could result in job loss and disciplinary actions from the licensure board, the hospital, and AOTA's Ethics Commission. Natasha might increase her criticism of Erin on her performance evaluation as retribution.

Note. AOTA = American Occupational Therapy Association. A variety of possible actions to address this situation and analyses of each are provided in this table; however, other actions or analyses are possible depending on the decision-making model and specific ethics theory or approach used (see Chapter 10, this volume).

ent can understand. Schwab (2006) noted that "obstacles to good decision making by patients are a serious concern in healthcare" and cited "a lack of information" as one of those obstacles (p. 575). Ethical practitioners need to be vigilant for other obstacles to effective communication as well, especially those under their control: Personal biases of the health care provider, time constraints for making decisions, and other barriers may influence communication in ways that limit the client's decision-making processes. In addition, effective communication among researchers, the profession, and the public is important to ensure that clients have an accurate understanding of data and research outcomes and avoid confusion and harm.

Occupational therapy practitioners need to ensure that communication with clients and their families is complete and thorough. For example, when discussing the possible use of constraint-induced therapy with a stroke survivor, the practitioner should describe the evidence available for both this approach and the other interventions used in stroke recovery. Likewise, practitioners' communication with parents who request sensory integration as the primary intervention for their child on the basis of stories they read on an online autism chat room also should draw on evidence-based reviews of sensory interventions with this population. The nature of the communication influences how the client and family make decisions about the client's care, so occupational therapy practitioners have a responsibility to communicate recommendations to clients in a fair and unbiased way—for example, by providing clients with a review of the literature on the effectiveness of the range of available interventions. The topic of communicating in a culturally appropriate way is exemplified in Case Study 5.2.

CASE STUDY 5.2. EXPLORING HEALTH COMMUNICATION ACROSS CULTURES

Terrance was an occupational therapist working with Hispanic clients with psychiatric disorders in a prevocational program. When he first began work with this population, he recognized that if he wanted to engage in client-centered, community-based practice, he would need to understand the issues unique to people in the Hispanic community. The first and most obvious issue was communication. Terrance needed to decide whether he would rely on an interpreter, learn the Spanish language, or use a combination of approaches. He ultimately used a combination of approaches depending on the situation and his increasing level of Spanish proficiency.

After 5 years of practice in this area, Terrance was ready for a new experience. He had learned much about himself and the issues that occupational therapy practitioners and other service providers face when working with the cultural issues embedded in the Hispanic community. He believed that he had developed the sensitivity to expand his interventions to immigrant populations with even greater cultural diversity. To improve his confidence, Terrance decided to review the available literature on communication and cultural competence. Several chapters in *Occupational Therapy Without Borders: Learning From the Spirit of Survivors* (Kronenberg, Algado, & Pollard, 2005) expanded his understanding of how communication influences the therapeutic process and were helpful to his journey. For example, Kronenberg and Pollard (2005) noted that language gaps and barriers make it difficult to fully understand a person's needs

in his or her cultural context and that family members should not be relied on to serve as translators because they may not accurately transmit the client's needs and desires, potentially leading to failed interventions. Thibeault (2005) observed that "occupational therapy is best practiced in a context where specific cultural environments are understood and respected, even if this translates into service delivery that is almost entirely defined and controlled by local stakeholders" (p. 236).

Terrance also discovered a book—*Race, Culture and Disability* (Balcazar, Suarez-Balcazar, Taylor-Ritzler, & Keys, 2010)—that he found helpful in making a connection between people with multicultural backgrounds and their need for autonomy and confidentiality. He located a program in his community that provided transition, counseling, and support services to immigrants, refugees, asylees, and other foreign-born people, some of whom had persistent mental illnesses (FIRN, n.d.). Terrance also learned from Cook, Razzano, and Jonikas (2010) that "different cultures have different likelihoods of help-seeking for mental illness and these may influence ways in which programs and providers handle engagement and the forging of effective therapeutic relationships" (p. 120).

The Code and Ethics Standards speak directly to occupational therapy practitioners' need to appreciate cultures and gain cultural competence in Principles 2K, 3I, and 4F. Terrance was confident that after taking these steps, he would be better equipped to provide competent and ethical occupational therapy services that recognized each person's right to autonomy and confidentiality. He also recognized that to serve these communities well and ensure his credibility, he must strictly adhere to Principle 3, Autonomy and Confidentiality, when visiting or working in community programs.

Cultural competency is particularly important to professionals serving diverse communities of people with psychiatric disorders. Terrance found through his reading of Cook et al. (2010) that methods of identifying and intervening with people with psychiatric disorders vary across cultures, necessitating education of professionals in the belief systems of the people and families served. He also learned that to expand his practice to work with diverse populations, he needed to network with multicultural groups and organizations like the one he found in his community and to gain additional knowledge and credibility. This learning needed to be a two-way street: Terrance also had to have something to offer the communities he was learning from. Finally, he reached out to AOTA's Multicultural Networking Groups (AOTA, 2011) to learn more about cultural diversity from an occupational therapy perspective.

Terrance thus developed a plan that he thought was viable and ethically grounded that would help him continue to expand his cultural competence through reading, networking, and volunteering with diverse individuals and organizations in and around his community and through developing relationships with Multicultural Networking Groups. In this way, he was able to increase his understanding of cultural differences and occupational therapy interventions in community-based settings.

CONSENT

Consent means "assent or approval" (Merriam-Webster, 2011, para. 1). Occupational therapy practitioners have an ethical obligation to obtain consent from clients or their representatives before initiating an evaluation or intervention, enrolling clients in research, or making information about their care available to third parties. Local, state, and federal regulations and institutional policies governing these activities reinforce this ethical obligation (see also Chapters 7 and 19, this volume). Supporting the client's wishes, sometimes over the preferences of family members, is of prime importance as long as the client's safety and well-being are not in jeopardy. Vignette 5.2 describes an occupational therapist's efforts to obtain parents' consent to discuss their child's occupational therapy priorities with his professional colleagues in order to meet the child's accessibility needs.

VIGNETTE 5.2. OBTAINING CONSENT FOR CONSULTATION

Elliott, an occupational therapist, was asked by the middle school where he delivered occupational therapy services to make recommendations for **Tara's** 504 plan (Section 504 of the Rehabilitation Act of 1973 ensures that schools provide students who have disabilities with reasonable accommodations to access

educational materials; U.S. Department of Education, 2011). Although Elliott had worked in school-based practice for 4 years, he was unfamiliar with how to contribute to a 504 plan for a student with developmental coordination disorder (DCD). Elliott reviewed the student record carefully and obtained brief information from team members, including Tara's mother. He continued to be unsure about assessing Tara's needs and making useful recommendations.

Elliott reviewed textbooks, read journal articles, and attended a webinar on DCD. In addition, he had general discussions with colleagues working with children and youths in other settings. He continued to feel that he needed more information to be helpful. Elliott consulted the Code and Ethics Standards, and after reading Principle 3B, Elliott recognized his obligation to keep the team, including Tara's parents, informed about his efforts and to obtain the parents' consent before discussing Tara's specific needs with another occupational therapist who had expertise in recommending assistive technology for students with DCD. Elliott knew this step was important in respecting Tara's and her family's confidentiality, which is supported by Principle 3G.

A corollary of the practitioner's obligation to obtain consent is the client's right to refuse treatment. Clients and research participants have the right to refuse an intervention or withdraw from research studies, as supported by Principles 3C and 3F. Although occupational therapy clients have the right to refuse an intervention (e.g., by informing the practitioner that they do not want to participate in occupational therapy for that session or day), the practitioner's ethical obligation to respect the clients' wishes does not preclude encouraging clients to participate in therapy as a way to achieve their established goals. Likewise, a practitioner should not attempt to restrain a client from leaving a session unless his or her departure could potentially harm the client or others or is against hospital or agency policies.

Clients who freely consent to participate in a research study (Principle 3E) may decide during the course of the study that they wish to withdraw. They may feel, for example, that participation requires too much time, that the benefit is not worth the risk, or simply that the process is boring. Although withdrawal from a research study may make life more complicated for the researcher, it is the participant's right to withdraw at any time for any reason.

COLLABORATION

Occupational therapy practice emphasizes collaboration between the occupational therapy practitioner and the client (AOTA, 2008, 2010). This partnership can extend to the immediate family, significant others, caregivers, or agencies as designated by the client or the law. AOTA (2008) presents this collaboration as a dynamic process between the occupational therapy practitioner and client: "Occupational therapy practitioners develop a collaborative relationship with clients in order to understand their experiences and desires for intervention" (p. 647).

Principle 3A of the Code and Ethics Standards obligates occupational therapy practitioners to establish collaborative relationships with clients and, as appropriate, their families, significant others, and caregivers. Before collaborating on setting goals and priorities, practitioners need to make sure they fully inform the client and designated others about the purpose of the intervention; benefits, risks, and potential outcomes, as well as any reasonable alternatives; the personnel who will provide the intervention; and timeframes for goal attainment. Vignette 5.3 describes an occupational therapy practitioner's efforts to involve the client and her family in learning about what the fall prevention assessment and intervention process has to offer and available options.

VIGNETTE 5.3. BALANCING AUTONOMY AND COLLABORATION

Clinton, an occupational therapist in private practice, had an exhibit at a senior expo in his county. He presented a poster and information focused on fall prevention and provided a screening tool for expo participants. **Felicia** was one of the older adults who visited Clinton's booth.

Felicia told Clinton that she'd had a recent fall that had shaken her confidence even though she wasn't seriously injured. She had reluctantly told her son and daughter-in-law about the incident, and she reported that they were now feeling very protective

of her, even suggesting that she move in with them or to assisted living. Felicia asked Clinton whether there was anything among his materials or in his practice experience that might help her. Clinton gave Felicia some fall prevention materials and links to evidence-based Web sites with additional information. He also told Felicia that most falls occur within the home and that sometimes an environmental assessment can identify human and environmental factors that contribute to falls. Felicia was excited to hear about this and wanted Clinton to come to her home the next day.

Clinton suggested that Felicia review the materials he had provided her and share this information with her son and daughter-in-law. He said that if, after reviewing this material, she still wanted him to conduct a home visit and environmental assessment, he would be pleased to work with her. Felicia called Clinton a few days later to say that she had discussed their conversation with her son and daughter-in-law and that they all agreed to move forward with the home visit.

Clinton's approach to work with Felicia respected her autonomy by establishing a collaborative relationship and explaining possible interventions (Principle 3A) and by obtaining her consent regarding the proposed assessment and sharing information with family members (Principle 3B). Clinton was pleased that Felicia had discussed fall prevention and an environmental assessment with her family; he had suggested having this discussion to encourage their collaboration and support for this potential process. Clinton also suggested that Felicia invite her son and daughter-in-law to their session, if Felicia wished, so they could learn more about the assessment process and what he might propose in terms of Felicia's safety and ability to age in place.

CONCLUSION

Adherence to Principle 3, Autonomy and Confidentiality, of the Code and Ethics Standards helps occupational therapy practitioners ensure that the services they provide are client centered and that interactions with clients are clear, are without bias, and allow the exercise of personal freedoms. Respect for the autonomy and confidentiality of both individual and collective clients is necessary to establish a sense of partnership, honesty, and understanding in occupational therapy practice.

REFERENCES

American Occupational Therapy Association. (2008). Occupational therapy practice framework: Domain and process (2nd ed.). *American Journal of Occupational Therapy*, 625–683. doi: 10.5014/ajot.62.6.625

American Occupational Therapy Association. (2010). Occupational therapy code of ethics and ethics standards (2010). *American Journal of Occupational Therapy*, 64(6 Suppl.), S17–S26. doi: 10.5014/ajot.2010.64S17

American Occupational Therapy Association. (2011). *Multicultural networking groups*. Retrieved from www.aota.org/Practitioners/Resources/Multicultural/Resources/37723.aspx

Balcazar, F. E., Suarez-Balcazar, Y., Taylor-Ritzler, T., & Keys, C. B. (Eds.). (2010). *Race, culture and disability: Rehabilitation science and practice*. Sudbury, MA: Jones & Bartlett.

Beauchamp, T. L., & Childress, J. F. (2009). *Principles of biomedical ethics* (6th ed.). New York: Oxford University Press.

Cook, J. A., Razzano, L. A., & Jonikas, J. A. (2010). Cultural diversity and how it may differ for programs and providers serving people with psychiatric disabilities. In F. E. Balcazar, Y. Suarez-Balcazar, T. Taylor-Ritzler, & C. B. Keys (Eds.), *Race, culture and disability: Rehabilitation science and practice* (pp. 115–135). Sudbury, MA: Jones & Bartlett.

FIRN. (n.d.) *What is FIRN?* Retrieved from www.firnonline.org/?page_id=27

Fremgen, B. F. (2012). *Medical law and ethics* (4th ed.). Upper Saddle River, NJ: Pearson Education.

Health Insurance Portability and Accountability Act of 1996, Pub. L. 104–191 110 Stat. 1936.

Kronenberg, F., Algado, S. S., & Pollard, N. (Eds.). (2005). *Occupational therapy without borders: Learning from the spirit of survivors*. Philadelphia: Elsevier.

Kronenberg, F., & Pollard, N. (2005). Overcoming occupational apartheid: A preliminary exploration of the political nature of occupational therapy. In F. Kronenberg, S. S. Algado, & N. Pollard (Eds.), *Occupational therapy without borders: Learning from the spirit of survivors*. (pp. 158–186). Philadelphia: Elsevier.

Merriam-Webster. (2011). Consent. Retrieved from www.merriam-webster.com/dictionary/consent

Patient Protection and Affordable Care Act, P. L. 111–148, § 3502, 124 Stat. 119, 124 (2010).

Rehabilitation Act of 1973, Pub. L. 93–112, 29 U.S.C. § 701 *et seq.*

Schwab, A. P. (2006). Formal and effective autonomy in healthcare. *Journal of Medical Ethics*, 575–579. doi: 10.1136/jme.2005.013391

Taylor, R. L. (2008). *The intentional relationship: Occupational therapy and use of self*. Philadelphia: F. A. Davis.

Thibeault, R. (2005). Connecting health and social justice: A Lebanese experience. In F. Kronenberg, S. S. Algado, & N. Pollard (Eds.), *Occupational therapy without borders: Learning from the spirit of survivors* (pp. 232–244). Philadelphia: Elsevier.

U.S. Department of Education. (2011). *Protecting students with disabilities*. Retrieved from www2.ed.gov/about/offices/list/ocr/504faq.html

U.S. Department of Health and Human Services. (n.d.). *Culture, language and health literacy*. Retrieved from www.hrsa.gov/culturalcompetence/index.html

Principle 4: Social Justice

6

S. Maggie Reitz, PhD, OTR/L, FAOTA, and
Stacey Harcum, MS, OTR/L, CBIS

SOCIAL JUSTICE

Principle 4. Occupational therapy personnel shall provide services in a fair and equitable manner.

Social justice, also called *distributive justice*, refers to the fair, equitable, and appropriate distribution of resources. The principle of social justice refers broadly to the distribution of all rights and responsibilities in society (Beauchamp & Childress, 2009). In general, the principle of social justice supports the concept of achieving justice in every aspect of society rather than merely the administration of law. The general idea is that individuals and groups should receive fair treatment and an impartial share of the benefits of society. Occupational therapy personnel have a vested interest in addressing unjust inequities that limit opportunities for participation in society (Braveman & Bass-Haugen, 2009). While opinions differ regarding the most ethical approach to addressing distribution of health care resources and reduction of health disparities, the issue of social justice continues to focus on limiting the impact of social inequality on health outcomes.

OCCUPATIONAL THERAPY PERSONNEL SHALL

A. Uphold the profession's altruistic responsibilities to help ensure the common good.
B. Take responsibility for educating the public and society about the value of occupational therapy services in promoting health and wellness and reducing the impact of disease and disability.
C. Make every effort to promote activities that benefit the health status of the community.
D. Advocate for just and fair treatment for all patients, clients, employees, and colleagues, and encourage employers and colleagues to abide by the highest standards of social justice and the ethical standards set forth by the occupational therapy profession.
E. Make efforts to advocate for recipients of occupational therapy services to obtain needed services through available means.
F. Provide services that reflect an understanding of how occupational therapy service delivery can be affected by factors such as economic status, age, ethnicity, race, geography, disability, marital status, sexual orientation, gender, gender identity, religion, culture, and political affiliation.

G. Consider offering *pro bono* ("for the good") or reduced-fee occupational therapy services for selected individuals when consistent with guidelines of the employer, third-party payer, and/or government agency.

Source. From the *Occupational Therapy Code of Ethics and Ethics Standards (2010)* (American Occupational Therapy Association, 2010a, pp. S21–S22).

The American Occupational Therapy Association (AOTA) revisited its roots in social activism when it added Principle 4, Social Justice, to the *Occupational Therapy Code of Ethics and Ethics Standards (2010)* (referred to as the "Code and Ethics Standards"; AOTA, 2010a). This new principle encourages occupational therapy practitioners to continue the commitment of the profession to those who need our services regardless of personal attributes or ability to pay. Although there is disagreement on how best to promote social justice in health care, efforts to achieve social justice frequently focus on "limiting the impact of social inequality on health outcomes" (AOTA, 2010a, p. S22).

The addition of this principle brings occupational therapy into alignment with other health professions. Because many have expressed an interest in how consistent AOTA's views on justice are with those of related health disciplines, we reviewed the ethics codes and policies of seven national professional organizations to determine whether they include the construct of social justice in their documents (see Table 6.1). All of these organizations have policies equivalent to the AOTA principle of Social Justice. Such policies or ethical principles discourage discrimination and encourage professional contribution to the greater welfare, often through offering services on a sliding scale or pro bono basis.

TABLE 6.1
Social Justice in Other National Professional Association Codes of Ethics

ASSOCIATION	POLICIES RELEVANT OR EQUIVALENT TO SOCIAL JUSTICE
American Counseling Association (2005)	"Counselors are encouraged to contribute to society by devoting a portion of their professional activity to services for which there is little or no financial return (pro bono publico)." (p. 4) "C.5. Nondiscrimination. Counselors do not condone or engage in discrimination based on age, culture, disability, ethnicity, race, religion/spirituality, gender, gender identity, sexual orientation, marital status/partnership, language preference, socioeconomic status, or any basis proscribed by law. Counselors do not discriminate against clients, students, employees, supervisees, or research participants in a manner that has a negative impact on these persons." (p. 10)
American Nurses Association (2001)	"Nursing has a distinguished history of concern for the welfare of the sick, injured, and vulnerable and for social justice." (p. 2)
American Physical Therapy Association (2009)	"Principle #8: Physical therapists shall participate in efforts to meet the health needs of people locally, nationally, or globally. (Core Value: Social Responsibility)" (p. 2) "8A. Physical therapists shall provide pro bono physical therapy services or support organizations that meet the health needs of people who are economically disadvantaged, uninsured, and underinsured." (p. 2)

(*continued*)

TABLE 6.1 (cont.)

ASSOCIATION	POLICIES RELEVANT OR EQUIVALENT TO SOCIAL JUSTICE
American Psychological Association (2010)	"Principle B: . . . Psychologists strive to contribute a portion of their professional time for little or no compensation or personal advantage." (p. 3) "Principle E: Respect for People's Rights and Dignity: Psychologists respect the dignity and worth of all people, and the rights of individuals to privacy, confidentiality, and self-determination. Psychologists are aware that special safeguards may be necessary to protect the rights and welfare of persons or communities whose vulnerabilities impair autonomous decision making. Psychologists are aware of and respect cultural, individual, and role differences, including those based on age, gender, gender identity, race, ethnicity, culture, national origin, religion, sexual orientation, disability, language, and socioeconomic status and consider these factors when working with members of such groups. Psychologists try to eliminate the effect on their work of biases based on those factors, and they do not knowingly participate in or condone activities of others based upon such prejudices." (p. 3)
American Speech–Language–Hearing Association (2010)	"Individuals shall not discriminate in the delivery of professional services or the conduct of research and scholarly activities on the basis of race or ethnicity, gender, gender identity/gender expression, age, religion, national origin, sexual orientation, or disability." (I. C.) "Individuals shall refer those served professionally solely on the basis of the interest of those being referred and not on any personal interest, financial or otherwise." (III. C.)
National Association of Social Workers (2008)	"Value: Service. Ethical Principle: Social workers' primary goal is to help people in need and to address social problems. Social workers elevate service to others above self interest. Social workers draw on their knowledge, values, and skills to help people in need and to address social problems. Social workers are encouraged to volunteer some portion of their professional skills with no expectation of significant financial return (pro bono service)." (paras. 2–3) "Value: Social Justice. Ethical Principle: Social workers challenge social injustice. Social workers pursue social change, particularly with and on behalf of vulnerable and oppressed individuals and groups of people. Social workers' social change efforts are focused primarily on issues of poverty, unemployment, discrimination, and other forms of social injustice. These activities seek to promote sensitivity to and knowledge about oppression and cultural and ethnic diversity. Social workers strive to ensure access to needed information, services, and resources; equality of opportunity; and meaningful participation in decision making for all people." (paras. 2–3)
Society for Public Health Education (2011)	"The Code of Ethics is grounded in fundamental ethical principles that underlie all health care services: respect for autonomy, promotion of social justice, active promotion of good, and avoidance of harm." (para. 2) "Section 2: Health Educators encourage actions and social policies that support and facilitate the best balance of benefits over harm for all affected parties." (para. 7)

This chapter describes the ways the Code and Ethics Standards support both current and expanded efforts by AOTA and individual practitioners to address social and occupational injustice. The chapter provides a historical review of the relationship of social justice to the profession's development and continued evolution and discusses strategies to promote adherence to this principle.

HISTORICAL LINKS

Social justice has been woven into the values and fabric of the profession since its inception. The term *social justice* originated in the work of social justice feminists in the United States, such as Jane Addams, and in Germany (Sklar, Schular, & Strasser, cited in Frank & Zemke, 2008). Jane Addams has been linked to the development of occupational therapy through her work at Hull House and the Chicago School of Civics and Philanthropy, where Eleanor Clarke Slagle took a course on Invalid Occupations (Breines, 1986; Frank & Zemke, 2008). The term *social justice* gained momentum before World War I "because it offered an alternative to charity as the justification for public policies that intervened in the relationships between capital and labor; and signified a redistribution of resources based on fairness rather than pity or fear" (Sklar et al., cited in Frank & Zemke, 2008, p. 127).

The profession of occupational therapy was developed by social activists who diligently addressed inequities and promoted social justice (Breines, 1986; Townsend, 1993; Townsend & Polatajko, 2007). In the early years of the profession, occupation was seen as being "as necessary to life as food and drink" (Dunton, quoted in Polatajko et al., 2007, p. 14). Following this line of thinking, limited opportunity to participate in occupations would result in a sort of occupational malnourishment; in essence, people would be starved of the opportunity to select and engage in occupations that bring meaning to their lives, their families, and their communities. Since the early days of the profession, this belief has evolved into the construct of occupational deprivation and a fledgling theory of occupational justice as conceived by Townsend and Wilcock (2004a, 2004b; see also Stadnyk, Townsend, & Wilcock, 2010).

Wilcock and Townsend saw occupational justice as being "likely a complementary extension of social justice" (cited in Townsend, 2003, p. 12). Although the terms are similar, there is a distinct difference; as Townsend (2003) described it,

whereas social justice adjudicates conditions so that everyone has equal access to education, or other possessions, occupational justice expresses a paradigm for recognizing that equality or sameness can produce injustices because of human and social differences. Social justice overlooks injustices related to participation in daily life occupations—injustices related to doing instead of having. (p. 12)

Social justice has been an integral part of the profession's ethics activities and documents starting with the first publication to specifically articulate the ethics of the profession. *Principles of Occupational Therapy Ethics* (AOTA, 1978) included 12 principles, one of which was entitled "Related to Bioethical Issues and Problems of Society." AOTA, through the 1979 revision of this document, encouraged occupational therapists to consider broader societal impacts on health and their relationship to service delivery (AOTA, 1984).

Through the years, associations and federations and other leaders in the profession have continued to develop and hone the profession's advocacy skills and to advocate for disadvantaged populations (AOTA, 2006; Kronenberg, Algado, & Pollard, 2005; Townsend, 1993; Townsend & Polatajko, 2007; World Federation of Occupational Therapists [WFOT], 2004, 2006). These actions have contributed to enhanced access to occupational therapy services and promoted justice around the globe. Persistent evidence of health disparities and occupational and social injustice, however, clearly indicate the need for continued dedication to these causes. Occupational therapy practitioners have the knowledge, skill, and ability to meet this need and join Townsend (1993) and others who remind us of our past values and need for future action:

Occupational therapy's social vision is founded on concepts and practice that are consistent with those working to build a just society. I believe that occupational therapy has tremendous potential which places the profession on a world stage with social movements oriented to peace and justice. (p. 182)

SOCIAL JUSTICE IN THE CODE AND ETHICS STANDARDS

Although the Code and Ethics Standards provide rules and guidance to encourage appropriate behavior, ethical conduct is far more than just following these rules; it includes "ethical action." *Ethical action* involves "mindful reflection" and is "a commitment to benefit others, to virtuous practice of artistry and science, to genuinely good behaviors, and to noble acts of courage" (AOTA, 2010a, p. S17).

The other six principles of the Code and Ethics Standards all relate in some way to promoting social justice and, at times, occupational justice as well, and of the six Principles 1 and 5 provide more direction than the others. Principle 1 is Beneficence, the desire and ability to do good work. Specifically, Principle 1B (provide evaluation and intervention plans specific to clients' needs) supports access to services (i.e., social justice) and obliges practitioners to customize services to meet clients' needs, which can also address occupational justice if the services assist with building a capacity for doing. Such services could take the form of facilitating occupations that had previously been denied or supporting the return to relinquished roles, routines, habits, or rituals (AOTA, 2008). Vignette 6.1 describes such services and exemplifies the potentially far reach of interventions that can serve not only an individual but also families and the greater community by enhancing access to occupation.

VIGNETTE 6.1. SUPPORTING A RETURN TO ROLES AND BENEFIT TO THE COMMUNITY

An occupational therapist and occupational therapy assistant team were working with **Simone**, a client with arthritis. If Simone had access to a wheelchair and other assistive devices, she could both resume paid employment as a bank clerk and participate in her favorite leisure occupation, feeding the ducks at the park across from the bank at lunchtime. The occupational therapy team investigated local resources and found an assistive technology loan closet where Simone could borrow and test devices before pur-

chase. Use of the loan closet, which was run by the local Arthritis Foundation, would allow her not only to see whether the device was worth the cost but also to schedule purchases as her budget allowed.

In addition, the occupational therapy team worked with Simone and the bank president to organize a benefit to raise money to purchase her wheelchair and park benches for others to use while enjoying the park and its waterfowl. Parents and grandparents found the additional benches particularly helpful, and increased park use was observed. The bank president also realized that although he was in technical compliance with the Americans With Disabilities Act of 1990, modifications to the bank entrance would enhance accessibility for Simone, as well as for the bank's aging customers and those with baby strollers. He contacted a construction company to perform the necessary modifications and received favorable feedback from his customers as a result.

Many opportunities exist in daily practice to ensure that clients are given every opportunity to resume or initiate participation in occupations that promote health and add quality to life. Although this level of care requires more effort on the part of occupational therapy practitioners, taking the extra steps for clients and the community should be a routine consideration in occupational therapy practice rather than the exception.

Principle 5, Procedural Justice, also supports both social and occupational justice. Specifically, Principle 5M reads, "Actively work with employers to prevent discrimination and unfair labor practices, and advocate for employees with disabilities to ensure the provision of reasonable accommodations" (AOTA, 2010a, p. S23). Many occupational therapy practitioners work in larger institutions such as hospitals and universities. The great potential to advocate for equal access to work for people with disabilities in these and other settings has yet to be fully realized.

SECURING JUSTICE AT THE INSTITUTION AND INDIVIDUAL LEVEL

Although growing numbers of occupational therapy practitioners are working in the community or delivering services at the population level, according to the latest AOTA workforce study (AOTA, 2010b, p. 18), two-thirds (67.7%) still work with individuals in some type of institution (e.g., hospital, school, long-term facility). Vignette 6.2 and Case Study 6.1 discuss ethical situations at this level of service delivery.

VIGNETTE 6.2. ENSURING RESPECT AND FAIRNESS DURING INTERVENTION

Dante, an occupational therapist, was the director of an acute inpatient rehabilitation unit in a large rural hospital. **Andrew**, age 21, was admitted for an anticipated 2- to 3-week stay for occupational and physical therapy services after a severe car crash. Andrew had suffered mild burns and numerous fractures. At the beginning of activity of daily living retraining, **Sally**, assigned to provide occupational therapy services to Andrew, discovered that Andrew was a transgender person. Unsure of how to proceed, Sally discussed Andrew's gender identity with the rest of the rehabilitation team, who all become wary of interacting with Andrew. The issue was brought to Dante's attention by a nurse on the unit who was concerned about the quality of Andrew's care.

Dante talked to his supervisor, the hospital's vice president for clinical services, about the situation without disclosing Andrew's name. They jointly agreed on three actions that upheld Principle 4, as well as aspects of six other ethical principles. First, the supervisor suggested that Dante contact Human Resources, which had excellent staff who could provide the rehabilitation team with in-service training regarding cultural competency and patients' rights. Second, they agreed that Dante would immediately replace Sally as Andrew's occupational therapist to give Sally a chance to reflect on the content of the workshop and her behavior and to protect Andrew from possible discriminatory care and Sally from potential continued unethical behaviors. Third, Dante would review the Code and Ethics Standards with Sally as part of an internal disciplinary action and in their ongoing supervisory meetings to stress the need for confidentiality, consideration of social justice, and appropriate use of the supervisory relationship.

CASE STUDY 6.1. PROMOTING ACCESS TO SERVICES

Brian was an occupational therapist working at an outpatient practice located in a small city. The practice employed administrative staff, occupational therapists, physical therapists, a part-time speech–language pathologist, and one physician, **Dr. Stanton**, who acted as director of the practice. The primary client base was older adults with various physical limitations, including rheumatic conditions, orthopedic injuries, cardiopulmonary conditions, and postsurgical follow-ups. In his current position, Brian evaluated new clients and provided one-to-one intervention. Additionally, he attended a multidisciplinary team meeting once a week to discuss clients' progress and performed home evaluations on an as-needed basis as determined by Dr. Stanton. The rehabilitation staff provided information and feedback regarding client needs and safety, but Dr. Stanton ultimately wrote the orders for assessment and continuation of therapy services.

Brian had been working with Dr. Stanton for just over a year and had begun to notice differential treatment for certain groups of clients. Many of the people he treated were well-to-do or had expensive private insurance, but Brian also treated clients from lower socioeconomic rungs who had less comprehensive insurance, if any at all, and often had to pay out of pocket for services. Because of the expense, clients with fewer financial resources typically had less frequent appointments than their wealthier counterparts, regardless of the severity of their needs. Brian also had recently noticed that significantly fewer home assessments were being ordered for these clients.

Brian decided to bring up the disparities he noticed in the next team meeting. When he did so, he was told not to worry about the less frequent appointments because "that's just the way the world works." Dr. Stanton also defended his decisions regarding orders for home assessments by stating that the clients Brian mentioned would not be able to afford most of the modifications he might recommend anyway; he also informed Brian that clients with little or no insurance did not have coverage for such an assessment. Brian was deeply troubled by the continued inequity he witnessed, but the rest of the staff seemed fine with the status quo. Other options that Brian considered to address this ethical issue appear in Table 6.2.

TABLE 6.2
Decision Table for Case Study 6.1

POSSIBLE ACTION	POSITIVE OUTCOMES	NEGATIVE CONSEQUENCES
No action	Brian avoids conflict and maintains comfortable relationships with his coworkers.	Some clients continue to receive substandard care, so this action does not uphold Principle 4 or Principles 1, 5, or 7.
Compile information on community resources for clients without financial resources	Brian avoids conflict and maintains comfortable relationships with his coworkers. Brian potentially provides some underserved clients the resources to bridge the gap and receive needed services. Brian attempts to uphold Principles 1 and 2.	Clients receive services from community sources whose employees are not as familiar with the clients and may be untrained. Some clients continue to receive substandard care. This action does not uphold Principle 4 or Principles 5 and 7.
Offer pro bono services to clients as necessary and in alignment with institutional policies	All of Brian's clients receive the occupational therapy services needed. This action upholds Principles 1 and 4 for Brian's clients.	Clients may still receive substandard care from other practitioners. The profit margin of the practice may decrease. Brian may cause conflict with other employees or management. This action fails to uphold Principles 5 and 7.
Suggest that the practice adopt a sliding-scale policy for clients without comprehensive insurance	All clients receive equitable care across disciplines. A large policy change sets the tone for all employees, not just Brian. This action upholds Principles 1, 4, and 7 and could bring Principle 5 into alignment with Principle 4.	The profit margin of the practice may decrease. A large policy change is difficult to initiate and pass.
Review Code and Ethics Standards with Dr. Stanton and ask for his support in establishing a task force to ensure equitable care	Dr. Stanton is given an opportunity to reflect on and change his behavior before being reported to entities with jurisdiction. This action may lead to upholding Principles 1 and 4 for all clients and Principle 7. This action may affect institutional rules related to Principle 5.	Brian may cause conflict with Dr. Stanton. Brian's job may be at risk. Brian must be prepared to report Dr. Stanton's behavior if Dr. Stanton refuses to review current practice.
Report Dr. Stanton's activities to the owners or board of directors of the practice	Dr. Stanton may be forced to treat clients equitably. This action may lead to upholding Principles 1 and 4 for all clients and may affect institutional rules related to Principle 5.	Brian's action may not follow the procedures and chain of command outlined by the practice. Brian may cause conflict with other employees. Brian's job may be at risk. This action may not uphold aspects of Principles 5 and 7.

(continued)

TABLE 6.2 (*cont.*)

Possible Action	Positive Outcomes	Negative Consequences
Report Dr. Stanton's activities to the ethics board with jurisdiction	Dr. Stanton may be held accountable for his actions and forced to treat clients equitably. Brian may report anonymously to avoid conflict. This action may encourage upholding Principles 1, 4, and 7.	Brian's action may not follow the procedures and chain of command outlined by the practice. If not reported anonymously, Brian's action may cause conflict with other employees. Brian's job may be at risk. This action may not uphold aspects of Principles 5 and 7.

Note. A variety of possible actions to address this situation and analyses of each are provided in this table; however, other actions or analyses are possible depending on the decision-making model and specific ethics theory or approach used (see Chapter 10, this volume).

SECURING JUSTICE AT THE POPULATION AND COMMUNITY LEVEL

Instances of grave injustice exist in many communities. People in immigrant communities (Ku, 2012), homeless shelters (Baggett, O'Connell, Singer, & Rigotti, 2010), and jails and prisons (Wilper et al., 2009), as well as people with disabilities (Centers for Disease Control and Prevention, 2011), have less access to health care compared with the general population. According to two reports by the U.S. Department of Health and Human Services (DHHS), Agency for Healthcare Research and Quality (DHHS, AHRQ; 2010a, 2010b), accelerated efforts are needed to improve access and equity in health care. These reports address the following themes:

- Health care quality and access are suboptimal, especially for minority and low-income groups.

- Quality is improving; access and disparities are not improving.

- Urgent attention is warranted to ensure improvements in quality and progress on reducing disparities with respect to certain services, geographic areas, and populations, including
  - Cancer screening and management of diabetes.
  - States in the central part of the country.
  - Residents of inner-city and rural areas.
  - Disparities in preventive services and access to care.

- Progress is uneven with respect to eight national priority areas:
  - Two are improving in quality: (1) Palliative and End-of-Life Care and (2) Patient and Family Engagement.
  - Three are lagging: (3) Population Health, (4) Safety, and (5) Access.
  - Three require more data to assess: (6) Care Coordination, (7) Overuse, and (8) Health System Infrastructure.
  - All eight priority areas showed disparities related to race, ethnicity, and socioeconomic status. (DHHS, AHRQ, 2010b, para. 8)

Whether because of the restrictive nature of the institution or lack of knowledge about choices or resources, people in these settings often experience social and occupational injustice. In fact, for people in restrictive settings such as prisons, social and occupational opportunities may be rescinded as punishment for misdeeds (e.g., solitary confinement). Vignette 6.3 describes an occupational therapy practitioner's efforts to address social injustice for immigrants.

VIGNETTE 6.3. EXTENDING SERVICES TO UNDERSERVED POPULATIONS

Maria was an occupational therapist working as a consultant at a nonprofit women's health center in an urban area. The center offered all of its services for free or on a sliding-scale basis. In her role there, Maria assisted in the development and implementation of educational programs and pamphlets about women's health issues.

Recently she had attended a continuing education course on the topic of cultural awareness and sensitivity. The course included an overview of the demographics in her city, which she learned had a significant population of relatively recent Asian immigrants, particularly from Southeast Asian nations such as Vietnam, Thailand, and the Philippines. On returning to work, Maria noticed that few or no Vietnamese, Thai, or Filipino women were taking advantage of the center's programs.

Maria was able to find several prominent and trusted members of the local Vietnamese, Thai, and Filipino communities who were willing to assist with recruitment of participants and the translation of marketing and educational materials. These volunteers also agreed to serve on a board of directors to assist the center in meeting the needs of the women in the community. This inexpensive strategy both addressed the disparity in those served and leveraged community stakeholders to assist in the identification of other needs of the community. This action upholds Principle 4, as well as Principles 1 (Beneficence), 2 (Nonmaleficence), and 31 (facilitation of meaningful communication).

Occupational injustice also occurs after disasters, which involve a unique set of ethical concerns, including the need to reflect on one's motivations, pursue relevant training and ensure competence, and seek a position with an authorized organization (AOTA, 2011). Ensuring that communities have procedures for evacuating all members in a safe and orderly way is one example of Principle 4 in action. Another example would be working to ensure that there are age-appropriate opportunities for occupational engagement at disaster shelters, an action that would also facilitate occupational justice. Vignette 6.4 describes how a real-life occupational therapist helped reestablish communications after a natural disaster.

VIGNETTE 6.4. PROMOTING OCCUPATIONAL JUSTICE AFTER A DISASTER

After Hurricane Katrina struck in August 2005, **Frank Pascarelli** used his occupational therapy skills to combat lack of access to basic communication

services in Pascagoula, Mississippi. Frank had greater ability to assist at a disaster site than most occupational therapy practitioners because of his unique, dual roles as an Air Force reservist and employee of the Centers for Disease Control and Prevention.

Frank decided to facilitate a low-cost method for affected people to communicate and reconnect with family and friends. Many people had lost their mailboxes in the storm, so Frank acquired and distributed replacement mailboxes and provided a cordless drill. Residents used the drill to attach their new mailbox to some physical structure remaining on their property (e.g., tree, fence post). The same cordless drill was passed from neighbor to neighbor, thus rebuilding a sense of community along with the communication system. Frank's next challenge was to assist in reclaiming a school playground to allow children to resume developmentally appropriate occupations (Hofmann, 2008).

Any citizen, including occupational therapy practitioners, can be prepared to help if a disaster occurs in his or her community, county, or state. Investigating local opportunities to volunteer and receive training as a responder before a disaster occurs gives people more options to serve if the circumstances arise. Readers are encouraged to locate the nearest Community Emergency Response Team (n.d.) training opportunity. Potential negative consequences of untrained attempts to provide aid in a disaster are described in Vignette 6.5.

VIGNETTE 6.5. GAINING COMPETENCY BEFORE A DISASTER

Portia was saddened and concerned about the eastern, rural portion of a neighboring state that had been hit that morning by a series of tornados. As an occupational therapist, she believed she could contribute to the disaster recovery efforts. She quickly packed some clothes and her dog into her car. As she drove east, a string of heavy thunderstorms resulted in flooded roads. She became lost in the darkness. The next day, she and her dog were rescued at taxpayers' expense.

CONCLUSION

The occupational therapy profession has a responsibility to confront instances of social and occupational injustice. Occupational therapy practitioners should seek ways to promote justice through advocacy and action to ensure that people, families, communities, and populations have the freedom to select and engage in occupations that promote health, well-being, and participation.

Although the case examples in this chapter focused on the delivery of occupational therapy interventions, the Code and Ethics Standards apply to all professional roles, including those of educator, scientist, and volunteer. For example, faculty and program directors are responsible for advocating for access to leisure occupations for all students, with and without disabilities, on their campuses. In addition, the Code and Ethics Standards urge scientists to ensure that their research does not consistently or systematically exclude specific populations.

Occupational therapy practitioners should develop the habit of monitoring the literature for research related to social justice and occupational justice (e.g., Riegel & Eglseder, 2009) and for other efforts to address health disparities (e.g., the curriculum initiative described by Ford, Waring, & Boggis, 2007). Practitioners should also regularly monitor the following Web sites to keep abreast of data related to health disparities at the local, state, national, and international levels:

- The Web sites of AOTA, WFOT, and the World Health Organization
- U.S. government Web sites such as *Healthy People 2020* (DHHS, Office of Disease Prevention and Health Promotion, 2010) and the *National Healthcare Disparities Report* (DHHS, AHRQ, 2010a)
- Applicable state Web sites.

Access to current information is essential in enabling practitioners to fulfill the ethical mandate of being competent providers of occupational therapy services in today's world.

The current magnitude of health disparities and limited access to occupation among different subgroups, groups, and populations within the United States require action from professional associations and their individual members. The Code and Ethics Standards reinforce the need to actively address these problems.

REFERENCES

American Counseling Association. (2005). *ACA code of ethics: As approved by the ACA Governing Council 2005*. Retrieved from www.counseling.org/Resources/CodeOfEthics/TP/Home/CT2.aspx

American Nurses Association. (2001). *Code of ethics for nurses with interpretive statements*. Retrieved from www.nursingworld.org/MainMenuCategories/EthicsStandards/CodeofEthicsforNurses/Code-of-Ethics.aspx

American Occupational Therapy Association. (1978). Principles of occupational therapy ethics. In H. L. Hopkins & H. D. Smith (Eds.), *Willard and Spackman's occupational therapy* (5th ed., pp. 709–710). Philadelphia: Lippincott.

American Occupational Therapy Association. (1984). Principles of occupational therapy ethics (revised 1979). *American Journal of Occupational Therapy, 38,* 799–802. doi: 10.5014/ajot.38.12.799

American Occupational Therapy Association. (2006). *AOTA's statement on health disparities.* Retrieved from www.aota.org/Practitioners/Official/SocietalStmts/39431.aspx

American Occupational Therapy Association. (2008). Occupational therapy practice framework: Domain and process (2nd ed.). *American Journal of Occupational Therapy, 62,* 625–683. doi: 10.5014/ajot.62.6.625

American Occupational Therapy Association. (2010a). Occupational therapy code of ethics and ethics standards (2010). *American Journal of Occupational Therapy, 64*(6 Suppl.), S17–S26. doi: 10:5014/ajot2010.62S17

American Occupational Therapy Association. (2010b). *2010 occupational therapy compensation and workforce study*. Bethesda, MD: AOTA Press.

American Occupational Therapy Association. (2011). The role of occupational therapy in disaster preparedness, response, and recovery. *American Journal of Occupational Therapy, 65*(6 Suppl.), S11–S25. doi: 10.5014/ajot.2011.65S11

American Physical Therapy Association. (2009). *Code of ethics for the physical therapist*. Retrieved from www.apta.org/AM/Template.cfm?Section=Policies_and_Bylaws1&TEMPLATE=/CM/ContentDisplay.cfm&CONTENTID=73012

American Psychological Association. (2010). *Ethical principles of psychologists and code of conduct* (2002, amended June 1, 2010). Retrieved from www.apa.org/ethics/code/index.aspx

American Speech–Language–Hearing Association. (2010). *Code of ethics* [Ethics]. Retrieved from www.asha.org/policy

Americans With Disabilities Act of 1990, Pub. L. 101–336, 42 U.S.C. § 12101.

Baggett, T. P., O'Connell, J. J., Singer, D. E., & Rigotti, N. A. (2010). The unmet health care needs of homeless adults: A national study. *American Journal of Public Health, 100,* 1326–1333. doi: 10.2105/AJPH.2009.180109

Beauchamp, T. L., & Childress, J. F. (2009). *Principles of biomedical ethics* (6th ed.). New York: Oxford University Press.

Braveman, B., & Bass-Haugen, J. D. (2009). Social justice and health disparities: An evolving discourse in occupational therapy research and intervention. *American Journal of Occupational Therapy, 63,* 7–12. doi: 10.5014/ajot.63.1.7

Breines, E. (1986). *Origins and adaptations: Philosophy of practice.* Lebanon, NJ: Geri-Rehab.

Centers for Disease Control and Prevention. (2011). *People with disabilities: Living healthy.* Retrieved from www.cdc.gov/Features/Disabilities/

Community Emergency Response Team. (n.d.). *Community Emergency Response Teams (CERT).* Retrieved from www.citizencorps.gov/cert/index.shtm

Ford, K., Waring, L., & Boggis, T. (2007, March 19). Living on the edge: The hidden voices of health disparities. *OT Practice, 12*(5), 17–22.

Frank, G., & Zemke, R. (2008). Occupational therapy foundations for political engagement and social transformation. In N. Pollard, D. Sakellariou, & F. Kronenberg (Eds.), *A political practice of occupational therapy* (pp. 111–143). London: Elsevier.

Hofmann, A. O. (2008, June 24). *Rebuilding lives: Occupational therapy and disaster relief.* Retrieved July 13, 2008, from www.aota.org/News/Consumer/Rebuilding.aspx

Kronenberg, F., Algado, S. S., & Pollard, N. (2005). *Occupational therapy without borders: Learning from the spirit of survivors.* Philadelphia: Elsevier.

Ku, L. (2012). Why immigrants lack adequate access to health care and health insurance. *Migration Information Source.* Retrieved from www.migrationinformation.org/Feature/display.cfm?ID=417

National Association of Social Workers. (2008). *Code of ethics of the National Association of Social Workers: Ethical principles.* Retrieved from www.naswdc.org/pubs/code/code.asp

Polatajko, H. J., Davis, J., Stewart, D., Cantin, N., Amoroso, B., Purdie, L., & Zimmerman, D. (2007). Specifying the domain of concern: Occupation as core. In E. A. Townsend & H. J. Polatajko (Eds.), *Enabling occupation II: Advancing an occupational therapy vision for health, well-being, and justice through occupation* (pp. 13–36). Ottawa, Ontario: Canadian Association of Occupational Therapists.

Riegel, S. K., & Eglseder, K. (2009). Occupational justice as a quality indicator for occupational therapy services. *Occupational Therapy in Health Care, 23,* 288–301.

Society for Public Health Education. (2011). *Code of ethics for the health education profession.* Retrieved from www.sophe.org/Ethics.cfm

Stadnyk, R. L., Townsend, E., & Wilcock, A. A. (2010). Occupational justice. In C. H. Christiansen & E. A. Townsend (Eds.), *Introduction to occupation: The art and science of living* (2nd ed., pp. 329–358). Upper Saddle River, NJ: Pearson Education.

Townsend, E. (1993). Occupational therapy's social vision (1993 Muriel Driver Memorial Lecture). *Canadian Journal of Occupational Therapy, 60*(4), 174–184.

Townsend, E. (2003, October). *Occupational justice: Ethical, moral and civic principles for an inclusive world.* Paper presented at the European Network of Occupational Therapy Educators, Prague, Czech Republic.

Townsend, E. A., & Polatajko, H. J. (Eds.). (2007). *Enabling occupation II: Advancing an occupational therapy vision for health, well-being, and justice through occupation.* Ottawa, Ontario: Canadian Association of Occupational Therapists.

Townsend, E., & Wilcock, A. (2004a). Occupational justice. In C. H. Christiansen & E. A. Townsend (Eds.), *Introduction to occupation: The art and science of living* (pp. 243–273). Upper Saddle River, NJ: Pearson Education.

Townsend, E. A., & Wilcock, A. A. (2004b). Occupational justice and client-centered practice: A dialogue in progress. *Canadian Journal of Occupational Therapy, 71*(2), 75–87.

U.S. Department of Health and Human Services, Agency for Healthcare Research and Quality. (2010a). *2010 National Healthcare Quality and Disparities Reports.* Retrieved from www.ahrq.gov/qual/qrdr10.htm

U.S. Department of Health and Human Services, Agency for Healthcare Research and Quality. (2010b). *Highlights from the National Healthcare Quality and Disparities Reports.* Retrieved from www.ahrq.gov/qual/nhdr10/Key.htm

U.S. Department of Health and Human Services, Office of Disease Prevention and Health Promotion. (2010). *Healthy People 2020* (ODPHP Publication No. B0132). Retrieved from www.healthypeople.gov/2020/TopicsObjectives2020/pdfs/HP2020_brochure.pdf

Wilper, A. P., Woolhandler, S., Boyd, J. W., Lasser, K. E., McCormick, D., Bor, D. H., & Himmelstein,

D. U. (2009). The health and health care of U.S. prisoners: A nationwide survey. *American Journal of Public Health, 99*, 666–672.

World Federation of Occupational Therapists. (2004). *World Federation of Occupational Therapists position statement: Community based reha-* *bilitation*. Retrieved from www.wfot.org/Resource Centre.aspx

World Federation of Occupational Therapists. (2006). *World Federation of Occupational Therapists position statement: Human rights*. Retrieved from www. wfot.org/ResourceCentre.aspx

Principle 5: Procedural Justice

7

Janie B. Scott, MA, OT/L, FAOTA

PROCEDURAL JUSTICE

Principle 5. Occupational therapy personnel shall comply with institutional rules, local, state, federal, and international laws and AOTA documents applicable to the profession of occupational therapy.

Procedural justice is concerned with making and implementing decisions according to fair processes that ensure "fair treatment" (Maiese, 2004). Rules must be impartially followed and consistently applied to generate an unbiased decision. The principle of procedural justice is based on the concept that procedures and processes are organized in a fair manner and that policies, regulations, and laws are followed. While *the law* and *ethics* are not synonymous terms, occupational therapy personnel have an ethical responsibility to uphold current reimbursement regulations and state/territorial laws governing the profession. In addition, occupational therapy personnel are ethically bound to be aware of organizational policies and practice guidelines set forth by regulatory agencies established to protect recipients of service, research participants, and the public.

OCCUPATIONAL THERAPY PERSONNEL SHALL

A. Be familiar with and apply the Code and Ethics Standards to the work setting, and share them with employers, other employees, colleagues, students, and researchers.
B. Be familiar with and seek to understand and abide by institutional rules, and when those rules conflict with ethical practice, take steps to resolve the conflict.
C. Be familiar with revisions in those laws and AOTA policies that apply to the profession of occupational therapy and inform employers, employees, colleagues, students, and researchers of those changes.
D. Be familiar with established policies and procedures for handling concerns about the Code and Ethics Standards, including familiarity with national, state, local, district, and territorial procedures for handling ethics complaints as well as policies and procedures created by AOTA and certification, licensing, and regulatory agencies.
E. Hold appropriate national, state, or other requisite credentials for the occupational therapy services they provide.

F. Take responsibility for maintaining high standards and continuing competence in practice, education, and research by participating in professional development and educational activities to improve and update knowledge and skills.

G. Ensure that all duties assumed by or assigned to other occupational therapy personnel match credentials, qualifications, experience, and scope of practice.

H. Provide appropriate supervision to individuals for whom they have supervisory responsibility in accordance with AOTA official documents and local, state, and federal or national laws, rules, regulations, policies, procedures, standards, and guidelines.

I. Obtain all necessary approvals prior to initiating research activities.

J. Report all gifts and remuneration from individuals, agencies, or companies in accordance with employer policies as well as state and federal guidelines.

K. Use funds for intended purposes, and avoid misappropriation of funds.

L. Take reasonable steps to ensure that employers are aware of occupational therapy's ethical obligations as set forth in this Code and Ethics Standards and of the implications of those obligations for occupational therapy practice, education, and research.

M. Actively work with employers to prevent discrimination and unfair labor practices, and advocate for employees with disabilities to ensure the provision of reasonable accommodations.

N. Actively participate with employers in the formulation of policies and procedures to ensure legal, regulatory, and ethical compliance.

O. Collect fees legally. Fees shall be fair, reasonable, and commensurate with services delivered. Fee schedules must be available and equitable regardless of actual payer reimbursements/contracts.

P. Maintain the ethical principles and standards of the profession when participating in a business arrangement as owner, stockholder, partner, or employee, and refrain from working for or doing business with organizations that engage in illegal or unethical business practices (e.g., fraudulent billing, providing occupational therapy services beyond the scope of occupational therapy practice).

Source. From the *Occupational Therapy Code of Ethics and Ethics Standards (2010)* (American Occupational Therapy Association, 2010b, pp. S22–S23).

Occupational therapy practice is regulated by the state or territory in which the practitioner works. Principle 5 of the *Occupational Therapy Code of Ethics and Ethics Standards (2010)* (referred to as the "Code and Ethics Standards"; American Occupational Therapy Association [AOTA], 2010b) focuses on *procedural justice*, which involves compliance with institutional rules; local, state, federal, and international laws; and AOTA documents applicable to the profession of occupational therapy (these are referred to collectively throughout this chapter as "regulations"). To meet the ethical obligation of procedural justice, occupational therapy practitioners are required to

- Obtain credentialing to ensure they are competent to practice

- Comply with licensure laws
- Abide by requirements established by third-party payers
- Meet specific expectations related to ethical conduct as established by the AOTA, the National Board for Certification in Occupational Therapy (NBCOT), and state regulatory boards (SRBs).

Concern about procedural justice is not limited to AOTA and occupational therapy practice. Other professions and professional organizations discuss procedural justice in their policies and codes of ethics. We reviewed codes and documents from eight health-related professional organizations, and all eight had language about procedural justice in their documents (see Table 7.1), as well as content about the importance of adherence to laws and policies governing practice, including continuing competence.

This chapter addresses four categories of obligation regarding the regulations that govern the practice of occupational therapy: (1) to fulfill credentialing and supervisory duties according to the regulations, (2) to maintain current knowledge of the regulations and to inform others about them, (3) to develop and adhere to institutional policies and procedures to ensure ethical practice, and (4) to ensure that financial and business relationships abide by the regulations.

CREDENTIALING AND SUPERVISORY DUTIES

Occupational therapy practitioners are obligated to have the appropriate credentials to practice in a particular state or jurisdiction and to keep these credentials current. For example, practitioners are responsible for notifying the state regulatory board when they change their residence. In addition, occupational therapy practitioners have the duty to verify the backgrounds, skill sets, and expertise of those they supervise (Reed, Ashe, & Slater, 2009). In providing adequate supervision, practitioners both adhere to local, state, and federal laws and regulations (Principle 5H) and fulfill the public trust (Principle 6E). In addition, many third-party payers have rules regarding not only what services they reimburse but also whom they consider as qualified to provide those services and at what level of supervision. Case Study 7.1 describes the impact of the failure to meet these responsibilities.

CASE STUDY 7.1. ADDRESSING A FAILURE TO MAINTAIN CREDENTIALS

Mary Jo had been an occupational therapist for 3½ years when she took maternity leave. Soon after the baby was born, she notified her employer that she would not be returning to her previous position in the near future. When the baby was 6 months old, Mary Jo and her new family moved to a larger home. Later that year, she applied for a new position with her previous employer and returned to work.

She had been back to work for almost a year when the time came for her annual performance review. Mary Jo had to provide evidence of her continuing education activities, a list of goals and accomplishments, and a copy of her current license to her supervisor, **Bill**. As Mary Jo and Bill reviewed her performance and related documentation covering the past year, they noticed that Mary Jo's license to practice occupational therapy had expired a year and a half ago and that she had been practicing with a lapsed license. Mary Jo realized that in the chaos of caring for a young child and moving, she had neglected to inform her state board of occupational therapy practice about her change of address and consequently did not receive her license renewal notice. Although Mary Jo had renewed her membership in AOTA, her membership in the state occupational therapy association had lapsed, and she consequently missed the notices this organization also had provided about licensure renewal.

Mary Jo and Bill were aware that occupational therapy practitioners are required to adhere to all state and national rules governing practice, including the principles of ethical practice. Mary Jo had a duty to practice occupational therapy in full compliance with her licensure law, which included language from AOTA's Code and Ethics Standards regarding ethical conduct. In addition, as an AOTA member, she had the duty to uphold the principles articulated in the Code and Ethics Standards. Mary Jo was in violation of Principle 5E, as well as Principles 6A (represent credentials accurately) and 6B (refrain from making false claims).

Even though Mary Jo's actions were not intentional, her neglect had serious consequences. Mary Jo's employer had billed Medicare and other third-party payers for services she had provided that required occupational therapy services to be provided by qualified therapists who met academic requirements for practice and adhered to the licensure regulations. The facility risked being fined, required to repay the reimbursed funds, and charged with fraudulent billing.

When Mary Jo approached her SRB to renew her occupational therapy license, the board reviewed her situation, placed her on probation for 1 year, and issued her a substantial fine. AOTA's Ethics Commission was informed of these actions and reviewed the circumstances surrounding Mary Jo's lapsed license; it issued her a *reprimand* ("a formal expression of disapproval of conduct communicated privately by letter that is nondisclosable and

TABLE 7.1
Policies Relevant or Equivalent to Procedural Justice

ASSOCIATION	POLICIES RELEVANT OR EQUIVALENT TO PROCEDURAL JUSTICE
American Counseling Association (ACA, 2005)	"Section C: Professional Responsibility. C.1. Knowledge of Standards. Counselors have a responsibility to read, understand, and follow the ACA Code of Ethics and adhere to applicable laws and regulations." (p. 9)
American Nurses Association (2001)	"Provision 5. The nurse owes the same duties to self as to others, including the responsibility to preserve integrity and safety, to maintain competence, and to continue personal and professional growth." (p. 1) "Provision 7.3. Advancing the profession through knowledge development, dissemination, and application to practice." (p. 12)
American Physical Therapy Association (2009)	"Principle #5: Physical therapists shall fulfill their legal and professional obligations. (Core Values: Professional Duty, Accountability)" (p. 2) "Principle #6: Physical therapists shall enhance their expertise through the lifelong acquisition and refinement of knowledge, skills, abilities, and professional behaviors. (Core Value: Excellence)" (p. 2)
American Psychological Association (2010)	"Principle B: Fidelity and Responsibility. Psychologists uphold professional standards of conduct, clarify their professional roles and obligations, accept appropriate responsibility for their behavior, and seek to manage conflicts of interest that could lead to exploitation or harm." (p. 3) "Principle C: Integrity. . . . Psychologists do not steal, cheat, or engage in fraud, subterfuge, or intentional misrepresentation of fact. . . ." (p. 3)
American Speech–Language–Hearing Association (2010)	"Principle of Ethics II. Individuals shall honor their responsibility to achieve and maintain the highest level of professional competence and performance." (p. 2) "Principle of Ethics III. Individuals shall honor their responsibility to the public by promoting public understanding of the professions, by supporting the development of services designed to fulfill the unmet needs of the public, and by providing accurate information in all communications involving any aspect of the professions, including the dissemination of research findings and scholarly activities, and the promotion, marketing, and advertising of products and services." (p. 3)
Board of Certification (BOC) for the Athletic Trainer (2006)	"Code 2: Competency. The Athletic Trainer or applicant: 2.1 Engages in lifelong, professional and continuing educational activities 2.2 Participates in continuous quality improvement activities 2.3 Complies with the most current BOC recertification policies and requirements." (p. 3) "Code 3: Professional Responsibility. The Athletic Trainer or applicant: 3.1 Practices in accordance with the most current BOC Practice Standards 3.2 Knows and complies with applicable local, state and/or federal rules, requirements, regulations and/or laws related to the practice of athletic training." (p. 3)

(continued)

TABLE 7.1 (*cont.*)

ASSOCIATION	POLICIES RELEVANT OR EQUIVALENT TO PROCEDURAL JUSTICE
National Association of Social Workers (2008)	"Ethical Principle: Social workers behave in a trustworthy manner. Social workers are continually aware of the profession's mission, values, ethical principles, and ethical standards and practice in a manner consistent with them. . . ." (para. 18)
	"Ethical Principle: Social workers practice within their areas of competence and develop and enhance their professional expertise. Social workers continually strive to increase their professional knowledge and skills and to apply them in practice. Social workers should aspire to contribute to the knowledge base of the profession." (para. 19)
Society for Public Health Education (2011)	"Article IV, . . . Section 2: Health Educators are informed of the latest advances in theory, research, and practice, and use strategies and methods that are grounded in and contribute to development of professional standards, theories, guidelines, statistics, and experience." (para. 30) "Article V: Responsibility in Research and Evaluation. Health Educators contribute to the health of the population and to the profession through research and evaluation activities. When planning and conducting research or evaluation, health educators do so in accordance with federal and state laws and regulations, organizational and institutional policies, and professional standards." (para. 34)

noncommunicative to other bodies"; AOTA, 2010a, p. S5). As Mary Jo's supervisor, Bill was subjected to disciplinary action by hospital administrators for his failure to verify that Mary Jo was licensed on her return to work. Table 7.2 summarizes the consequences and outcomes of Mary Jo's failure to maintain her credentials.

As a result of her experience, Mary Jo helped Bill develop a tracking and notification system to help the other occupational therapy practitioners in the department keep abreast of their license renewal dates and acquisition of continuing education credits. She also presented an in-service to occupational therapy staff on the importance of keeping the SRB apprised of any changes in their home address and contact information.

CURRENT KNOWLEDGE OF THE REGULATIONS

Principle 5 of the Code and Ethics Standards obligates occupational therapy practitioners not only to maintain current knowledge regarding regulations governing occupational therapy practice but also to inform employers and occupational therapy employees, students, and others about those regulations and any changes to them. To meet this obligation, occupational therapy practitioners must continually update their knowledge about the regulations that pertain to practice. In Vignette 7.1, an occupational therapist and occupational therapy assistant inform a supervisor about the regulations regarding the supervision of an occupational therapy assistant.

VIGNETTE 7.1. FULFILLING THE DUTY TO INFORM OTHERS

Connie, a occupational therapy supervisor, submitted her resignation to her immediate supervisor. Connie located an occupational therapist who was willing to contract with the hospital to supervise the department's occupational therapy assistant, **Kelly**, and communicated this information to the assistant program director before leaving her position. Months later, Connie learned that Kelly had not received occupational therapy supervision since her departure.

Connie communicated the seriousness of the situation to the assistant program director on at least two occasions and offered suggestions and solutions.

TABLE 7.2
Issues in Addressing a Failure to Maintain Credentials

ISSUE	CONSEQUENCES	OUTCOMES
Failure to notify the state regulatory board of address change	The board of occupational therapy practice reviewed Mary Jo's application for licensure renewal because she had been practicing without a license. Principle 5E requires practitioners to hold appropriate credentials.	The board of occupational therapy practice issued Mary Jo a license to practice occupational therapy but placed her on 1 year of probation and issued her a fine. Mary Jo agreed to provide occupational therapy staff with an in-service regarding the SRB's requirement to notify the practice board of changes in personal information.
Bill's failure to verify Mary Jo's credentials	Bill and Mary Jo recognized their responsibilities and the violation of Principle 5G.	Bill and Mary Jo developed a tracking and notification system to help occupational therapy practitioners at the facility keep abreast of license renewal dates and continuing education credits.
Mary Jo's use of the OT/L credential	Signing documentation as an OT/L was a misrepresentation in communications to the public and third-party payers and thus a violation of Principle 6A.	The AOTA Ethics Commission reviewed Mary Jo's case for violations of Principles 5E, 5G, 6A, and 6B and issued her a letter of reprimand. The administration of Mary Jo's facility instructed her to review all policies and procedures related to credentialing and documentation and the code of conduct. Mary Jo agreed to take continuing education courses on ethics.
Use of inaccurate information in billing to Medicare and third-party payers	Medicare views these actions as abuse rather than intentional fraud. This action violated Principle 6B.	The facility agreed to work with Medicare and Mary Jo to negotiate a settlement.
Bill's failure to adhere to the *Guidelines for Supervision, Roles, and Responsibilities During the Delivery of Occupational Therapy Services* (AOTA, 2009)	Because of Bill's lack of familiarity with policies and guidelines of the profession, Bill, his staff, and ultimately the hospital violated organizational policies and federal regulations.	Bill reviewed the *Guidelines* document and attended continuing education courses related to supervision.

Note. AOTA = American Occupational Therapy Association.

Connie no longer wanted to be involved, but she wanted to be responsible and ethical. She obtained copies of the supervision requirements from the SRB and *Guidelines for Supervision, Roles, and Responsibilities During the Delivery of Occupational Therapy Services* (AOTA, 2009) and mailed them to Kelly and the assistant program director. She also telephoned Kelly to discuss the situation and her concerns directly with him, noting that Kelly's license might be jeopardized if he continued to practice without adequate supervision. She suggested to Kelly that he consider contacting the state board of occupational therapy practice and reporting the situation and that he investigate whether third-party payers had rules about whom they considered to be qualified to provide services. Kelly gathered the results of his research and met with the assistant program director to reiterate his need for supervision by an occupational therapist under the Code and Ethics Standards, state licensure laws, and third-party payer requirements.

The principle of Procedural Justice emphasizes the duty of occupational therapy practitioners to comply with the documentation requirements of third-party payers and their employers' institutional policies. Occupational therapy documentation should accurately reflect the services delivered and the outcomes and should be of the kind and quality that satisfy the scrutiny of peer reviews, legal proceedings, and accrediting agencies. Inaccurate documentation is a violation of the Code and Ethics Standards, which states that occupational therapy practitioners should not use any form of communication that is false, fraudulent, or deceptive. Vignette 7.2 describes an occupational therapist's efforts to inform herself and her supervisor about regulations regarding documentation.

VIGNETTE 7.2. COMPLYING WITH INSTITUTIONAL REGULATIONS

Amelia recently passed the NBCOT certification exam and began working at a state facility serving people with developmental disabilities. Her supervisor, **José**, who was also new to the facility, discovered that many of the client records did not have any occupational therapy progress notes. José suggested that he and Amelia re-create notes for all of the charts using the sign-in sheets documenting client attendance.

Amelia wanted to please José and keep her new job, but she was uncertain whether she should agree with José's request. She was concerned about whether her compliance would be legal and ethical and, if so, whether to take time away from client care or come in on the weekends to complete the documentation.

Amelia reviewed the Code and Ethics Standards for guidance. In addition to Principles 5A, 5L, and 5N, all of which address responsibilities for educating others about and adhering to regulations, she discovered that Principle 6, Veracity, also applied—particularly Principles 6B (refrain from participating in deceptive communication), 6C (record and report accurately and timely), and 6D (ensure that documentation is done in accordance with regulations). She also reviewed institutional policies regarding coming in to work when not scheduled and denying current clients the services they need and expect. She decided that it would be inappropriate and unprofessional to comply with José's request and made an appointment to discuss her concerns with José (Scott, 2002b).

POLICIES AND PROCEDURES TO ENSURE ETHICAL PRACTICE

The principle of Procedural Justice obligates occupational therapy practitioners to work to resolve potential breaches of the Code and Ethics Standards. The first attempts at resolution should take place locally (see Principle 7D)—for example, with the immediate supervisor or fieldwork coordinator. Consulting the code of conduct established by the institution is the next step. If these strategies do not bear fruit, practitioners should explore the relative jurisdictions of the SRB, NBCOT, and AOTA and file complaints with the appropriate board or organization; jurisdictional issues are discussed in Chapter 2 of this volume. Vignette 7.3 describes the attempts of a fieldwork student to resolve his lack of adequate supervision.

VIGNETTE 7.3. ADDRESSING FAILURE TO PROVIDE ADEQUATE SUPERVISION

Paul, an occupational therapy student in a fieldwork placement, was concerned about the limited supervision he was receiving. He reviewed the Code and Ethics Standards and found that by failing to provide him with adequate supervision, his immediate supervisor may have breached Principles 5B, 5G, and 5H. Paul's supervisor may also have violated state laws and regulations that address the responsibilities of a licensed occupational therapist in supervising occupational therapy assistants, students, and other personnel. According to Principle 7C, Paul realized, he had an obligation under the Code and Ethics Standards to report the suspected breaches of his supervisor's ethical conduct; Principle 7C reads, "Occupational therapy personnel shall take adequate measures to discourage, prevent, expose, and correct any breaches of the Code and Ethics Standards, and report any breaches of the former to the appropriate authorities" (AOTA, 2010b, p. S25).

Paul considered the appropriate lines of communication to follow. He decided that a meeting with his immediate fieldwork supervisor to discuss his concerns and needs was the first step, so he made an appointment with her. If this conversation did not result in the desired outcome, he resolved to consult with university faculty. If these efforts did not result in additional supervision, Paul would contact his academic fieldwork coordinator to see whether she would agree to provide more regular and direct supervision to enhance Paul's educational experience and to help safeguard the clients on his caseload.

If these strategies failed, Paul discovered, he could file a complaint with the SRB, NBCOT, or AOTA. His SRB had specific regulations addressing supervision of nonlicensed personnel. If his occupational therapy fieldwork supervisor held current certification with NBCOT, he could file a complaint with that organization to help ensure consumer protection. Finally, if Paul's fieldwork supervisor was an AOTA member, he could file an ethics complaint citing the principles of the Code and Ethics Standards that he believed were violated (Scott, 2002a).

FINANCIAL AND BUSINESS RELATIONSHIPS

Financial accountability extends to all work roles and contexts in which occupational therapy services are delivered. This obligation exists for practitioners in clinics, long-term care facilities,

independent practice, and any other setting in which monetary compensation is involved. There is a strong correlation between the principles of Procedural Justice and Veracity. Both principles embody the expectation that occupational therapy practitioners will follow established policies and procedures to accurately document and bill.

Many occupational therapy practitioners with an entrepreneurial spirit establish a private practice based on their expertise, often with children and youth, injured workers, or older adults who wish to age in place (Bureau of Labor Statistics, U.S. Department of Labor, 2012; Herz, Bondoc, Richmond, Richman, & Kroll, 2005). Principle 5P guides private practitioners to "maintain the ethical principles and standards of the profession" (AOTA, 2010b, p. S23) in all business arrangements. Vignette 7.4 describes a situation in which an occupational therapist in private practice fails to meet these obligations.

VIGNETTE 7.4. ADDRESSING FAILURE TO MAINTAIN ETHICAL PRINCIPLES IN PRIVATE PRACTICE

Pamela Pediatrics, a company owned by Pamela, an occupational therapist, provided occupational therapy services to preschool children with special needs in a clinic setting. Pamela had been a clinical fieldwork supervisor for 8 years, and although the practice was busy and the clinic's staffing level was low, she currently had three Level I fieldwork students. The students were concerned that the children were receiving inadequate care and that the students were receiving inadequate supervision.

The students consulted the Code and Ethics Standards and discovered that Principle 1, Beneficence, was violated because understaffing could lead to a lack of safety for both the children and the students. Principle 5H, regarding the provision of appropriate supervision by those with supervisory responsibility, was also relevant. Principle 5P, they realized, held Pamela to the same obligations to her clients and fieldwork students in her private practice as she would have in an institution. Pamela was responsible both for providing competent services to the children, who may have been at increased risk for injury, and for supervising the students according to relevant guidelines (e.g., Accreditation Council for Occupational Therapy Education, 2012). The students contacted their school for guidance.

CONCLUSION

Laws, rules, and guidelines are created to help ensure that the public is protected from harm by unqualified practitioners. Principle 5 of the Code and Ethics Standards outlines the duty of occupational therapy practitioners to abide by regulations established to protect consumers of occupational therapy services, employers, third-party payers, students, the profession, and society at large. Practitioners must continually update their knowledge about applicable laws, rules, and regulations governing practice.

REFERENCES

Accreditation Council for Occupational Therapy Education. (2012). 2011 Accreditation Council for Occupational Therapy Education (ACOTE®) standards. *American Journal of Occupational Therapy, 66* (6 Suppl.), S6–S74. doi: 10.5014/ajot.2012.66S6

American Counseling Association. (2005). *ACA code of ethics: As approved by the ACA Governing Council 2005.* Retrieved December 6, 2010, from www.counseling.org/Resources/CodeOfEthics/TP/Home/CT2.aspx

American Nurses Association. (2001). *Code of ethics for nurses with interpretive statements.* Retrieved December 9, 2010, from www.nursingworld.org/MainMenuCategories/EthicsStandards/CodeofEthicsforNurses/Code-of-Ethics.aspx

American Occupational Therapy Association. (2009). Guidelines for supervision, roles, and responsibilities during the delivery of occupational therapy services. *American Journal of Occupational Therapy, 63,* 797–803. doi: 10.5014/ajot.63.6.797

American Occupational Therapy Association. (2010a). Enforcement procedures for the *Occupational Therapy Code of Ethics and Ethics Standards. American Journal of Occupational Therapy, 64*(6 Suppl.), S4–S16. doi: 10.5014/ajot.2010.64S4

American Occupational Therapy Association. (2010b). Occupational therapy code of ethics and ethics standards (2010). *American Journal of Occupational Therapy, 64*(6 Suppl.), S17–S26. doi: 10.5014/ajot.2010.64S17

American Physical Therapy Association. (2009). *Code of ethics for the physical therapist.* Retrieved December 9, 2010, From www.apta.org/AM/Template.cfm?Section=Policies_and_Bylaws1&TEMPLATE=/CM/ContentDisplay.cfm&CONTENTID=73012

American Psychological Association. (2010). *Ethical principles of psychologists and code of conduct* (2002, amended June 1, 2010). Retrieved December 9, 2010, from www.apa.org/ethics/code/index.aspx

American Speech–Language–Hearing Association. (2010). *Code of ethics [Ethics].* Retrieved December 9, 2010, from www.asha.org/policy

Board of Certification for the Athletic Trainer. (2006). *BOC standards of professional practice.* Retrieved from www.bocatc.org/index.php?option=com_content&view=article&id=51&Itemid=111

Bureau of Labor Statistics, U.S. Department of Labor. (2012). *Occupational outlook handbook: Occupational therapists.* Retrieved from www.bls.gov/oco/ocos078.htm

Herz, N., Bondoc, S., Richmond, T., Richman, N., & Kroll, C. (2005, March). Becoming an entrepreneur. *Administration and Management Special Interest Section Quarterly, 21,* 1–3.

Maiese, M. (2004). *Procedural justice.* Retrieved from www.beyondintractability.org/essay/procedural_justice/

National Association of Social Workers. (2008). *Code of ethics of the National Association of Social Workers.* Retrieved from www.naswdc.org/pubs/code/code.asp

Reed, K. L., Ashe, A. M., & Slater, D. Y. (2009, April). *Everyday ethics: Ethical challenges in emerging practice.* Slide show presented at the AOTA Annual Conference & Expo, Houston.

Scott, J. B. (2002a, January 14). Everyday ethics: Clarifying concerns and remedies. *OT Practice, 7*(1), 9.

Scott, J. B. (2002b, May 13). Everyday ethics: Recreating notes. *OT Practice, 7*(5), 7.

Society for Public Health Education. (2011). *Code of ethics for the health education profession.* Retrieved from www.sophe.org/Ethics.cfm

Principle 6: Veracity

8

Janie B. Scott, MA, OT/L, FAOTA

VERACITY

Principle 6. Occupational therapy personnel shall provide comprehensive, accurate, and objective information when representing the profession.

Veracity is based on the virtues of truthfulness, candor, and honesty. The principle of *veracity* in health care refers to comprehensive, accurate, and objective transmission of information and includes fostering the client's understanding of such information (Beauchamp & Childress, 2009). Veracity is based on respect owed to others. In communicating with others, occupational therapy personnel implicitly promise to speak truthfully and not deceive the listener. By entering into a relationship in care or research, the recipient of service or research participant enters into a contract that includes a right to truthful information (Beauchamp & Childress, 2009). In addition, transmission of information is incomplete without also ensuring that the recipient or participant understands the information provided. Concepts of veracity must be carefully balanced with other potentially competing ethical principles, cultural beliefs, and organizational policies. Veracity ultimately is valued as a means to establish trust and strengthen professional relationships. Therefore, adherence to the Principle also requires thoughtful analysis of how full disclosure of information may impact outcomes.

OCCUPATIONAL THERAPY PERSONNEL SHALL

A. Represent the credentials, qualifications, education, experience, training, roles, duties, competence, views, contributions, and findings accurately in all forms of communication about recipients of service, students, employees, research participants, and colleagues.
B. Refrain from using or participating in the use of any form of communication that contains false, fraudulent, deceptive, misleading, or unfair statements or claims.
C. Record and report in an accurate and timely manner, and in accordance with applicable regulations, all information related to professional activities.
D. Ensure that documentation for reimbursement purposes is done in accordance with applicable laws, guidelines, and regulations.

E. Accept responsibility for any action that reduces the public's trust in occupational therapy.
F. Ensure that all marketing and advertising are truthful, accurate, and carefully presented to avoid misleading recipients of service, students, research participants, or the public.
G. Describe the type and duration of occupational therapy services accurately in professional contracts, including the duties and responsibilities of all involved parties.
H. Be honest, fair, accurate, respectful, and timely in gathering and reporting fact-based information regarding employee job performance and student performance.
I. Give credit and recognition when using the work of others in written, oral, or electronic media.
J. Not plagiarize the work of others.

Source. From the *Occupational Therapy Code of Ethics and Ethics Standards (2010)* (American Occupational Therapy Association, 2010b, pp. S23–S24).

The obligation of Veracity is detailed in Principle 6 of the *Occupational Therapy Code of Ethics and Ethics Standards (2010)* (referred to as the "Code and Ethics Standards"; American Occupational Therapy Association [AOTA], 2010b). This obligation extends to all areas of professional and public communication, including marketing, "professional relationships, documentation standards, billing practices, risk management, peer review, community relations, and regulatory reporting and compliance" (Bennett-Woods, 2005, p. 11). According to Beauchamp and Childress (2009), neither the Hippocratic Oath (see Chapter 1 of this volume) nor the early versions of the *Principles of Medical Ethics* (the first version of the American Medical Association's [AMA's] code of ethics) made reference to veracity. The AMA created the *Code of Medical Ethics* in 1847, and the title was changed to the *Principles of Medical Ethics* in 1903 (AMA, n.d.). Beginning in the 1980s, however, the *Principles of Medical Ethics* began to include language regarding the duty to be honest with both patients and colleagues.

As Beauchamp and Childress (2009) observed, "Obligations of veracity are based on respect owed to others" (p. 289). Veracity, trust, autonomy, and fidelity are closely linked, particularly as they relate to the relationships and obligations that occupational therapy practitioners have involving their clients, colleagues, and the public. Three primary categories of behavior are covered by Principle 6, Veracity: truthful communication with others (public duty), documentation, and attribution (AOTA, 2010b, p. S24).

COMMUNICATION WITH THE PUBLIC

Occupational therapy practitioners have a public duty to be honest in all oral and written communication within the profession and with external audiences, including students, colleagues, clients, and the public (AOTA, 2010b). When practitioners present information in a way that is unclear or dishonest, harm may occur to the recipient, and the public perception of the occupational therapy profession may be damaged. Principles 6A, 6B, 6E, 6F, and 6H address Veracity as a public duty. Conducting oneself in a way that deviates from these standards is a violation of Principle 6 of the Code and Ethics Standards, as well as of many requirements established by state occupational therapy regulatory boards (SBRs) and the National Board of Certification in Occupational Therapy (NBCOT). As physician and social work pioneer Richard Clark Cabot (1915) observed nearly a century ago, "To fool a patient is tyranny, not guidance" (p. ix).

An example from the medical literature serves to illustrate the harm caused by failure to uphold the principle of Veracity. Dr. Andrew Wakefield and his colleagues (1998) published research in *Lancet* purporting to provide evidence of a connection between the measles, mumps, and rubella (MMR) vaccine and the onset of autism. The veracity of Wakefield's claims could not be substantiated, and he was required to retract his reports of study outcomes (Godlee & Smith, 2011), was convicted of misconduct and ethics breaches, and had his medical license revoked

(General Medical Council, 2010). Because of the fraudulent information he communicated to the public, rates of immunization with the MMR vaccine dropped, potentially leading to a public health problem. Wakefield continued to stand behind his fraudulent reporting, meaning that his miscommunication has continued to spread fear. Wakefield violated his public duty to be honest and truthful in his communications, a major violation of the ethics principle of Veracity.

This example highlights the ethical obligation of all health care professionals to fulfill the public duty of Veracity to avoid direct or indirect harm to patients. Principle 1F enlists occupational therapy practitioners to make sure that interventions are evidence based to the extent possible, and Principle 1G obligates us to ensure our competence to avoid inflicting harm directly or indirectly. Occupational therapy practitioners have an obligation to be aware of retracted research by staying current with developments in the literature and to debunk myths and prevent further harm by ensuring that clients have up-to-date knowledge. Additionally, the Code and Ethics Standards place the expectation on practitioners to be objective in their practice (Principle 2G) and to maintain high standards of competence (Principle 5F) to ensure the safety and well-being of those served. Adherence to these principles helps occupational therapy practitioners remain alert to innovations in practice and ensure that they deliver competent services so that information and interventions provided are efficacious.

In her 2011 American Occupational Therapy Foundation Breakfast With a Scholar lecture, Ruth Purtilo spoke about *moral courage*—the importance of having confidence in one's decisions and a reasonable belief that the course of action one takes is the correct one. Moral courage is required when facing an ethical dilemma and is possible only when one has the competence and the confidence to make the best possible judgment or decision. For example, an occupational therapy practitioner who receives a referral for a client whose condition is unfamiliar must assess his or her skills and abilities in the context of the client's needs and determine whether it would be in the client's best interest to refer him or her to another practitioner with expertise in that prac-

tice or specialty area. Occupational therapy practitioners must have the moral courage to make the best choice for the client, which is ultimately the best choice for the practitioner, too. In Case Study 8.1, the practitioners have the moral courage to review their behaviors and choose ethical actions.

CASE STUDY 8.1. EXHIBITING MORAL COURAGE TO ADDRESS A LACK OF VERACITY

Joel and **Monica** were occupational therapists who had worked together for 4 years with older adults in an inpatient subacute unit of a long-term care facility. They had had limited opportunities to provide caregiver education to their patients' families to help them anticipate the needs of the family member after discharge and adapt their home environment for greater accessibility. Joel and Monica thought their patients and families needed these services to experience successful transitions back home.

Joel and Monica began planning a business venture that would enable them to provide caregiver education, environmental assessment, and care coordination for patients being discharged from hospital and acute care settings to home and to their families. They planned a transition from full-time employment to private practice. Joel and Monica constructed a business plan, conducted a needs assessment, created an office location initially in one of their homes, and promoted their practice through brochures directed to patients and families and to the professional community (e.g., doctors, rehabilitation professionals, area agencies on aging). As a part of the process, Monica investigated AOTA's Specialty Certification in Environmental Modification, and Joel planned to obtain special certification through the National Association of Home Builders (NAHB). They understood that to be successful in their business, they had to fulfill a need that wasn't currently being met in their community and to promote themselves as experts in the area of aging in place (Scott, 2009).

The promotional materials Joel and Monica developed listed the services they would offer, including aging-in-place consultation, environmental assessments, caregiver education, and care coordination. In their bios, they listed the following skills and experience: 8 years of experience in inpatient occupational therapy service delivery, discharge planning with patients and families, caregiver education and training, and home safety evaluations. They included the following certifications: certification by NBCOT, state licensure in occupational therapy, and certification in home modifications. Joel and Monica knew, as they were creating these materials, that they had initial certification by NBCOT; however, this certification was not current, and the certification in home modifications they listed was what they hoped to acquire before they officially opened their business.

Joel and Monica decided to get a head start on their outreach campaign and shared their publicity materials with the agency's social worker, a physical therapist friend, and staff at the local area agency on aging. Once the information got out, however, people began to question the veracity of the statements they made in their materials. Joel and Monica knew with moral certainty that they needed to review the misstatements they had made in the brochures and other documents they had distributed, examine the ramifications and impact of having this information go public, and develop strategies to retract the materials. They also realized that they would have to reexamine their entire plan of implementation.

Joel and Monica used the Code and Ethics Standards to help structure their reflection on the facts in their situation and to begin their remediation plan. Their reflection led to the following realizations:

- Joel and Monica had misrepresented their credentials—NBCOT certification, AOTA specialty certification, and NAHB certification—in violation of Principle 6A. In particular, they realized, their use of a federally registered trademark with NBCOT could potentially involve them in fraud litigation, which could be communicated to their SRB and the Disciplinary Action Information Exchange Network (see Chapter 2, this volume).
- They had published information suggesting that they had far more experience than was accurate, violating Principle 6B.
- They made a commitment to revise their materials and their business plan in an effort to restore the public's trust in them as practitioners and in the profession in general.

Failure to do so would have resulted in a violation of Principle 6E.

Joel and Monica were overwhelmed by the scope of their errors, but they had the moral courage to face and rectify them. They decided to personally contact each person and agency that had received their material with a written apology and a request that the recipient destroy the brochures they had received. They thought this was an important step in respecting their public duty to be ethical. Additionally, Joel and Monica decided to delay publicizing their private practice until they had obtained the certifications and gained the expertise they needed to be successful, competent, and ethical occupational therapists.

Occupational therapy students have reported observations from their fieldwork Level II experiences about patients who received a doctor's referral for occupational therapy but who were not aware of why they were referred and the outcomes they should expect from these interventions. When occupational therapists do not review the evaluation results, plan of care, expected length of intervention, and anticipated outcomes with their patients, patients' trust in the services and provider wavers. In Case Study 8.2 and Vignette 8.1, occupational therapists must take steps to fulfill the duty of Veracity in communicating with patients.

CASE STUDY 8.2. IMPROVING VERACITY IN CLIENT COMMUNICATION

Caroline was an occupational therapist with 20 years of experience specializing in interventions for patients recovering from hand surgery and traumas of the hand and upper extremity. After undergoing hand surgery and four occupational therapy sessions, **Deborah**, a patient, asked Caroline about her prognosis. Although Caroline was aware of the outcomes that would likely result from the intervention, she told Deborah, "I'm really not sure; you should ask your doctor."

Later, Caroline reflected on her actions regarding sharing information with this and other patients. She realized she was afraid that if she replied honestly, Deborah might terminate care early, reducing the potential benefits of the intervention. Caroline also questioned whether she had been operating from a position of paternalism by taking away Deborah's opportunity to make decisions about her care. Caroline consulted the Code and Ethics Standards and found direction that would be helpful in her patient interactions.

Under Principle 3A, Caroline found her obligation to fully disclose to Deborah the benefits, risks, and potential outcomes of the interventions offered. She also noted her responsibility to keep Deborah informed about her progress toward established goals (Principle 3B). Caroline identified the ethical duty articulated in Principle 1H regarding her responsibility to terminate occupational therapy services in collaboration with Deborah or when Deborah had achieved maximum benefits. If Caroline had any doubts about whether Deborah could understand the information regarding the assessments, interventions, and potential risks and benefits (Principle 3J), Caroline would need to take steps to make sure that this information was clear and delivered in a way that Deborah could comprehend. Regarding the duty of Veracity, if Caroline withheld information or provided the patient with communication that was vague, false, or deceptive, she would be in violation of Principle 6B. Caroline recognized that she needed to be clear and accurate when presenting information to Deborah and her other patients. Finally, Caroline reflected that if she did not share her assessment of Deborah's progress with her, it might reduce Deborah's belief in the benefits of the interventions she was receiving.

Caroline decided to contact the referring doctor and explain Deborah's concerns regarding her care and prognosis. She also informed the doctor of her own intention to more fully share her assessment and anticipated outcomes with Deborah during their next session. They agreed that Caroline would encourage Deborah to speak with the surgeon if she had any additional questions. Caroline felt freer after sharing her dilemma with the surgeon and clarifying her responsibilities to her patient. These actions helped her maintain compliance with the Code and Ethics Standards.

VIGNETTE 8.1. ENSURING VERACITY IN MULTIPLE ROLES

Bruce worked for a pediatric inpatient rehabilitation facility and provided services to survivors of

brain and spinal cord injuries. He also made and sold pediatric furniture and adaptive equipment through his home business. Bruce wanted to know whether it would be ethical for him to tell his patients' parents about his business and the opportunity for them to buy furniture or adaptive equipment created especially for them. Bruce knew he had an obligation to adhere to the policies and guidelines of the institution in which he worked and to federal and state laws and regulations. He also consulted Principle 6 of the Code and Ethics Standards, his employer's guidelines on employees' referrals to their own businesses (Principles 6B and 6F), and an advisory opinion for the Ethics Commission by Austin (2006). Austin described the ethical conflicts that can exist when occupational therapists provide direct service to clients and also sell products to them from a company in which they have invested or from which they receive a commission.

What subprinciples of Principle 6, Veracity, of the Code and Ethics Standards are applicable to this situation? Are there any potential problems if Bruce bills a third party (e.g., the state Medical Assistance program) for these contractual services? In addition, as Austin (2006) asked, "Would the objective therapeutic relationship be compromised? . . . The trust so critical to a therapeutic relationship may be breached and ultimately reflect negatively on the profession of occupational therapy and those that provide services (Principle 6D)" (p. 138).

DOCUMENTATION

All facets of occupational therapy practice, research, and education require documentation, and Principles 6C, 6D, and 6G refer specifically to documentation. The information occupational therapy practitioners and students supply to local, state, and federal agencies must be accurate and in accordance with stated regulations. Failure to ensure veracity in documentation violates Principle 6, as well as laws and regulations established to govern occupational therapy and protect clients.

Ethical practice requires the documentation of assessments, progress, and number of minutes or units spent in interventions for billing purposes. Those whose practice includes consultation must provide documentation according to the specifications of the agreed-on work. Whether documentation is required for the purposes of billing, recording gains and losses, or supplying evidence to standard setters, compliance is required on a consistent basis.

Third-party payers (e.g., Medicare) have specific stipulations about the type and timing of documentation that must be submitted to receive reimbursement. Documentation standards and requirements established by Medicare are often followed by other payers. In addition, the SRBs (see Chapter 2 of this volume) and NBCOT (2011) have established standards requiring the professionals they regulate to be accurate and truthful and to respect the privacy of the clients they serve. The *NBCOT Candidate/Certificant Code of Conduct* articulates two principles that are consistent with the language and expectations in the Code and Ethics Standards:

> Principle 3. Certificants shall be accurate, truthful, and complete in any and all communications, direct or indirect, with any client, employer, regulatory agency, or other parties as relates to their professional work, education, professional credentials, research and contributions to the field of O.T.

> Principle 4. Certificants shall comply with laws, regulations, and statutes governing the practice of occupational therapy. (NBCOT, 2011, p. 2)

As described in Case Study 8.3, the accuracy of documentation for billing purposes (Principle 6D) has both ethical and legal implications.

CASE STUDY 8.3. ENSURING VERACITY IN DOCUMENTATION

Madison was an occupational therapist working in a not-for-profit teaching hospital on an inpatient rehabilitation unit. The pace was fast, and the productivity requirements kept all of the rehabilitation professionals moving quickly to meet the established standards. On a regular basis, however, patients were not ready or available or refused to come to the unit for their therapy sessions. When this occurred, the competition for patients increased between occupational therapy and physical therapy; whoever could get to the patient first was able to get their minutes in. Madison and **Jonah**, a physical therapist, agreed that when schedules got tight and it was feasible, they would co-treat so that patients would get some amount of services and the therapists' productivity numbers wouldn't be too low, which would get them in trouble.

Jonah approached Madison at lunch one day when their workloads were particularly heavy. Jonah proposed that they co-treat Mr. Pitts in the afternoon and each bill for the standard three units of service. By the time Jonah and Madison saw Mr. Pitts, though, it was late in the day, and there wasn't enough time for them to see him for the full three units. Even though Madison was able to provide only two units of occupational therapy service to Mr. Pitts, Madison and Jonah agreed that they would each bill for the full three units of time, and Madison would make up the time with Mr. Pitts the next day. Madison wasn't totally comfortable with this plan but didn't want to get in trouble with their supervisor, so she documented the intervention as three units. This same situation occurred several times over a period of 3 months until Jonah was reassigned to another unit. During all of this time, Madison neglected to think about the legal and ethical implications of her actions.

Late one evening, Madison reflected on her day and became uncomfortable with the decisions she and Jonah had been making regarding billing. At first she told herself not to worry about it, that occupational therapists and physical therapists did this kind of thing all the time and it wasn't a big deal. However, she remembered that she had recently read about Medicare fraud investigations and worried that she could fall into this legal and ethical abyss. Madison consulted the Code and Ethics Standards and went to Medicare.gov, the Centers for Medicaid and Medicare Services Web site, to review how her behaviors might be interpreted. The first thing Madison saw on Medicare.gov (n.d.) was, "What is fraud and abuse? Medicare fraud happens when Medicare is billed for services or supplies you never got." The more she read, the more she realized that what she and Jonah had done had placed them, their licenses, and the hospital in jeopardy.

Madison's review of the Code and Ethics Standards led her to see that her behaviors violated

Principle 6D, "Ensure that documentation for reimbursement purposes is done in accordance with applicable laws, guidelines, and regulations" (AOTA, 2010, p. S24). She also found that Principle 5, Procedural Justice, had been violated: "Occupational therapy personnel shall comply with institutional rules, local, state, federal, and international laws and AOTA documents applicable to the profession of occupational therapy" (AOTA, 2010, p. S22).

Madison realized that in the worst-case scenario, she could lose her job and her license to practice occupational therapy and could be sued. She considered her potential courses of action, which included saying and doing nothing, contacting the family lawyer to get guidance on the situation, or making an appointment to meet with her supervisor and be honest about what had happened and work with her toward resolution. Madison chose the latter option. Some of the options and the possible results she considered are reflected in Table 8.1.

Madison met with her supervisor, and they then met with the hospital's legal counsel. Under the Code and Ethics Standards, her supervisor had an ethical obligation (Principles 1M and 7C) to report this situation to AOTA and the licensure board. Madison shared all of the information she had discovered in the Code and Ethics Standards and at Medicare.gov in an effort to be transparent. At the end of many meetings, Madison wasn't fired; however, she was disciplined by the AOTA Ethics Commission as an AOTA member and by the state licensure board. In addition, she arranged a way to achieve financial restitution with the hospital and Medicare. All agencies involved were somewhat lenient because Madison voluntarily came forward to disclose her actions rather than waiting to see whether her actions would be discovered.

Occupational therapy practitioners involved in research also must abide by the ethical principle of Veracity. They must obtain approval from the appropriate institutional review board and secure consent from research participants. If occupational therapy practitioners misrepresent their research and outcomes, they potentially endanger both their clients and the profession. Chapter 19 of this volume discusses the need for concern in the accuracy and veracity of reports of findings in occupational therapy research, including ensuring that the work reported is accurate and reflects the author's own work unless specified otherwise.

Occupational therapy educators are bound by the principle of Veracity in developing a syllabus that articulates performance expectations by which student and faculty are judged and provides guidelines for integrity. In addition, syllabi should be constructed to meet the standards approved by the Accreditation Council for Occupational Therapy Education (ACOTE). Faculty must be honest and forthcoming regarding course-specific details, such as learning activities, and more broadly communicate how a particular course is related to the curriculum design to be in compliance with the following standard:

> The program must have written syllabi for each course that include course objectives and learning activities that, in total, reflect all course content required by the Standards. Instructional methods (e.g., presentations, demonstrations, discussion) and materials used to accomplish course objectives must be documented. Programs must also demonstrate the consistency between course syllabi and the curriculum design. (AOTE, 2012, p. S32)

Similarly, Principle 6C requires occupational therapy practitioners to accurately document the continuing education they obtain for licensure or certification renewal and for continuing competence. Practitioners must maintain a record of continuing education courses and activities in accordance with the standard-setting body, typically to include the name of the course, dates, number of contact hours, and evidence of attendance or participation. The organization or SRB may require that these records be submitted at the time of license or certification renewal or in the event of an audit. Practitioners should be aware of documentation retention policies; those whose documentation is reviewed and considered to be incomplete may face disciplinary action or a delay in license or certification renewal.

ATTRIBUTION

Principles 6I and 6J focus on *attribution,* or the explicit recognition of others as the originators of ideas. Occupational therapy students and

TABLE 8.1
Decision Table for Case Study 8.3

POSSIBLE ACTION	POSITIVE OUTCOMES	NEGATIVE CONSEQUENCES
No action	Madison avoids discomfort and embarrassment.	Madison continues the behaviors and places her license in jeopardy. Jonah continues his billing practices. Madison violates state and federal laws and hospital policies. Madison violates her responsibility as an AOTA member to uphold ethics principles (Principles 5 and 6D).
Cease behavior but take no additional action	Madison avoids discomfort and embarrassment. Madison avoids committing additional fraudulent billing.	Jonah continues his billing practices. Madison and Jonah continue to violate state and federal laws and hospital policies. Madison violates her responsibility as an AOTA member to uphold ethics principles (Principles 5 and 6D).
Discuss the issues with her supervisor	Madison feels relief from her emotional tension when she discloses her behaviors and concerns to her supervisor. Both Madison and her supervisor have an obligation to report to the authorities any acts that appear unethical or illegal (Principle 1M). Madison's supervisor also contacts Jonah's supervisor to provide information and seek appropriate legal and ethical action (Principles 5 and 6D).	Madison's supervisor is obligated under Principle 7C to prevent breaches of the Code and Ethics Standards. The hospital may fire or discipline Madison and her supervisor. Jonah may be angry that he is also disciplined. Medicare may fine the hospital. Madison may face civil penalties from Medicare and the SRB, may lose her license to practice, and may be disciplined by AOTA's Ethics Commission.
Inform Medicare	Madison upholds her duty under Principles 1M, 5, and 6D to address her violations of these principles. Madison gains a greater understanding of her legal and ethical obligations regarding billing and reimbursement.	Medicare reports these breaches of policy and ethics to the National Practitioner Data Bank. Madison negotiates repayment of debt with Medicare. The SRB disciplines Madison by placing her on probation and requiring her to pay a fine and take ethics education courses.

Note. A variety of possible actions to address this situation and analyses of each are provided in this table; however, other actions or analyses are possible depending on the decision-making model and specific ethics theory or approach used (see Chapter 10, this volume). AOTA = American Occupational Therapy Association; SRB = state regulatory board.

practitioners have a duty to provide attribution when they use the words and thoughts of others. This topic is relevant not only for students and researchers but also for clinicians who develop inservices, policy manuals, and screening tools and for consultants who create surveys and reports for people, communities, organizations, and agencies. This obligation applies both to word-for-word duplications and to summaries of others' ideas that are incorporated into one's own work.

Two advisory opinions have been published on *plagiarism*, which is the failure to provide adequate attribution for the ideas one uses from other sources (Ashe, 2011; Kornblau, 2000). Kornblau (2000) noted, "The sources can include printed or formally published works, electronic media, presentations or workshops, videotaped or audiotaped materials, and information obtained from the Internet" (p. 205). Ashe's (2011) advisory opinion expanded on Kornblau's:

> The concept of plagiarism encompasses not only material that has been copyrighted and published but also unpublished works, speeches, tweets, blogs, photographs, drawings, and the like. . . . Information available to all on the Internet is not necessarily in the public domain. (p. 219)

When reproducing the words and thoughts of others, ignorance is not a legitimate defense. All students and occupational therapy practitioners have a responsibility under the Code and Ethics Standards, institutional rules, and copyright law to clearly state when ideas, words, and images are not their own. Vignette 8.2 describes circumstances in which occupational therapy practitioners decide to use others' work without attribution.

VIGNETTE 8.2. FAILING TO ENSURE VERACITY IN ATTRIBUTION

Lisa, an occupational therapist, and **Peter**, an occupational therapy assistant, received funding from the occupational therapy department where they worked to attend a national conference. As a condition of receiving this funding, their supervisor, **Dominique**, made two requests. First, they were to attend sessions relevant to the hospital's interest in increasing its health and wellness programming, particularly sessions focused on mental health; productive aging; and rehabilitation, participation, and disability. Second, after the conference, they were to provide a series of five staff in-services about the sessions they attended and recommend ways the department could translate this new information into innovative health and wellness programming to be offered to outpatients and the community. Lisa and Peter enthusiastically agreed to these requirements and appreciated the opportunity they had been offered.

Lisa and Peter had an excellent time at the conference. They attended a variety of sessions and special events and were reunited with many of their friends from occupational therapy school, past positions, and recent conferences. Unfortunately, Lisa and Peter lost their focus on Dominique's assignment. They attended a couple of sessions on health and wellness but none on mental health or rehabilitation, participation, and disability. Lisa and Peter decided to download the handouts from the sessions they had missed from the conference Web site and combine this information to develop several of their in-services. They also put together a presentation for staff about the wellness activities they had learned about relative to productive aging. In putting together their in-service presentations, however, they neglected to provide reference citations to the content they shared or otherwise credit the conference presenters.

If Lisa and Peter downloaded mental health slides from the conference Web site and presented this information to staff as if they had been in attendance, was this a violation of the ethical principle of Veracity? If yes, what subprinciples are applicable? Also, did the fact that their presentation materials did not provide full attributions to their sources constitute an ethics violation?

CONCLUSION

Occupational therapy students and practitioners have an obligation to be truthful when they present information to their clients, organizations, agencies, and the public. Veracity is an ethical principle that helps occupational therapy practitioners focus on the ongoing importance of candor in their written and oral communications to fulfill their public duty of truthful communication, be honest in documentation, and ensure that attributions are accurate.

REFERENCES

Accreditation Council for Occupational Therapy Education. (2012). 2011 Accrediataion Council for Occupational Therapy Education (ACOTE®) standards. *American Journal of Occupational Therapy,* 66(6 Suppl.), S6–S74. doi: 10.5014/ajot.2012.66S6

American Medical Association. (n.d.). *Ethics timeline: 1847–1940*. Retrieved from www.ama-assn.org/ama/pub/physician-resources/medical-ethics/code-medical-ethics/history-ama-ethics/ethics-timeline-1847-1940.page

American Occupational Therapy Association. (2010). Occupational therapy code of ethics and ethics standards (2010). *American Journal of Occupational Therapy, 64*(6 Suppl.), S17–S26. doi: 10.5014/ajot.2010.64S17

Ashe, A. M. (2011). Avoiding plagiarism in the electronic age. In D. Y. Slater (Ed.), *Reference guide to the Occupational Therapy Code of Ethics and Ethics Standards* (2010 ed., pp. 219–222). Bethesda, MD: AOTA Press.

Austin, D. (2006). Ethical considerations when occupational therapists engage in business transactions with clients. In D. Y. Slater (Ed.), *Reference guide to the Occupational Therapy Code of Ethics and Ethics Standards* (2010 ed., pp. 135–139). Bethesda, MD: AOTA Press.

Beauchamp, T. L., & Childress, J. F. (2009). *Principles of biomedical ethics* (6th ed.). New York: Oxford University Press.

Bennett-Woods, D. (2005). *Ethics at a glance: Veracity*. Denver: Regis University. Retrieved from http://rhchp.regis.edu/HCE/EthicsAtAGlance/Veracity/Veracity.pdf

Cabot, R. C. (1915). *Social service and the art of healing*. New York: Moffat, Yard.

General Medical Council. (2010, May 24). *Determination on serious professional misconduct (SPM) and sanction*. Retrieved from www.gmc-uk.org/wakefield_SPM_and_Sanction.pdf_32595267.pdf

Godlee, F., & Smith, J. (2011). Wakefield's article linking MMR vaccine and autism was fraudulent. *British Medical Journal, 342*, c7452.

Kornblau, B. L. (2000). Plagiarism. In D. Y. Slater (Ed.), *Reference guide to the Occupational Therapy Code of Ethics and Ethics Standards* (2010 ed., pp. 205–208). Bethesda, MD: AOTA Press.

Medicare.gov. (n.d.). *Fraud and abuse*. Retrieved from www.medicare.gov/navigation/help-and-support/fraud-and-abuse/fraud-and-abuse-overview.aspx

National Board for Certification in Occupational Therapy. (2011). *NBCOT candidate/certificant code of conduct*. Retrieved from www.nbcot.org/pdf/Candidate-Certificant-Code-of-Conduct.pdf?phpMyAdmin=3710605fd34365e380b9ab41a5078545

Purtilo, R. (2011, April). *A conversation about moral courage*. Lecture presented at the AOTA Annual Conference & Expo, Philadelphia.

Scott, J. B. (2009). Consultation. In E. B. Crepeau, E. S. Cohn, & B. A. B. Schell (Eds.), *Willard and Spackman's occupational therapy* (11th ed., pp. 964–972). Philadelphia: Lippincott Williams & Wilkins.

Wakefield, A. J., Murch, S. H., Anthony, A., Linnell, J., Casson, D. M., Milik, M., . . . Walker-Smith, J. A. (1998). Ileal-lymphoid-nodular hyperplasia, non-specific colitis, and pervasive developmental disorder in children. *Lancet, 351*, 637–641.

Principle 7: Fidelity

9

S. Maggie Reitz, PhD, OTR/L, FAOTA

FIDELITY

Principle 7. Occupational therapy personnel shall treat colleagues and other professionals with respect, fairness, discretion, and integrity.

The principle of fidelity comes from the Latin root *fidelis* meaning loyal. *Fidelity* refers to being faithful, which includes obligations of loyalty and the keeping of promises and commitments (Veatch & Flack, 1997). In the health professions, fidelity refers to maintaining good-faith relationships between various service providers and recipients. While respecting fidelity requires occupational therapy personnel to meet the client's reasonable expectations (Purtilo, 2005), Principle 7 specifically addresses fidelity as it relates to maintaining collegial and organizational relationships. Professional relationships are greatly influenced by the complexity of the environment in which occupational therapy personnel work. Practitioners, educators, and researchers alike must consistently balance their duties to service recipients, students, research participants, and other professionals as well as to organizations that may influence decision making and professional practice.

OCCUPATIONAL THERAPY PERSONNEL SHALL

A. Respect the traditions, practices, competencies, and responsibilities of their own and other professions, as well as those of the institutions and agencies that constitute the working environment.
B. Preserve, respect, and safeguard private information about employees, colleagues, and students unless otherwise mandated by national, state, or local laws or permission to disclose is given by the individual.
C. Take adequate measures to discourage, prevent, expose, and correct any breaches of the Code and Ethics Standards, and report any breaches of the former to the appropriate authorities.
D. Attempt to resolve perceived institutional violations of the Code and Ethics Standards by utilizing internal resources first.
E. Avoid conflicts of interest or conflicts of commitment in employment, volunteer roles, or research.

F. Avoid using one's position (employee or volunteer) or knowledge gained from that position in such a manner that gives rise to real or perceived conflict of interest among the person, the employer, other Association members, and/or other organizations.

G. Use conflict resolution and/or alternative dispute resolution resources to resolve organizational and interpersonal conflicts.

H. Be diligent stewards of human, financial, and material resources of their employers, and refrain from exploiting these resources for personal gain.

Source. From the *Occupational Therapy Code of Ethics and Ethics Standards (2010)* (American Occupational Therapy Association, 2010, pp. S24–S25).

Fidelity has been defined as the "faithful fulfillment of vows, promises, and agreements and discharge of fiduciary responsibilities" (Slater, 2011, p. 226). Principle 7, Fidelity, of the *Occupational Therapy Code of Ethics and Ethics Standards (2010)* (referred to as the "Code and Ethics Standards"; American Occupational Therapy Association [AOTA], 2010) focuses on professional relationships and faithfulness and loyalty within these relationships. *Professional relationships* include those with clients, colleagues across the institution, employers, and institution administrators (AOTA, 2010; Purtilo & Doherty, 2011).

In discussions of fidelity, the term *fiduciary* often appears. *Fiduciary* refers to a person—in our profession, an occupational therapy practitioner—who is

> often in a position of authority, who obligates himself or herself to act on the behalf of another (as in managing money or property) and assumes a duty to act in good faith and with care, candor, and loyalty in fulfilling the obligation. (Slater, 2011, p. 226)

In ways beyond merely managing physical objects or money, occupational therapy practitioners are obligated to clients, students, peers, employers, and employees, as well as fellow board members and fellow volunteers on professional committees or commissions or in other groups. We are obligated to their care and the fulfillment of their *occupational potential,* defined by Wilcock (2006) as the "future capability to engage in occupation toward needs, goals, and dreams for health,

material requirement, happiness, and well being" (p. 343).

Although occupational therapy practitioners are obligated to their clients as well as their colleagues and students, the focus of Principle 7 is on the importance of maintaining and nurturing professional relationships to facilitate the ultimate goal of enhanced client care. Professional behaviors related to the principle of Fidelity can be categorized as respect (Principles 7A and 7B), prevention and analysis of potential ethical breaches (Principles 7C, 7D, and 7G), prevention of possible conflicts (Principles 7E and 7F), and stewardship of resources (Principle 7H).

When examining any ethical issue, it is important to review all principles and then weigh the possible conflicting values before taking action. Within the principle of fidelity, balance also is stressed; occupational therapy practitioners have a duty to balance loyalty to clients with loyalty to colleagues, employers, and institutions. (The importance of finding the appropriate balance is discussed further in Chapter 20 of this volume.)

HISTORY OF FIDELITY IN OCCUPATIONAL THERAPY

The focus of the ethical principles articulated by the profession at its founding was on the provision of ethical and competent care, not professional relationships. The profession addressed the value and importance of professional relationships at a later date. The spirit of the current Principle 7 first appeared in *Principles of Occu-*

pational Therapy Ethics (AOTA, 1978) under two separate principles:

IV. Related to Intra-professional Colleagues

The occupational therapist shall function with discretion and integrity in relations with other members of the profession and shall be concerned with the quality of their services. Upon becoming aware of objective evidence of a breach of ethics or substandard service the occupational therapist shall take action according to established procedure.

V. Related to Other Personnel

The occupational therapist shall function with discretion and integrity in relations with personnel and cooperates with them as may be appropriate. Similarly, the occupational therapist expects others to demonstrate a high level of competence. Upon becoming aware of objective evidence of a breach of ethics or substandard service the occupational therapist shall take action according to established procedure (p. 710).

When the principles were organized into the *Occupational Therapy Code of Ethics* in 1988, only one of these two principles remained: Principle 5, which was renamed "Professional Relationships" (AOTA, 1988). Six years later, when the *Code of Ethics* was again revised, the term *fidelity* first appeared in Principle 6 (AOTA, 1994, p. 1038): "Occupational therapy personnel shall treat colleagues and other professionals with fairness, discretion, and integrity (fidelity, veracity)." In the 2000 revision of the *Code of Ethics*, *veracity* and *fidelity* were separated into two distinct principles. Principle 6 focused on truthfulness, whereas Principle 7 primarily addressed fidelity; the wording of the principle remained the same except for the removal of *veracity* (AOTA, 2000). In the 2005 revision, the word *respect* was added to Principle 7, and that wording remains in effect in the current *Code and Ethics Standards*: "Occupational therapy personnel shall treat colleagues and other professionals with respect, fairness, discretion, and integrity" (AOTA, 2010, p. S24).

RESPECT

Calls for *civility*, an outward display of respect, have been increasing in recent times in business, politics, education, and health care and within communities. The American Medical Association (2011) recently announced that about 20% of graduating medical students reported being mistreated and that the association would take action to lower this figure. The most frequent type of mistreatment medical students reported was humiliation and belittlement by faculty, residents, and fellow students. Respect is the topic of Vignette 9.1, which takes place in an occupational therapy education classroom, and Vignette 9.2, which unfolds in an academic setting. Situations similar to those described in these vignettes could easily occur in other practice settings.

VIGNETTE 9.1. SHOWING RESPECT

Carmen was excited about starting her first faculty position. The semester was going well, and she felt well prepared to share her expertise with her students. A few weeks later, however, she became concerned when a student, **Mary**, started leaving the class for 10-minute intervals on a regular basis. Carmen thought this unusual and was concerned about Mary's inability to remain seated for the 50-minute lectures. She also was concerned because Mary's frequent departures caused Carmen to lose her focus and also disrupted the other students' attention. Carmen could tell by observing their nonverbal communication, including unprofessional behaviors such as rolling their eyes and making sidebar comments, that the rest of the class were frustrated by Mary's behavior. Carmen knew she needed to take action before the situation further deteriorated, but she was unsure what to do.

After class, Carmen scheduled a meeting to discuss the situation with the program director, **Kurt**. At the meeting, they both agreed that Mary's and the other students' behaviors were disrespectful but that Mary's behavior should be addressed first. Carmen e-mailed Mary and asked her to meet before class. Carmen told Mary that her behavior of frequently leaving class was disruptive and disrespectful to both the class and to her as the professor. Mary was mortified and said that she had not realized the impact of her behavior on others and that she was not intentionally being disrespectful. Using the problem-solving and activity analysis skills she was learning, Mary determined that she needed to wake up earlier so she had time to find a parking spot and visit the restroom before class. Mary thanked Carmen for bringing this to her attention and asked if she could apologize to the class. Carmen agreed, and they went to class together.

VIGNETTE 9.2. PROMOTING A CLIMATE OF CIVILITY

Amanda was a graduate assistant for **Dr. Howell**. She was working on a literature review for a project of Dr. Howell's and had a question. Amanda approached the faculty office hallway and overheard Dr. Howell and another faculty member talking about a third faculty member in very disparaging terms. Amanda coughed to alert them to her presence, but after acknowledging her presence they continued their conversation in a similar manner. She then returned to the graduate assistant office and sat there feeling awkward, wondering what she should do.

In the days that followed, Amanda was frozen in nonaction and felt ill and sick to her stomach. She started missing classes, calling in sick, and missing work hours with Dr. Howell. Dr. Howell became frustrated because she was working on a deadline for a complex grant application, and she fired Amanda. Amanda considered warning Dr. Howell's newly hired graduate assistant about the inappropriate behavior of the faculty. Amanda was concerned, however, that this behavior, like Dr. Howell's, would be disrespectful, so she abandoned that plan.

Instead, Amanda sought out the program director, **Dr. Casey**, and reported her observations and her concern that if she reported Dr. Howell's behavior, it might appear to be in retaliation for being fired. Although not excusing Dr. Howell's behavior, Dr. Casey shared that the faculty were under a great deal of stress because of statewide budget cuts and that she was planning to address the level of stress and adaptive versus maladaptive coping strategies at the next faculty meeting. Dr. Casey also reminded Amanda that if she saw a repeat of Dr. Howell's behavior, she should be prepared to address her concerns directly with Dr. Howell. Dr. Casey offered to

mentor Amanda on how to approach Dr. Howell if this situation was to recur.

Dr. Casey followed through with her plan to discuss adaptive stress reduction techniques at the faculty meeting and reminded faculty about the importance of role modeling professional behavior and collegiality. Which principles are supported by this action? Does this action violate any of the principles? What other actions could or should Dr. Casey take?

PREVENTION AND ANALYSIS OF POTENTIAL ETHICAL BREACHES

The need to be vigilant in identifying potential ethical issues and to prevent breaches if at all possible is one of the themes woven throughout Principle 7. If an ethical breach cannot be prevented, occupational therapy practitioners need to take steps to resolve the issue directly without escalating the issue to other levels unless necessary. Sometimes the behavior warrants the involvement of other entities, however. Vigilance is required to see and address unethical behaviors before they become entrenched in individuals or organizations. Addressing potential unethical behavior can be challenging and uncomfortable but is the necessary and preferred action because it can prevent harm to clients, coworkers, the institution, and profession. An example of how an occupational therapist identified a potential problem and addressed it without escalation is provided in Case Study 9.1.

CASE STUDY 9.1. ANALYZING AND PREVENTING A POTENTIAL ETHICS BREACH

Noemi, the occupational therapy supervisor at a skilled nursing facility, was excited to learn that **Bonnie**, one of the occupational therapy staff, was presenting at the state association conference. Noemi arrived early to the session to be sure to get a good seat and wish Bonnie well, but Bonnie was not in the room. As time passed, Noemi double-checked her conference schedule to make sure she was in the correct room. Finally, Bonnie arrived. Noemi overheard someone in the audience say, "Oh, the presenter was in that group having so much fun in the bar last night with that guy **Don**. I could never drink before presenting; I would wait to celebrate after I had presented! If she partied that hard last night, I wonder what she will do tonight?"

When it was time for Bonnie to begin her presentation, she dropped her notes, became flustered, and stated, "I wish someone would bring me a drink to settle my nerves." She continued with the presentation, frequently apologizing for not being prepared. After the presentation was over, Noemi waited for the other audience participants to leave and approached Bonnie. Bonnie said, "I am glad that's over; let's go get drinks." Noemi agreed to go with Bonnie but said that she wanted to talk to her about her presentation. Although Noemi was worried about the health and well-being of Bonnie, she also was concerned for the reputation of her staff and facility.

Once they were seated, Noemi asked Bonnie some open-ended questions to have Bonnie reflect on her performance. As the conversation unfolded, Bonnie told of unexpectedly meeting a group of occupational therapy school alums the night before and losing track of time as she enjoyed the impromptu reunion and reconnected with Don, an "old flame." Noemi then shared the comment she had heard before the presentation started about Bonnie's behavior at the bar. Bonnie was embarrassed and declined a second drink offer from the server, saying she needed to get home.

When Noemi returned to work the following week, she reviewed the Code and Ethics Standards, particularly Principle 2, Nonmaleficence; Principle 5, Procedural Justice; and Principle 7, Fidelity. She was concerned that Bonnie might have an evolving substance abuse problem or other personal issues that could affect both client care and Bonnie's own well-being. Noemi reviewed the time records and productivity measures for all five occupational therapists who reported to her. She discovered that Bonnie had a pattern of arriving late to work most Fridays.

When Noemi met with Bonnie, Bonnie at first was angry and wanted to know why she was being picked on. Noemi explained that she had reviewed the records of all five therapists. Bonnie then admitted that she regularly went to a happy hour on Thursday nights at a bar that was a favorite among out-of-town young businessmen. The happy hours and related socialization kept her up quite late. The

businessmen only had to fly home the next day, but Bonnie had to wake up early and go to work. Noemi was sympathetic about Bonnie wanting a social life; however, Noemi told Bonnie that her attendance pattern had to be modified if she wanted to keep her job. In addition, she provided Bonnie with materials from human resources about their employee assistance program.

The following Friday, Bonnie reported to work early, brought Noemi her favorite muffin, and thanked her for taking the time to address the issue before it escalated further. If Bonnie's behavior had continued and adversely affected client care, Noemi had been prepared to report Bonnie to the appropriate institution officials and, if needed, the appropriate professional regulatory bodies. Soon thereafter, Noemi was relieved to see that Bonnie was making adjustments to ensure that her personal lifestyle did not affect her punctuality and job performance.

PREVENTION OF POSSIBLE CONFLICTS

Although open communication and transparency can assist in preventing conflicts, not all conflicts can or should be prevented. For example, failure to confront an individual or group regarding unethical behavior because of fear of a potential conflict is a violation of the Code and Ethics Standards, specifically Principles 5B, 5D, 5L, 6E, 6H, and 7C. If the potential for a conflict is known, however, occupational therapy practitioners can take steps to resolve it quickly before the conflict has a chance to expand and take important time away from other institutional priorities. (Avoidance of conflicts of interest and commitment were discussed in Chapter 4 on nonmaleficence; see Vignettes 4.4 and 4.6.) In Case Study 9.2, an occupational therapist deals with conflict provoked by a lack of transparency.

CASE STUDY 9.2. PREVENTING CONFLICT BY PROMOTING TRANSPARENCY

Candace was a 30-year-old computer programmer with chronic schizophrenia. Following an acute episode of psychosis and subsequent hospitalization, Candace lost her job. When she got out of the hospital, she joined a local clubhouse to ease back into community responsibilities and find a new job. There she met **Eleanor**, a clubhouse staff member, who provided her with an orientation to the clubhouse model and a tour of the facility. At the end of the orientation, Eleanor asked Candace how she had learned about the program and whether she had any questions. Candace explained that her inpatient occupational therapist had recommended the clubhouse. She also said that she had been very reluctant to join the clubhouse but that the occupational therapist had convinced her to join by telling her that she could get paid for duties such as assisting with upgrading the computers at the facility and that they would find her a permanent full-time job. Eleanor had to inform Candace that it was not possible for the clubhouse to pay members for their duties at the facility; however, she also explained that they could train her and find her a temporary position, but it was up to Candace to find permanent employment for herself with the support of clubhouse staff.

Eleanor was familiar with many of the occupational therapists at the hospital where Candace disclosed she had been admitted, so Eleanor decided to call and make sure the hospital staff had accurate information about the clubhouse model and available services. She spoke with **Hannah**, the director of the occupational therapy department, which provided services to clients with both mental illness and physical dysfunctions. Hannah explained that sometimes they chose to misinform clients or exaggerate what the clubhouse offered to get people to become members. In the course of the conversation, it became apparent that Hannah, who specialized in stroke rehabilitation, did not have much concern for or knowledge about the importance of transitional mental health services. When Eleanor suggested to the director that exaggerating the services offered at the clubhouse might raise ethical concerns, Hannah became very defensive and stated that she was more experienced and had a more advanced degree than Eleanor. She told Eleanor to "forget the whole thing."

Eleanor had followed the guidance of Principle 7 and had attempted to handle the situation locally without escalating the situation and involving more people than needed. Hannah, however, chose to be confrontational and obstructive. Instead of forgetting about the whole thing, as Hannah had directed, Eleanor reflected on the options available to her to

ensure that clients were told the truth about the clubhouse and the available services while minimizing potential conflict, if possible. After a period of reflection and review of the Code and Ethics Standards, Eleanor considered her options. The potential actions and an analysis of the pros and cons of each appear in Table 9.1. *(Case study developed by Stacey Harcum, MS, OTR/L, CBIS)*

STEWARDSHIP OF RESOURCES

Occupational therapy personnel in supervisory positions are stewards of a variety of resources, including equipment, supplies, and time. The largest expense in an occupational therapy department budget is usually salaries. Occupational therapy practitioners and their supervisors must be ethical in their time use because this is a valuable (and therefore expensive) resource. Depending on the circumstances, misuse of time may constitute merely inefficiency, or it may constitute fraud.

Social interaction among team members while on the job is essential to team building and collaboration. Occupational therapy practitioners need to network and spend time communicating with colleagues both within and external to the department. They are obligated, however, to ensure that this networking supports both collegiality and client care. Frequent socialization at the expense of the performance of other job duties or persistent use of work time to perform personal life tasks is inappropriate and unethical. An incident involving the fraudulent use of time by an employee is detailed in Vignette 9.3.

VIGNETTE 9.3. ADDRESSING MISUSE OF RESOURCES

Ralph, an occupational therapy supervisor for the past 5 years, was proud of his department's productivity and ability to positively influence clients' lives. **Miranda**, a head nurse, stopped him in the hall one day and asked to speak to him. He was surprised when she reported that the new graduate they had just hired, **Tim**, was playing online poker and flirting at the nursing station. Although Ralph was aware

TABLE 9.1
Decision Table for Case Study 9.1: Conflicts

Possible Action	Positive Outcomes	Negative Consequences
No action	Eleanor avoids potential conflicts with Hannah and the occupational therapy staff.	Patients continue to be lied to at the hospital. This action does not uphold Principle 7 and also fails to uphold Principles 1, 2, 5, and 6.
Review the memorandum of understanding (MOU) between the clubhouse and the hospital and discuss with Hannah	Eleanor seeks to bring hospital policies into line with ethical practice. Hannah may provide more accurate information to potential clients.	Patients may continue to be lied to at the hospital. Eleanor may cause conflict with Hannah and hospital staff. This action does not uphold Principle 7 and also fails to uphold Principles 1, 2, 5, and 6.
Review current clubhouse marketing materials, both printed and on the Web site, work with clubhouse members to make edits to ensure clarity, and send updated material to Hannah	Eleanor seeks to bring hospital policies into line with ethical practice. Hannah may provide more accurate information to potential clients. This action upholds Principles 3, 4, and 6, especially 6F.	Patients may continue to be lied to at the hospital. This action fails to uphold Principles 1, 2, and 5.
Request a formal meeting with Hannah and a clubhouse member to review the current MOU and to review the updated marketing materials	Eleanor opens an honest dialogue that is client centered. If the meeting is successful, this action upholds all principles.	Hannah could refuse to meet, and this might distress the Clubhouse member. If the meeting is not held, Eleanor fails to uphold Principles 1, 2, 5, 6, and 7. Patients would continue to be lied to at the hospital, resulting in failure to uphold Principles 1, 2, and 5.
Request a meeting with the clubhouse executive board for guidance	Because of the care taken to try other local, direct strategies first, this action upholds Principle 7A. Eleanor's action follows the chain of command at the clubhouse.	Eleanor may cause conflict with other hospital employees. Patients may continue to be lied to at the hospital.
Report Hannah to appropriate regulatory bodies	Eleanor seeks to bring hospital occupational therapy practices into line with the Code and Ethics Standards. Eleanor's action follows the chain of command at her place of employment. This action may encourage the upholding of all principles.	Eleanor may cause conflict with Hannah and other hospital employees.

Note. A variety of possible actions to address this situation and analyses of each are provided in this table; however, other actions or analyses are possible depending on the decision-making model and specific ethics theory or approach used (see Chapter 10, this volume).

that Tim spent a good deal of time networking on the nursing units, he believed this to be a positive behavior. Now he was concerned that Tim's behavior was having a negative impact on clients.

Ralph decided to collect more information because he did not want to confront Tim on the basis of only one person's perception. Unfortunately, the three unit head nurses reported similar behavior. In addition, as Ralph left the office of one of the head nurses, he saw Tim playing a video. Because it was near lunchtime, Ralph asked Tim if he would like to join him for lunch.

Ralph opened the lunchtime discussion by asking Tim how he was balancing the need for productivity with his enjoyment of the social milieu of the hospital. As the discussion unfolded, Tim confirmed that he was having difficulty with that balance. He had been rounding up his documented productivity minutes, as he had seen done while at his Level II fieldwork placement.

Ralph informed Tim that this was unethical behavior, as was his use of work time to play games, and that he would be placed on a more intensive mentoring program. Ralph further explained that charging patients for services not rendered was fraud and could jeopardize both Tim's job and his license. Ralph also informed Tim that he would arrange a meeting with the hospital's accountant and lawyer to determine what corrective actions were needed. Ralph then strongly encouraged Tim to report his actions and planned remediation to the state regulatory board as soon as possible, because it would be in his best interest to self-report his behavior than for Ralph to contact the board.

CONCLUSION

Occupational therapy practitioners are human and, therefore, fallible. Principle 7, Fidelity, encourages practitioners to acknowledge this fact and seek to minimize ethical violations and their repercussions through preventive action. Occupational therapy practitioners need to be proactive and strengthen collegiality to promote the well-being of our clients, colleagues, and employers. By concentrating on developing a positive, respectful climate and instituting other preventive strategies, practitioners can diminish the severity and frequency of unprofessional behaviors. However, if unprofessional behaviors are evidenced and are egregious or frequent, Principle 7 also provides guidance as to the necessary next steps.

REFERENCES

American Medical Association. (2011, August). One in five medical school grads report mistreatment; AMA taking action. *AMA MedEd Update*. Retrieved from www.ama-assn.org/ama/pub/meded/2011-august/ 2011-august.shtml

American Occupational Therapy Association. (1978). Principles of occupational therapy ethics. In H. L. Hopkins & H. D. Smith (Eds.), *Willard and Spackman's occupational therapy* (5th ed., pp. 709–710). Philadelphia: Lippincott.

American Occupational Therapy Association. (1988). Occupational therapy code of ethics. *American Journal of Occupational Therapy, 42,* 795–796. doi: 10.5014/ajot.42.12.795

American Occupational Therapy Association. (1994). Occupational therapy code of ethics. *American Journal of Occupational Therapy, 48,* 1037–1038. doi: 10.5014/ajot.48.11.1037

American Occupational Therapy Association. (2000). Occupational therapy code of ethics. *American Journal of Occupational Therapy, 54,* 614–616. doi: 10.5014/ajot.54.6.614

American Occupational Therapy Association. (2005). Occupational therapy code of ethics (2005). *American Journal of Occupational Therapy, 59,* 639–642. doi: 10.5014/ajot.59.6.639

American Occupational Therapy Association. (2010). Occupational therapy code of ethics and ethics standards (2010). *American Journal of Occupational Therapy, 64*(6 Suppl.), S17–S26. doi: 10.5014/ ajot2010.62S17

Purtilo, R. (2005). *Ethical dimensions in the health professions* (4th ed.). Philadelphia: W.B. Saunders.

Purtilo, R. B., & Doherty, R. F. (2011). *Ethical dimensions in the health professions* (5th ed.). St. Louis, MO: Elsevier Saunders.

Slater, D. L. (Ed.). (2011). Glossary. In *Reference guide to the Occupational Therapy Code of Ethics and Ethics Standards* (pp. 225–227). Bethesda, MD: AOTA Press.

Veatch, R. M., & Flack, H. E. (1997). *Case studies in allied health ethics.* Upper Saddle River, NJ: Prentice Hall.

Wilcock, A. A. (2006). *An occupational perspective of health* (2nd ed.). Thorofare, NJ: Slack.

Part III. Models

Introduction

Janie B. Scott, MA, OT/L, FAOTA

Part I provided readers with an overview of the evolution of the *Occupational Therapy Code of Ethics and Ethics Standards (2010)* (referred to as the "Code and Ethics Standards"; American Occupational Therapy Association [AOTA], 2010) in response to societal changes. In Part II, all of the ethical principles in the Code and Ethics Standards were defined in the context of occupational therapy across various roles and practice settings. In the case studies and vignettes of chapters in Part II, the authors provided strategies to resolve a variety of ethical dilemmas.

Part III introduces ethical decision-making models, drawing on the work of ethics experts and occupational therapy authors. Readers will learn a four-step decision-making process that is synthesized from the work of these authors and that provides a way to explore the ethical dilemmas practitioners face in occupational therapy practice. This four-step model, together with the resources available through their own institutions, AOTA, their state regulatory board, and the National Board for Certification in Occupational Therapy, will help readers address ethical situations in an appropriate manner.

Reference

American Occupational Therapy Association. (2010). Occupational therapy code of ethics and ethics standards (2010). *American Journal of Occupational Therapy, 64*(6 Suppl.), S17–S26. doi: 10.5014/ajot2010.64S17

Solving Ethical Dilemmas

10

Janie B. Scott, MA, OT/L, FAOTA

An *ethical dilemma* is a conflict between two divergent moral challenges that one must resolve in deciding on the proper course of action. Some have defined an *ethical dilemma* as a struggle in deciding between good and evil (Beauchamp & Childress, 2009; Hansen, 1988; Purtilo & Doherty, 2011), but most situations health care practitioners face involve subtler distinctions: "As occupational therapists we face dilemmas in day-to-day practice that may not be as dramatic as those discussed in the media, however, to the individual patients and families involved they are crucial" (Hansen, 1988, p. 279).

When occupational therapy practitioners identify an ethical situation that is difficult to resolve, a decision-making model can help them analyze the situation, determine the appropriate course of action, and reach an equitable solution. A four-step process for use in solving ethical dilemmas is described in this chapter. This process draws from models that reflect both thinking within occupational therapy and perspectives from medicine and nursing.

BACKGROUND

A variety of decision-making models are available in the literature to assist occupational therapy practitioners and other health professionals in resolving ethical dilemmas. The sections that follow briefly examine a selection of the many available models.

Occupational Therapy Ethical Decision-Making Models

Morris (2010) proposed a three-step model for evaluating ethical dilemmas in occupational therapy practice: ascertain whether an ethical dilemma is being faced, analyze possible courses of action to arrive at a proposed course of action, and evaluate the proposed course of action at different levels of moral reasoning (see Figure 10.1). Purtilo and Doherty (2011) identified a six-step model for solving ethical dilemmas:

- Step 1: Gather relevant information.
- Step 2: Identify the type of ethical problem.
- Step 3: Analyze the problem using ethics theories or approaches.
- Step 4: Explore the practical alternatives.
- Step 5: Act.
- Step 6: Evaluate the process and outcome.

Purtilo and Doherty's and Morris's models are similar; both underscore the importance of gathering all relevant data, articulating which ethical issues may apply following a review of ethical principles, defining a plan of action, and evaluating

Am I facing an ethical dilemma?

1. What are the relevant facts, values, and beliefs?

2. Who are the key people involved?

3. State the dilemma clearly.

Analyze

1. What are the possible courses of action?

2. What conflicts could arise from each action?

3. Proposed course of action:

Evaluate

1. Code and Ethics Standards, Level III

2. Social Roles, Level II

3. Self-Interests, Level I

Does your proposed course of action lead to *consensus?* If yes, then proceed. If no, contact the appropriate resource for guidance: AOTA, NBCOT, or your State Regulatory Board.

FIGURE 10.1

Morris's (2003) ethical decision-making model.

Note. AOTA = American Occupational Therapy Association; NBCOT = National Board for Certification in Occupational Therapy.
Source. From "Is It Possible to Be Ethical?" by J. Morris, February 24, 2003, *OT Practice, 8*(4), pp. 18–23. Copyright © 2003 by the American Occupational Therapy Association. Adapted with permission.

the potential outcomes of the plan. Purtilo and Doherty's model, however, includes a final step of evaluating the process and outcomes after action has been taken. This evaluative component can promote the practitioner's competence in solving future ethical dilemmas.

Slater and Bogenrief (2010) presented a framework for ethical decision making (see Box 10.1) that consists of specific questions to help practitioners process situations that contain ethical dilemmas. The additional detail may help some practitioners better understand the full

---

BOX 10.1

Framework for Ethical Decision Making

1. How do I name and frame the problem?
2. Does the problem constitute ethical distress or an ethical dilemma (or something else)? *Ethical distress* exists when the individual knows the appropriate course of action, but institutional rules pose barriers to following what the individual believes to be correct (AOTA, 2007; Purtilo, 2005). An *ethical dilemma* occurs when the occupational therapy practitioner encounters a situation in which there are two or more ethical answers to a question or two or more equally incorrect actions that would violate ethical conduct. The dilemma involves choosing from ethical actions that may be equally similar or dissimilar (AOTA, 2007; Purtilo, 2005). When questions arise that are neither moral nor ethical in nature but are difficult to resolve, it may not have a basis in morality or ethics.
3. Who are the players?
4. What information do I have? What other information do I need?
5. What resources are available to assist me?
6. What are my options, and what are the likely consequences of each?
7. How do I prioritize my moral values?
8. What is the best action for me to take?
9. Which action will I choose?
10. How will I defend my action?
11. When I evaluate and reflect on the outcome, what conclusions can I draw?
12. Will I do it differently next time?

Source. Slater and Bogenrief (2010).

---

context of the dilemma, consider additional options for action, evaluate potential consequences of an action, analyze outcomes, and use the experience to improve future decisions.

Ethical Decision-Making Models From Other Professions

Fairchild (2010) developed an ethical decision-making model to assist nurses in processing ethical dilemmas. The Nurses' Ethical Reasoning Skills (NERS) model includes "reflection (critically reflective consciousness), reasoning (dialectic reasoning), and review of competing values" (Fairchild, 2010, p. 356). The NERS model highlights the importance of using intuition and reflection to support the process of ethical decision making. Fairchild discussed the responsibility nurses have to be moral, particularly in complex health care environments in which there are multiple duties

(e.g., to administration, patient, family). She acknowledged that although caring comes from within the individual practitioner, caring also is expected from leadership and the health delivery system itself. In addition, she noted, practitioners evaluate each situation as a whole, examining the context and the values, motivations, and perspectives of the stakeholders in making decisions or evaluating complex situations. The ultimate outcome of the process is to avoid conflict and open a dialogue to promote understanding between the parties involved.

Hundert (2003) proposed an ethical problem-solving model for use within medicine in response to an identified lack of models available to physicians:

The model . . . attempts to fill this void by developing a conceptual understanding of the nature of moral dilemmas that can be applied to both theoretical and practical problems in medicine. . . . A difficult problem becomes a "dilemma" when we are quite sure that we will be making a big mistake regardless of whatever path we choose. (p. 427)

Hundert's descriptive model involves the following steps:

- Identification of conflicting values (make lists)
- Value balancing—that is, weighting of each value (consider the consequences of actions; weigh legal responsibilities, cultural expectations, and institutional policies; and identify personal vs. professional values)
- Reflective equilibrium (identify alternate actions)
- Review for consistency.

As Hundert noted, decision making provokes anxiety in many people because it involves weighing their own values against competing perspectives (moral principles). His recommendation was to retain lists of conflicting values and decisions and review them to help understand and expand the ethical reasoning processes.

A FOUR-STEP PROCESS FOR ETHICAL DECISION MAKING

Regardless of the specific ethical decision-making model one uses, the process should contain at least four elements: (1) gather the facts, and specify the dilemma; (2) analyze possible courses of action, taking into account both a set of principles and potential consequences; (3) select and implement a course of action; and (4) evaluate the results of the action. It is beneficial to use the same model whenever dilemmas arise; consistent use of one model can help practitioners gain competence and ensure that their decisions are ethical.

Step 1: Gather the Facts, and Specify the Dilemma

The first step is to reflect on the facts of the situation and decide whether they constitute an ethical dilemma as opposed to a misunderstanding, a potential legal issue, or a personnel issue (Morris, 2010). It is useful at this stage to identify the

personal values and beliefs of the key people involved and their bearing on the dilemma. These key people, or stakeholders, could include the client and his or her family members, internal influencers (e.g., supervisor, institutional rules; see Chapter 20, this volume), and external influencers (e.g., third-party payers, state regulatory boards; see Chapter 21, this volume).

It is important to identify the primary, secondary, and tertiary stakeholders and examine their relationships and obligations. The *primary stakeholder* may be a company, agency, or organization around whom the ethical situation pivots. The primary stakeholder is the key figure who is directly affected by the ethical dilemma. *Secondary stakeholders* are close to the situation and indirectly affected. Finally, *tertiary stakeholders* have a distant, external involvement and relationship with the key people involved in the dilemma but potentially can be affected by a decision (McCurtis, 2008).

Step 2: Analyze Possible Courses of Action

Evaluating the facts of a dilemma against existing principles and regulations helps occupational therapy practitioners analyze their options and select the appropriate course of action. In addition to the *Occupational Therapy Code of Ethics and Ethics Standards (2010)* (referred to as the "Code and Ethics Standards"; American Occupational Therapy Association [AOTA], 2010a), practitioners are obligated to abide by federal and state laws, the policies of their employers, and regulations established by state regulatory boards (SRBs) governing practice in their state or jurisdiction. State regulations, national certifications, and organizational policies help guide practitioners in their behaviors, choices, and approaches to ethical decision making (see Chapter 2, this volume). For example, the responsibilities of occupational therapy assistants are dictated by SRB practice acts and the profession's standards of practice. Occupational therapy assistants may contribute to a client's evaluation, but an occupational therapist has the primary responsibility to evaluate clients, interpret the findings, and develop a plan of intervention (AOTA, 2009, 2010b, 2010c). An occupational therapy assistant asked to complete an evaluation, for example, would know that refusing to complete the evaluation is both legally and ethically correct.

Step 3: Select and Implement a Course of Action

Once the best way to resolve the ethical dilemma is clear, the occupational therapy practitioner takes action. For example, he or she may attempt to remediate the problem locally (e.g., through direct communication with the person involved) or file a complaint through the SRB, National Board for Certification in Occupational Therapy (NBCOT), or AOTA (jurisdiction guidelines are provided in Chapter 2, this volume).

The "best" course of action is situation specific; what works in one situation may be ineffective in another. In general, the best course of action may be for the stakeholders to discuss the situation, the issues that are involved, and ways to identify a satisfactory resolution. This step may include the primary stakeholder agreeing to take an ethics course or engage in other remediation activities to reduce the potential of reoccurrences. This strategy is most likely to be effective when no one was harmed and no laws or regulations were broken.

Step 4: Evaluate the Results of the Action

Purtilo and Doherty (2011), Hundert (2003), Morris (2010), and others included a step in their models focusing on the importance of evaluating the conclusions that were drawn at the end of a deliberative process. During reflection, the practitioner should review whether the recommendations made were consistent with ethical standards, laws, and institutional policies; were reached by consensus; and stood the test of time. The final question to be considered is, If disciplinary actions were recommended, were they consistent with action taken previously when similar infractions occurred? In Case Study 10.1, an occupational therapist must disentangle her obligation to safeguard the client's right to privacy from her duty to report a potential danger to the community.

CASE STUDY 10.1. ADDRESSING THE DUTY TO REPORT VS. THE RIGHT TO PRIVACY

Keith was hospitalized following a stroke and received occupational therapy and physical therapy services. Before his stroke, Keith had led an active life working part-time, socializing with friends, providing transportation for family and friends, and maintaining his own apartment. Keith shared with his occupational therapist, **Carolyn**, that he believed he was ready to return to his "old life" and to reestablish familiar routines. Carolyn was committed to supporting Keith's health and participation in familiar and meaningful occupations, a role consistent with that described in AOTA's *Occupational Therapy Practice Framework: Domain and Process* (AOTA, 2008). She and Keith agreed to complete a series of formal and informal assessments to determine his level of occupational performance before he returned to his previous occupations, including driving. These assessments raised concerns about Keith's readiness to return to driving, and Carolyn recommended a comprehensive driving evaluation through a driver rehabilitation program.

Carolyn believed that her primary duty was to Keith, but she was uncertain about her ethical obligation to report her misgivings about his driving to the state motor vehicle administration (MVA), to her employer (who might be liable if Keith caused a car crash following discharge), and to Keith's family. Carolyn used the four-step ethical decision-making process to analyze the situation and determine a course of action.

Step 1: Gather the Facts, and Specify the Dilemma. Keith had had a stroke. Carolyn's assessment revealed possible deficits in Keith's judgment, reaction time, and attention. Carolyn recommended a comprehensive driver evaluation because she believed Keith or the community might be at risk if he returned to driving now, and she also believed that she could collaborate with Keith to enable his return to his prior roles in the community. The key people involved included Keith, Keith's family, Carolyn, her employer, the state medical advisory board, and the community. Carolyn identified her dilemma as the following: Did she have an ethical obligation to inform others about her concerns regarding Keith's ability to drive safely?

Step 2: Analyze Possible Courses of Action. Carolyn considered the following possible actions:

- Inform Keith of the outcome of the formal and informal assessments and reiterate her recommendations.
- Investigate state regulations, Health Insurance Portability and Accountability Act (HIPAA) guidelines, the Code and Ethics Standards, and institutional rules that might relate to this situation. Contact the medical advisory board (MAB) of the MVA regarding their reporting requirements.
- Inform Keith's family of her concerns.
- Do nothing.

Carolyn also considered the potential consequences of these actions. Carolyn might discover that legal, ethical, and policy rules obligated her to report her doubts about Keith's driving. If she fulfilled this obligation, Keith might discontinue his occupational therapy intervention. If Keith failed to obtain a comprehensive driver evaluation, his family might take away his car keys without justifiable evidence. If Carolyn reported Keith, he might claim that she had violated HIPAA provisions (i.e., that Carolyn had no right to discuss the outcome of her evaluations with third parties). Doing nothing, however, had the potential to cause harm and to violate laws and ethical principles.

Carolyn reviewed the Code and Ethics Standards and discovered that the following principles were relevant: Principle 1, Beneficence, especially Principle 1A (refer to specialists solely on the basis of the client's needs); Principle 3, Autonomy and Confidentiality, especially Principles 3A (establish a collaborative relationship with clients and others as appropriate), 3G (respect confidentiality and right to privacy), and 3H (maintain confidentiality of all communications); and Principle 5, Procedural Justice, especially Principles 5A (apply and share the Code of Ethics) and 5B (abide by institutional rules). At the social roles level, Keith's family and friends relied on him to live independently, do errands for others, and give friends rides as needed.

Carolyn's social roles involved her professional membership and identity. She had an obligation to practice occupational therapy ethically and competently. Carolyn also was a member of the same community as Keith and wanted to maintain her reputation. Carolyn's self-interest was focused on her desire to be respected in the workplace and in the community. The outcome of this was important to her for altruistic reasons, for employment security, and as an opportunity to give occupational therapy increased public visibility.

Step 3: Select and Implement a Course of Action. Carolyn contacted her state MVA's MAB. She learned that people with certain conditions (e.g., autism, epilepsy, multiple sclerosis, stroke) must notify the MVA when they have a new occurrence of one of these conditions or when applying for or renewing a driver's license (e.g., Maryland Motor Vehicle Administration, 2012). The MAB receives reports from physicians and health care providers when they treat a patient who has one of the reportable conditions. Carolyn decided to present Keith with the results of the assessments and reiterate her recommendation to obtain the comprehensive driver evaluation. She explained to him that she had ethical and legal responsibilities to act on his and the community's behalf, particularly if he did not follow her recommendations. Carolyn revealed the outcome of her research with the MVA, which created an obligation for her to report her concerns to the state for their action. She also reinforced that following through with the driver assessment did not necessarily mean that he would have to retire from driving. Carolyn let Keith know that assessment and intervention might result in several years of continued driving, continuation of his role as driver for his friends, and reassurance to his family of his confirmed safe driver status.

Step 4: Evaluate the Results of the Action. At the conclusion of this analytical process, Carolyn was confident that her proposed course of action was ethical and in compliance with state regulations. She provided Keith, the primary stakeholder, encouragement to act on his own behalf in a way that would ensure that he and the community would be safe and that he would maintain his roles with family and friends. Reaching a collaborative decision with Keith to have the driver evaluation enabled Carolyn to stay within ethical guidelines, state MVA requirements, and federal HIPAA regulations.

Case Study 10.2 describes the conflict between the duty to maintain appropriate professional boundaries and the desire to avoid harming the client.

CASE STUDY 10.2. PROTECTING PROFESSIONAL BOUNDARIES

Diego was an occupational therapy assistant employed at a rural community hospital. His primary responsibility was service delivery to an inpatient rehabilitation population. Diego was occasionally asked to work with outpatient clients when there were staff shortages. Diego enjoyed the opportunity to work in both areas because he was able to work with clients over a longer period of time and observe their progress.

One client with whom Diego was familiar was **Petra**, who had been treated for a brain injury. She had been a client on both the inpatient and the outpatient physical rehabilitation caseloads and later for depression on the behavioral health unit. Diego had implemented the intervention plan for Petra in both settings. Because he had worked with Petra for so long, they usually chatted when they saw each other. Diego shared some of his personal history with Petra, part of which he considered to be a therapeutic use of self. He tried to stay within the boundaries of professional behavior.

Diego terminated his employment with the community hospital and began to work at an outpatient rehabilitation facility nearby. Before leaving the hospital, Diego said good-bye to the clients and staff with whom he was most familiar, including Petra, and wished them well. After he left, to his surprise Petra stopped by his new job to say hello on several occasions. Diego attempted to handle the situation by professionally greeting Petra and letting her know that his new job kept him busy. Shortly thereafter, however, Petra began calling and driving by Diego's house. The phone calls disturbed Diego's spouse. Petra also had left a note for Diego on his front door and tried to reach him through social media.

He did not want to be friends with Petra and was uncertain how to appropriately end contact with her without hurting her feelings. His spouse grew concerned about his safety and urged him to take action, but he had difficulty deciding whether this was a personal, professional (ethical), or legal situation. He decided to take the time to use the four-step ethical decision-making process to determine his next steps.

Step 1. Gather the Facts, and Specify the Dilemma. Petra was visiting Diego's place of employment and contacting him at home. Diego valued his privacy. He also valued equality and wanted to treat Petra and himself fairly. Diego had an obligation to adhere to applicable laws and regulations that governed his practice. Finally, he did not want to act precipitously and violate Petra's dignity. The key people involved were Diego, Petra, Diego's employer, and Diego's family.

Diego's dilemma was as follows: Did Diego owe Petra a duty to protect her from disappointment, which might exacerbate her behavioral health condition, by taking assertive steps to get her to stop visiting him at home and work without invitation?

Step 2. Analyze Possible Courses of Action. Diego considered the following courses of action:

- Tell Petra again verbally and in writing to cease contacting him.
- Contact his new supervisor at work for guidance because Petra's visits were disruptive at his place of employment.
- Consult the Code and Ethics Standards to see whether ethical principles apply to his situation.
- Contact the local police and report his concerns that Petra was stalking him.
- Do nothing and hope Petra would get bored or find another love interest.

Diego also considered the potential consequences of these actions. Petra might not understand Diego's intention and might feel that he was harassing her. Diego's supervisor might say that because Petra is not one of their clients, Diego needs to take care of this problem himself quickly or his probation status might be jeopardized. Diego reviewed the Code and Ethics Standards to attempt to clarify whether under these values and guidelines he owed a duty to Petra since she was no longer his client.

Step 3: Select and Implement a Course of Action. The next time Diego saw Petra, he told her directly that they no longer had a therapeutic relationship and that he did not want to be her friend. He also stated clearly that if she did not stop contacting him, he would contact the police and obtain a restraining order.

What values and principles apply to this situation? How might Diego's social roles be affected by his actions? Whose self-interests are being served? Does the proposed course of action lead to consensus? If not, what resource is most appropriate to contact for guidance (AOTA, NBCOT, or SRB)?

In Case Study 10.3, occupational therapy practitioners must take immediate steps to rectify an ethics breach involving competence. Questions are provided to prompt readers to analyze the ethical dilemmas themselves.

CASE STUDY 10.3. TAKING RESPONSIBILITY FOR ENSURING COMPETENCE

Diane was a registered occupational therapist with 3 years of experience in hospital-based physical rehabilitation. The census at the hospital had decreased in the past year because of downsizing in local industries. Diane's position changed from full-time to part-time. To supplement her income, she began working in an outpatient clinic.

When Diane first accepted the position at the outpatient clinic, she was unaware that many of the clients needed hand therapy. During a typical session with a client requiring hand therapy, Diane used electrical and superficial (e.g., hot packs) physical agent modalities (PAMs). During a weekly supervision meeting, Diane asked whether the clinic would pay for her to take classes so she could learn the proper administration of PAMs. **Jayne**, Diane's supervisor, was shocked to learn that Diane hadn't already taken these courses as required by the SRB. She told Diane to see no more hand clients until she had taken the appropriate courses and had the required supervision in place.

Jayne reflected on her conversation with Diane and felt conflicted about whether further action was appropriate and necessary. Fortunately, no one had been injured by Diane's use of PAMs; however, the potential for injury had existed. Was educating Diane about the licensure requirements regarding PAMs enough? Because Diane was an AOTA member, possessed current certification through NBCOT, and was licensed through the SRB, did Jayne have an obligation to report her discovery to the organizations and to the SRB? Moreover, did Jayne have an obligation to verify Diane's competence in the use of PAMs before assigning her to see hand clients? If yes, what is the appropriate course of action for her to take?

Use the first two steps of the four-step decision-making process to help Jayne determine her possible courses of action. Review Figure 2.2 to establish jurisdiction for this case. After you have completed this analysis, decide which course of action you would select.

CONCLUSION

A variety of approaches to solving ethical dilemmas are available to occupational therapy practitioners using models that have been proposed within occupational therapy, medicine, and nursing. These models, and the four-step process discussed in this chapter, can help practitioners analyze ethical dilemmas to find the solution that best matches the context.

Some ethical dilemmas are easy and straightforward to resolve. Others, however, involve reflection, research, and thoughtful analysis. Practitioners should remember that in difficult situations, resources are available through the SRB, AOTA, and NBCOT. For dilemmas that cannot be solved on the local or direct level, these organizations and agencies function as stakeholders to protect the professional and the public.

The question "Is it possible to be ethical?" (Morris, 2010) has no easy answer. Each ethical dilemma is unique; the people, stakeholders, and nuances differ from case to case. With this in mind, consistent use of a decision-making model will help occupational therapy practitioners identify potential courses of action. There are no black-and-white answers to most ethical dilemmas, but with patience, research, and objectivity, occupational therapy practitioners will successfully solve their difficult ethical questions.

REFERENCES

American Occupational Therapy Association. (2007). *Everyday ethics: Core knowledge for occupational therapy practitioners and educators.* Bethesda, MD: AOTA Press.

American Occupational Therapy Association. (2008). Occupational therapy practice framework: Domain and process (2nd ed.). *American Journal of Occupational Therapy, 62,* 625–683. doi: 10.5014/ajot.62.6.625

American Occupational Therapy Association. (2009). Guidelines for supervision, roles, and responsibilities during the delivery of occupational therapy services. *American Journal of Occupational Therapy, 63,* 797–803. doi: 10.5014/ajot.63.6.797

American Occupational Therapy Association. (2010a). Occupational therapy code of ethics and ethics standards (2010). *American Journal of Occupational Therapy, 64*(6 Suppl.), S17–S26. doi: 10.5014/ajot.2010.64S17

American Occupational Therapy Association. (2010b). Scope of practice. *American Journal of Occupational Therapy, 64*(6 Suppl.), S70–S77. doi: 10.5014/ajot.2010.64S70

American Occupational Therapy Association. (2010c). Standards of practice for occupational therapy. *American Journal of Occupational Therapy, 64* (6 Suppl.), S106–S111. doi: 10.5014/ajot.2010.64S106

Beauchamp, T. L., & Childress, J. F. (2009). *Principles of biomedical ethics* (6th ed.). New York: Oxford University Press.

Fairchild, R. M. (2010). Practical ethical theory for nurses responding to complexity in care. *Nursing Ethics, 17,* 353–362.

Hansen, R. A. (1988). Nationally speaking: Ethics is the issue. *American Journal of Occupational Therapy, 42,* 279–281. doi: 10.5014/ajot.42.5.279

Health Insurance Portability and Accountability Act of 1996, Pub. L. 104–191 110 Stat. 1936.

Hundert, E. M. (2003). A model for ethical problem solving in medicine, with practical applications. *Focus, 1,* 427–435.

Maryland Motor Vehicle Administration. (2012). *MVA's Medical Advisory Board.* Retrieved from www.mva.maryland.gov/Driver-Safety/Older/mva-medical-advisory-board.htm#reasons-for-referrals-medical-advisory-board-review

McCurtis, B. (2008). *Primary, secondary, tertiary stakeholders . . . Oh my!* Retrieved from www.stakeholderguide.com/?p=261

Morris, J. F. (2010). Is it possible to be ethical? In D. Y. Slater (Ed.), *Reference guide to the Occupational Therapy Code of Ethics and Ethics Standards* (2010 ed., pp. 73–80). Bethesda, MD: AOTA Press.

Purtilo, R. B. (2005). *Ethical dimensions in the health professions.* St. Louis, MO: Elsevier.

Purtilo, R., & Doherty, R. F. (2011). *Ethical dimensions in the health professions* (5th ed.). St. Louis, MO: Elsevier.

Slater, D. Y., & Bogenrief, J. (2010, April). *Doing the right thing: Ethical and legal practice.* Presentation at the AOTA Annual Conference & Expo, Orlando, FL.

Part IV.
Applications

Introduction

Janie B. Scott, MA, OT/L, FAOTA, and S. Maggie Reitz, PhD, OTR/L, FAOTA

The chapters in Part IV each focus on a specific area of practice. Chapters 11 through 16 address the American Occupational Therapy Association's (AOTA's) six *Centennial Vision* themes: mental health; productive aging; children and youth; health promotion and wellness; work and industry; and participation, disability, and rehabilitation (AOTA, 2007). In addition, Chapter 17 addresses ethics in administration and private practice, Chapter 18 ethics in higher education, and Chapter 19 ethics in occupational therapy research, and Chapters 20 and 21 discuss ethical issues in internal (within-institution) and external (between-institution) relationships.

When reviewing the case studies and vignettes in Part IV and addressing their own ethical dilemmas, readers are encouraged to remember and use their knowledge base as occupational therapy practitioners. Occupational therapy practitioners' and students' academic knowledge of activity analysis, human performance, and the other elements of competent practice provides them with the skills and ability to analyze and solve ethical dilemmas. After examining the variety of situations and different ways to approach dilemma resolution presented in Part IV, readers will increase their confidence in their own ability to personally take action, when necessary, for the good of the client and the profession.

Reference

American Occupational Therapy Association. (2007). AOTA's *Centennial Vision* and executive summary. *American Journal of Occupational Therapy, 61,* 613–614. doi: 10.5014/ajot.61.6.613

Ethics in Diverse Mental Health Settings

11

*Susan Haiman, MPS, OTR/L, FAOTA, and
Deborah Yarett Slater, MS, OT/L, FAOTA*

The practice of psychiatry and treatment standards for people with mental illness have evolved considerably over the past 50 years. Within the world of mental health and mental illness, occupational therapy practitioners have faced many challenges both to keep current with innovations and to take leadership roles in creating change. As practitioners have faced evolving models of care, they have confronted new ethical questions. Consider the following examples. In 1970, people admitted for treatment to a university medical center noted for its excellence might be taken off all medication for several weeks to "see how they looked" before a regimen of new medication was begun. The result was that many people lost control, were taken forcefully to a seclusion room, and were medicated against their will. Then occupational therapy practitioners were asked to enter the seclusion room to do art with highly agitated clients, confronting the practitioners with a potential ethical challenge: How were they to respond when asked to participate in interventions that they had a professional obligation to provide to benefit the client but that also could result in injury to themselves or property?

In the same era, it was not unusual for clients to be encouraged to "talk their way" through depression before being prescribed antidepressant medication. Participation in occupation was be-

lieved to be the best way to motivate clients to reach beyond their depression, and practitioners of all disciplines would forcefully "encourage" them to get out of bed to attend these sessions. At the time, this was standard intervention. Yet with current knowledge about the biological basis of illnesses and professional commitment to client-centered practice, would this be considered ethical practice today (or even legal, given the potential for coercion and the client's right to refuse intervention)?

In this chapter, we review the current state of occupational therapy practice with people who have been diagnosed with mental illness and in settings where mental health services are routinely provided. We then examine common ethical dilemmas and issues that have occurred in the recent past as paradigm shifts have occurred across mental health service delivery models.

MENTAL HEALTH PRACTICE TODAY

Since the era of deinstitutionalization of clients, the percentage of mental health practitioners nationwide has continued to shrink, as have the financial resources allocated for therapy services and the number of beds on inpatient units (Treatment Advocacy Center, 2009). There are many reasons for this shift, not the least of which is the upheaval of the 1990s health care "revolution" during which the number of for-profit hospitals and health maintenance organizations rose. Capitated insurance payment models led to both shortened stays and a reduction in the daily reimbursement rate that covered hospital-based occupational therapy services. Today, although the percentage of occupational therapy practitioners working exclusively in mental health or "behavioral health" settings has dwindled (American Occupational Therapy Association [AOTA], 2010b), practitioners continue to work with clients who exhibit deficits in occupational performance. These deficits can result in vocational disruption, inability to manage illness, extreme stress reactions, limited social skills, and homelessness.

Current settings where occupational therapy practitioners might work, generally from the most to the least restrictive environment, include but are not limited to

- Hospitals (acute inpatient units in state or community hospitals, university medical centers, or military hospitals)
- Partial hospitalization programs (self-contained or part of a mental health system)
- Military fields of operation (war or combat zones)
- Assertive community teams
- Outpatient clinics or private practices
- Community-based clubhouses
- Consumer- or peer-run organizations
- Health promotion and wellness programs.

Although the settings may have changed, the need for occupational therapy intervention to address mental health issues remains.

PROFESSIONAL ETHICS IN MENTAL HEALTH PRACTICE

The challenges of providing ethical, client-focused care in the current health care environment continue to escalate, and mental health settings are no exception. General ethical principles that apply to occupational therapy service provision

in other practice areas also are relevant in the mental health continuum of care. The primary concerns for practitioners in mental health practice regarding each principle of the *Occupational Therapy Code of Ethics and Ethics Standards (2010)* (referred to as the "Code and Ethics Standards"; AOTA, 2010a) are provided in Table 11.1 and illustrated in the case studies and vignettes in this chapter. Prominent issues in mental health with possible ethical implications include (but are not limited to)

- Competence and supervision
- Reimbursement and its role in guiding practice
- Scope of practice for occupational therapy and other professions (e.g., state licensure laws and regulations)
- Therapeutic relationships
- Service delivery models.

Competence and Supervision

A trend in practice settings, also related to scope of practice (and perhaps reimbursement and staffing efficiency), is the pressure to have professionals train aides in technical skills related to client care. *Aides* also may be referred to as "rehabilitation or restorative aides, extenders, paraprofessionals, and rehab techs" depending on the setting (AOTA, 2009, p. 801). Because this level of personnel is less expensive than licensed professionals, lower labor cost is certainly one incentive for this practice. What are the implications, though, of teaching others knowledge and skills that occupational therapy practitioners have acquired through an intensive educational and fieldwork program and for which they have been certified via examination to vouch for their expertise? Are there limits to what can and should be done by aides or nonprofessional staff (i.e., people trained to assist occupational therapy practitioners but who are not licensed in the field) or colleagues in other disciplines to make staff more interchangeable and "efficient"? This may be a pragmatic management approach to limited staffing and reimbursement, but the most important consideration is whether this model benefits

TABLE 11.1
Ethical Principles Across the Mental Health Continuum

PRINCIPLE	PRIMARY CONCERN FOR PRACTITIONERS
1. Beneficence	To be competent and exercise clinical reasoning skills and professional judgment to ensure they are providing services that can reasonably be expected to benefit their clients
2. Nonmaleficence	To not harm clients
3. Autonomy, Confidentiality	To support clients in exercising their autonomy to make decisions, provided the clients are capable of doing so without harm to themselves or others. To maintain the confidentiality of client information and communication, except when laws mandate disclosure for reasons of safety
4. Social Justice	To advocate for clients to receive needed services, particularly when resources are limited and fair allocation presents ethical challenges
5. Procedural Justice	To comply with applicable laws and regulations. State licensure laws define the legal scope of practice, but in a mental health setting where much intervention occurs through groups, the blurring of professional roles can present specific challenges to maintaining and promoting the unique perspective of occupational therapy within the multidisciplinary team.
6. Veracity	To provide accurate and objective information in all forms of communication
7. Fidelity	To "treat colleagues and other professionals with respect, fairness, discretion, and integrity" (AOTA, 2010b, p. S24).

Source. American Occupational Therapy Association (2010a).

clients, whose well-being should be the primary concern.

It is unlikely that clients know the difference between the credentials and training of various health care providers. The onus is on the providers to fulfill professional and ethical responsibilities to ensure that client needs are met by qualified, competent providers, whether the occupational therapist is delegating tasks, cross-training others, or supervising. These responsibilities must be met to uphold Principles 5G (ensure that duties assigned match credentials, qualifications, experience, and scope of practice) and 5H (provide appropriate supervision) of the Code and Ethics Standards. Given that a team approach is common in service provision in most mental health settings, issues of competence and supervision are important. Although these issues may be relevant in other health care settings, much of mental health care is provided outside of the traditional medical model, leading to a possible increase in role blurring and diffusion of professional identities.

Reimbursement

Sometimes, appropriate training of nonprofessionals can provide support to a limited occupational therapy staff and enable them to provide services to a larger number of clients. However, the language in state practice acts must be considered before training and assigning any tasks to unlicensed personnel. Some states do not allow the use of aides, and some payers (e.g., Medicare) will not reimburse for occupational therapy services provided by unlicensed personnel.

Occupational therapy practitioners also may be asked to teach colleagues in other disciplines to "do what we do" because their services are reimbursable and occupational therapy is not. This activity can have scope-of-practice implications when people who are not licensed as occupational therapists or occupational therapy assistants are providing services identified as occupational therapy and billing for those services as occupational therapy. Administrative directives that appear to be reimbursement driven must be carefully evaluated, whether they relate to levels of personnel providing services or the decision to provide group versus individual therapy sessions. If administrators issue improper mandates to staff or students, practitioners can cite Principle 2I of the Code and Ethics Standards: "Occupational therapy personnel shall avoid compromising client rights or well-being based on arbitrary administrative directives by exercising professional judgment and critical analysis" (AOTA, 2010a, p. S20). The potential for harm and failure to benefit from therapy exists when administrative directives replace professional judgment backed by data from an occupational profile and assessments. Providing more therapy than clients can tolerate to boost reimbursement also can contribute to harm and violates Principle 2, Nonmaleficence, of the Code and Ethics Standards.

Both the *Occupational Therapy Practice Framework: Domain and Process* (AOTA, 2008) and the *Standards of Practice for Occupational Therapy* (AOTA, 2010c) outline processes for service provision that start with an evaluation, consistent with Principle 1B (provide appropriate evaluation and a plan of intervention for all clients) of the Code and Ethics Standards. However, the model in many mental health settings, both inpatient and outpatient, is to refer clients to groups on the basis of a team assessment of their needs; the occupational therapist, in this model, should take an active role in making recommendations. Clients then receive intervention in a group format, likely along with individual counseling by a psychologist, social worker, or other qualified mental health professional. Goals may be developed and addressed by the team as a whole, individually by each discipline, or both. The occupational therapist is a part of the team, but an individualized occupation-based evaluation, perhaps including standardized or other assessments, with collaborative goals and a plan of care to achieve them may not be part of this model. In some settings, this model may cause perceived conflicts for occupational therapy practitioners, who may feel they are not in compliance with their professional standards of practice, which outline a more prescribed evalu-

ation process. In this situation, practitioners are encouraged to assert their ethical and professional responsibilities to meet with the client to at least screen or obtain preliminary data for an assessment that will guide interventions from an occupational therapy perspective.

An evaluation can be defined in different ways and encompass variable methods of obtaining data. From an ethical perspective, practitioners should choose assessment tools that are current and provide targeted information to delineate performance deficits; the results of such assessments guide the development of collaborative goals and the selection of service delivery methods. Close attention to applicable laws and to the qualifications of test or assessment administrators should guide the judgment of occupational therapists as to whether or not they can ethically complete the Mini-Mental Status Exam (Scheiber, 2004), for example, or teach a non–occupational therapy practitioner how to complete the Test of Grocery Shopping Skills (Brown, Rempfer, & Hamera, 2009).

Scope of Practice

State licensure laws include a legal definition of the occupational therapy scope of practice. Language in these practice acts is often quite general and typically does not enumerate specific interventions within the scope of occupational therapy practice. More important, occupational therapy practitioners do not exclusively "own" the interventions included in those laws. It is not uncommon for nurses, physical therapists, and occasionally others to address deficits in, for example, activities of daily living or community reintegration skills. Instrumental activities of daily living and community reintegration skills are often a strong focus of a variety of practitioners working with mental health clients, who may require remediation in these areas to successfully hold a job or live independently. Moreover, in mental health settings, many interventions occur in a group context with various members of the therapeutic team, one of whom is likely to be an occupational therapy practitioner.

Often a mental health practitioner will lead a group with a colleague from another discipline, and other staff members also may move in and out of group leadership roles depending on the daily schedule and needs of the unit. This practice can result in a blurring of roles, making the responsibilities of occupational therapy less well defined and its contributions potentially less clear. The boundaries of a professional scope of practice can be difficult for clients, as well as for others, to discern. Maintaining a strong role and identity can be challenging for occupational therapy practitioners in mental health settings, where services are often billed as part of a total aggregate rate rather than by individual discipline and where participation in multidisciplinary teams is common. However, the emphasis on addressing occupational performance deficits in the context of barriers to participation is central to the philosophy of occupational therapy and can be promoted as a unique contribution to the team management of the client.

Therapeutic Relationships

The essence of a constructive therapeutic relationship is trust; clients who are in a vulnerable state by virtue of requiring help to regain their health and abilities trust that their providers will act in their best interests, protect them from harm, and prevent unauthorized sharing of their private information. The majority of principles in the Code and Ethics Standards contain language that addresses one or more aspects of the therapeutic relationship. Examples include

- Requiring competence in providing services (Principle 1E)
- Referring to a practitioner who can best meet the client's needs (Principle 1I)
- Refusing to provide unnecessary services (Principle 1H)
- Ensuring that clients are not abandoned in the course of their treatment (Principle 2B)
- Avoiding relationships that exploit recipients of service and/or interfere with professional judgment and objectivity (Principle 2C)
- Avoiding sexual relationships (Principle 2D)
- Obtaining consent before providing services (Principle 3B)
- Respecting the client's right to refuse services (Principle 3C)

- Conversing openly and collaboratively with clients to ensure they comprehend services, risks, and benefits (Principle 3J)
- Advocating for needed services for clients through available means (Principle 4E)
- Delegating tasks to other personnel that are within their competence or scope of practice and providing appropriate supervision (Principles 5G and 5H)
- Ensuring that communication and information conveyed is accurate and not false, fraudulent, deceptive, or misleading (Principles 6B and 6C).

Nowhere is honest communication more important than in a mental health setting, where clients' dysfunction may result from or be exacerbated by betrayals of trust in previous relationships and circumstances. These clients also may be more vulnerable and exhibit more impaired judgment because of the nature of their illnesses.

Adhering to ethical principles in a therapeutic relationship can be challenging in settings in which the practitioner's own safety may be jeopardized, such as in corrections facilities or, at times, homeless shelters. Clients in these settings are more likely to be aggressive and impulsive and to have a history of violence than those in more traditional mental health settings, who are often voluntary residents (Castaneda, 2010). Maintaining continuity of care, focusing on the client's safety and well-being, and protecting the client from harm or exploitation, all ethical mandates, are more difficult when practitioners themselves have received threats or have experienced actual physical or psychological harm. In these situations, practitioners need to mindfully protect the confidentiality of clients' disclosures and abide by laws related to reporting potential harm and danger directed toward themselves or others.

Service Delivery Models

Given the wide array of settings in which mental health practitioners practice, use of a case-based approach to identify and analyze ethical dilemmas can be helpful. The following sections briefly describe several such settings and include an ethical dilemma that might occur in each setting. Although the settings themselves are important, the population served and roles of other staff, if any, working with clients are equally significant, whether within a community-based facility, a medical setting, a consumer-run entity, a school, or a private practice.

Inpatient Services

Inpatient units can vary in size, focus of care, age of clients, and diagnoses of clients, or they can be general in nature. Some may include specific units dedicated to the care of people with anxiety or mood disorders, eating disorders, substance abuse, geriatric psychiatric disorders and dementia, or substance abuse. Although not unique to inpatient settings, the acute or "crisis" nature of the services often intensifies the sense of urgency a practitioner experiences. Unfortunately, little time is available for deliberation and procedural reasoning when an ethical dilemma arises. Consider the dilemma faced by the occupational therapist in Case Study 11.1. In reading the case study, keep in mind that the professional community is a small world, and just as social networking Web sites link people in predictable and unpredictable ways, it is not uncommon to find a mix of personal and professional connections in practice (Newman, Barabási, & Watts, 2006). Case Study 11.1 describes the difficulty of maintaining confidentiality when personal relationships are involved.

CASE STUDY 11.1. ADDRESSING A CONFIDENTIALITY BREACH IN AN INPATIENT FACILITY

Anna was the supervising therapist at a private psychiatric hospital that provided services to inpatients, outpatients attending work readiness programs, and adolescents participating in a partial hospitalization program. She supervised three occupational therapists but had no caseload on the inpatient units. Outside of work, she was dating a psychiatrist, **Martin**, from another health system. The relationship had been a tempestuous one, punctuated by unexplained disappearances by Martin lasting for weeks at a time. After a series of these disappearing acts, Martin dis-

closed that he had bipolar disorder and had managed to get out of town during most of his manic episodes. He sought to protect Anna, his family, and his clients from his illness by leaving the area.

Unfortunately, he became unable to contain his behavior during the latest episode, and the hospital where he had admitting privileges became involved. To support this talented and successful man, the hospital administration stated that Martin needed to get care immediately, and if he did so, they would not move to have his medical license revoked. Desperate to save his career, Martin found the best possible therapy with **Dr. Wizer**, an elderly, highly esteemed professor of traditional psychoanalysis. He told Anna of this plan and his confidence that he would find stability from this therapy.

Two weeks later, Anna began noticing that Martin was becoming increasingly psychotic and suicidal. Martin informed her that he had gotten a call that his therapist, Dr. Wizer, was ill and would be out of work for an undetermined amount of time. At work the next day, one of Anna's supervisees approached her and said, "I have a new patient admitted with symptoms of depression and severe psychosis who is an elderly, highly esteemed professor of traditional psychoanalysis. How do I go about treating someone who is already an expert in the field in which I am treating him?" Anna's first response was to ask her supervisee, "What's his name?" The occupational therapist answered, "Dr. Wizer." Anna immediately realized that her break in adherence to Principle 3G opened an ethical dilemma with the potential for additional ethical violations to occur.

What should Anna do? Inform the unit staff of her dilemma or maintain confidentiality? Try to convince her boyfriend to see another doctor without being able to explain why? In analyzing the case, Anna must first ascertain the exact nature of the problem or problems. Second, she should identify the players involved, the ethical principles that may guide possible actions, the consequences of each of those actions, and, finally, the best option and why.

The central problem presented to Anna was how to handle an individual like Dr. Wizer, essentially a celebrity, who was now in the patient role in a clinical arena in which others generally considered him to be an expert. The situation was further complicated by the fact that Dr. Wizer also had a professional, clinical relationship with Anna's boyfriend, Martin. So much of the complexity revolved around the mixing of personal and professional relationships, often the source of ethical dilemmas. The primary parties were Anna, her staff, Martin, and Dr. Wizer. The critical issues appeared to revolve around Autonomy and Confidentiality (Principle 3), as well as Nonmaleficence (Principle 2), particularly 2C ("avoid relationships that exploit the recipient of services . . . physically, emotionally, psychologically . . . or in any other manner that conflicts or interferes with professional judgment and objectivity"; AOTA, 2010a, p. S20) and 2G ("avoid situations in which a practitioner . . . is unable to maintain clear professional boundaries or objectivity to ensure the safety and well-being of recipients of service"; p. S20).

On one hand, the simple answer to Anna's supervisee's original question is that she should treat Dr. Wizer no differently than any other patient—that is, with respect and dignity, protecting his confidentiality and privacy. Anna, on the other hand, had a potentially conflicted professional relationship with Dr. Wizer because he was her boyfriend's therapist. Therefore, she needed to recuse herself from any care or professional interaction with him to avoid a conflict of interest. She did not need to state a specific reason, but she did need to clarify her role and ensure that professional boundaries were clearly enforced.

Because Dr. Wizer was her boyfriend's therapist (and was now unavailable), Anna wanted to ensure that Martin's mental health issues were addressed, but her personal relationship with him again blurred her roles. She needed to be able to parse out her role as girlfriend to Martin from her role as a mental health professional. Given the potential conflict of interest, Anna could suggest that Martin explore alternative options for continuing treatment on the basis of the undetermined length of Dr. Wizer's absence. Ultimately, Martin would have to decide how to proceed with his treatment.

Although this case occurred in a mental health setting, issues of professional boundaries, conflict of interest, and confidentiality are applicable to any context where an occupational therapy practitioner may encounter someone he or she knows in a professional capacity transposed to a client role.

Partial Hospitalization Programs

Partial hospitalization programs (PHPs) are full-day programs within a psychiatric hospital, behavioral health department of a hospital, or community setting. They provide an intermediate level of care for people with mental illness. Programs generally are open for 6 to 8 hours on weekdays, with formal programming being delivered for about 6 hours. Clients may use personal transportation, or the setting may offer a van service to facilitate attendance. Services provided by multidisciplinary teams often include

- Comprehensive, skills-based treatment to stabilize clients and improve functioning
- Case management and aftercare planning
- Individual skills training emphasizing cognitive behavior therapy, dialectical behavior therapy, and life skills training
- Prevocational rehabilitation and vocational counseling
- Medication consultation and treatment. (McLean Hospital, 2010, para. 1)

Clients in PHPs have a wide range of diagnoses. However, some PHPs are set up for specific client populations, such as those with eating disorders, addictions, or borderline personality disorders. PHPs also can be used to provide clients with an intensive level of intervention and services in an effort to prevent hospitalization. Vignette 11.1 describes the balancing of two important ethical principles in a PHP.

VIGNETTE 11.1. BALANCING CONFIDENTIALITY WITH A CLIENT ORIENTATION IN A PARTIAL HOSPITALIZATION PROGRAM

DeWayne, a client recently discharged from a PHP, proudly informed **Danielle**, one of the occupational therapists, that he had started a new job. He thanked Danielle for all the help in vocational planning and work readiness that the program provided. He then asked, "How would it be if I came back to the program to share my success story with other clients? Maybe they'd get some ideas from me and maybe some motivation."

Which of the following responses might be most appropriate?

1. "That's a very nice offer, and you have every right to be proud of your accomplishment, but privacy rules prevent us from allowing you to return, as we have to protect the confidentiality of the current client group."
2. "Great idea. Could you come by today at 1:00 p.m.?"
3. "That's a good idea. Why don't I ask our clients how they feel about you joining us for a Return to Work Group? If they are OK with you returning, I'll call you and set it up for the end of this week."

This scenario is common in mental health practice: Proud of their successes, clients often want to share them with others. The issue is whether it is ethical to allow the client to return to the intervention environment. Principle 3G guides occupational therapy practitioners to "ensure that confidentiality and the right to privacy are respected and maintained regarding all information obtained about recipients of service, students, research participants, colleagues or employees" (AOTA, 2010a, p. S21). From a legal standpoint, a stringent adherence to Health Insurance Portability and Accountability Act of 1996 (U.S. Department of Health and Human Services, 1996) guidelines would make Answer 1 the correct one. However, there is a way to balance adherence to this policy and the values and goals of today's mental health practice, in which consumer-driven programs abound. Peer support is considered key to management of and recovery from mental illness. Thus, it is not at all unusual for clients to share experiences or serve as role models or counselors.

In keeping with the recovery model, which emphasizes a support network, adaptive skills, and the right to self-determination or autonomy (also part of Principle 3 of the Code and Ethics Standards), Answer 3 is the preferred ethical response to this issue. Clients in the group will have the opportunity to weigh the pros of potentially increased insight and motivation against the cons of a possible breach in their confidentiality. By obtaining a written release from all program participants, Danielle allows the

clients to choose to hear from a peer who is on the mend. She must then ensure that the experience is safe and productive by working with DeWayne to review the rules of the program and to tailor his content to the setting. Danielle also must commit to being present for the entire onsite experience.

Community-Based Practice: Clubhouse Model

Community-based practice calls on occupational therapy practitioners to fulfill varied roles, some of which may be outside their comfort zone. As in home health practice, practitioners may find themselves in clients' homes, boardinghouses, or apartments where the environment may be uncomfortable, disorganized, or odiferous. These environments may provide evidence of a client's lack of home management skills, even in clients who are able to socialize or work. Alternatively, the occupational therapist may be working in a psychosocial clubhouse, which is typically characterized by client-centered goals and shared responsibilities and experiences. The International Center for Clubhouse Development (ICCD; 2009) has described the clubhouse model as follows:

ICCD Clubhouses provide members with opportunities to build long-term relationships that, in turn, support them in obtaining employment, education and housing. They are community centers that offer members:

- A work-ordered day in which the talents and abilities of members are recognized and utilized within the Clubhouse;
- Participation in consensus-based decision-making regarding all important matters relating to the running of the Clubhouse;
- Opportunities to obtain paid employment in mainstream businesses and industries through a Clubhouse-created Transitional Employment Program. In addition, members participate in Clubhouse-supported and independent programs;
- Assistance in accessing community-based educational resources;

- Access to crisis intervention services when needed;
- Evening/weekend social and recreational events; and
- Assistance in securing and sustaining safe, decent and affordable housing. (para. 1).

The clubhouse and recovery models may raise dilemmas for occupational therapy practitioners. For the most part, clubhouse staff members are not trained in the neuroscience of psychiatric disorders or the cognitive and psychosocial sequelae. They also do not have training in activity analysis and adaptation or knowledge of the impact of person, environment, and occupational choices on occupational performance. Clubhouse staff are generally college graduates with diverse academic backgrounds, but they are not required to have education focused on mental health practices. Many clubhouse staff members are certified through a national examination administered by the U.S. Psychiatric Rehabilitation Association (USPRA) as a Certified Psychiatric Rehabilitation Professional, but the pathway to that certification exam is variable, with no standardized curriculum (USPRA, 2010). As a result, an occupational therapy practitioner employed by a clubhouse may face dilemmas regarding whether to intervene when concerns arise about the ability of unlicensed staff to appropriately and competently assess the person–environment–occupation fit to meet the complex needs of the clients. This important ability is needed in this setting but is not within the skill set of the nonprofessionals most likely to work in a clubhouse, whose training is not standardized. Vignette 11.2 describes an ethical dilemma encountered by an occupational therapy assistant in a clubhouse.

VIGNETTE 11.2. ADHERING TO COMPETENCE REQUIREMENTS AT A CLUBHOUSE

The management of a clubhouse recently hired **Su-Lin**, an occupational therapy assistant. Money was tight, but the management valued occupational therapy expertise in the analysis of activity demands and occupational performance and believed that an occupational therapy assistant could provide these types of service better than other staff at the agency and at less cost than an occupational therapist. Analysis of activity demands and occupational performance was considered an important benefit in facilitating client function in daily work and life skills. The clubhouse director was concerned about impending dementia in one of the clients and asked Su-Lin to administer the Lowenstein Occupational Therapy Cognitive Assessment (Lowenstein et al., 1989), a cognitive–perceptual evaluation.

This scenario presents both legal and ethical issues. A profession's scope of practice is legally defined in state licensure laws, and some states have very specific language related to occupational therapy assistants. In Massachusetts, for example, state regulations do not permit occupational therapy assistants to complete any part of a screening, evaluation, or assessment. Principle 5, Procedural Justice, of the Code and Ethics Standards obligates occupational therapy practitioners to comply with institutional rules; local, state, federal, and international laws; and Association documents applicable to the profession of occupational therapy. In addition, Su-Lin was practicing without supervision. The requirement for supervision of occupational therapy assistants by an occupational therapist, as well as the roles and scope of practice for the occupational therapy assistant, are detailed in two AOTA official documents: *Guidelines for Supervision, Roles, and Responsibilities During the Delivery of Occupational Therapy Services* (AOTA, 2009) and *Standards of Practice for Occupational Therapy* (AOTA, 2010c).

Furthermore, Principle 5G of the Code and Ethics Standards mandates that "duties assumed by or assigned to other occupational therapy personnel match credentials, qualifications, experience, and scope of practice" (AOTA, 2010a, p. S23), and Principle 5H requires that practitioners "provide appropriate supervision to individuals for whom they have supervisory responsibility" (p. S23). Although the clubhouse management may have had good intentions, Su-Lin was in jeopardy because of noncompliance with legal and ethical requirements. In addition, there was potential for client harm; Su-Lin had not been deemed competent by an occupational therapy supervisor to administer or interpret this assessment (even if state law permitted), so the score and recommendations would not be valid.

Private Practice

Private practice in mental health can take many forms. Occupational therapy practitioners may see clients in a professional office setting or may provide services through contracted home care agencies. Clients can also contract directly with occupational therapy practitioners if no physician referral is required in the state or they are not seeking insurance reimbursement. Additionally, practitioners may see clients in a variety of community settings (e.g., grocery stores, restaurants, libraries, or potential apartments) to facilitate their community integration. Intervention occurs in any setting where clients can engage in authentic occupational participation. Case Study 11.2 describes an ethical dilemma in the context of the private practice of occupational therapy.

CASE STUDY 11.2. UNRAVELING ETHICAL PRIORITIES IN PRIVATE PRACTICE

Barbara demonstrated significant performance problems in instrumental activities of daily living and extreme vulnerability to stress. Her anxiety interfered with everything, from tracking expenses to even considering volunteer work. Barbara currently lived in an apartment with her sister, **Janet**, who also had marked occupational performance limitations, especially in the areas of initiating activities and maintaining engagement in occupations. Barbara had been diagnosed with bipolar disorder and Janet with depression and an eating disorder. The clients' family had sufficient resources to pay privately for needed services.

Following the crisis hospitalization of Janet, the family believed the sisters needed an onsite daily caregiver. They hired a companion, **Denise**, for Barbara and Janet 4 days per week from early morning through dinner. Denise assumed many roles, which the sisters passively allowed. Among these roles were answering the phone, cooking dinner, and driving by herself on shopping excursions to distances the sisters would not normally travel. Before Denise had been hired, the sisters' world was narrowed by their symptoms, but they managed to see friends, travel to their favorite stores, and shop independently. Instead of enhancing the functional

level of the sisters, the companion in reality was having the opposite effect.

During a regularly scheduled meeting, Barbara told **Cindy**, the occupational therapist, that Denise had suffered a slight stroke over the weekend but was now "fine" and back to work. This was the second report of a health incident during which Denise had "fainted." When Cindy asked if she or her sister had told their family about these incidents, Barbara said no. When Cindy mentioned her concern about the safety of the situation, Barbara was most worried about Denise not losing the job. She had never considered the situation as being potentially unsafe.

Two major ethical concerns are at play in this situation. The first is related to the safety and the health and well-being of the both the companion and the sisters. The second is the diminished autonomy of the sisters and, as a consequence, a further restriction of their participation in the community. Cindy's obligation under Principle 1 (Beneficence) was to "demonstrate a concern for the well-being and safety" of the sisters and to prevent foreseeable harm to them and their companion, which might require action on her part. Given that Barbara disclosed incidents that had the potential to compromise the sisters' safety, Cindy needed to create a viable solution. She needed to assess the safety of the situation and request a letter from the companion's doctor indicating whether it was safe for her to continue in the companion role.

Considerations regarding the sisters' autonomy should include an assessment of the specific tasks someone in a companion role is expected to perform and the skills needed to accomplish these tasks. A "job description" could be written with input from the sisters and agreed to by all involved parties to identify the parameters of the actual job and prevent a more informal use of the companion. Although the sisters may have mental health disorders, respect for client autonomy and self-determination, if they are judged to be mentally competent, must be part of an ethical solution. Such activities also support Principle 3A of the Code and Ethics Standards, calling for a collaborative relationship with clients, and Principle 3J, mandating that practitioners "make every effort to facilitate open and collaborative dialogue with clients and/or responsible parties to facilitate comprehension of services and their potential risks/benefits" (AOTA, 2010a, p. S21). Paramount in Cindy's concerns must be addressing the sisters' performance skills and patterns (with or without assistance) safely and effectively to allow them to live independently and participate in necessary and desired occupations.

Consumer-Run Organizations

Client centeredness and self-determination are expressions of autonomy supported by Principle 3, Autonomy and Confidentiality, of the Code and Ethics Standards. Nowhere are client centeredness and self-determination more evident than in the development of client-run organizations. These consumer- or family-driven grassroots organizations emerged as a result of dissatisfaction with professional attitudes toward families and people with mental illness. The National Alliance on Mental Illness and the National Mental Health Association are among the best-known consumer-run organizations. Over many years, occupational therapy practitioners have joined these types of organizations, which use models based on collaboration and partnership (Haiman, 1995, 2004). In Vignette 11.3, an occupational therapist confronts a direct order to engage in unethical practice.

VIGNETTE 11.3. DEFENDING THE NEED FOR ETHICAL PRACTICE IN A CONSUMER-RUN ORGANIZATION

A consumer-run organization formed by parents to provide social and emotional support for their adult children hired an occupational therapist, **Hali**, to run programs and coordinate the central office. She was to do this with the help of two of the organization's participants, who had been working as office assistants for 2 years before Hali's arrival.

Several parents on the organization's board suddenly raised the issue of "fairness" in the office arrangement; they stated that other participants might want the same opportunity to improve their work skills. They asked Hali to immediately tell the two workers that their jobs were being terminated at the end of that week. Hali stated that it was unreasonable and unethical to abruptly change the program without warning or preparation for the transition to another meaningful work-related

occupation. The parents, whose true motive was to make those positions available to their own children, nevertheless demanded that the practitioner follow their orders. Instead of following the directive, Hali proposed a smooth transition over a few weeks, stating, "I cannot ethically agree to mistreat these consumers in this way. If you want them to go within the week, you will have to tell them yourselves." As a result of Hali's advocacy and determination to find an ethical resolution, the parents backed down. The workers were given notice, and a 4-week transitional work program was developed. The original workers and others who followed in this new program were able to transition to new employment over a 4-week period.

This case study illustrates several critical points. One is the professional responsibility of occupational therapy practitioners to be familiar with and take action based on the Code and Ethics Standards. Language in Principle 4, Social Justice, supports the ethical obligation of occupational therapy personnel to "advocate for just and fair treatment for all patients [and] clients . . . and encourage employers and colleagues to abide by the highest standards of social justice and the ethical standards set forth by the occupational therapy profession" (AOTA, 2010a, Principle 4D, p. S22). Practitioners also are obligated to "advocate for recipients of occupational therapy services to obtain needed services through available means" (Principle 4E, p. S22). Although these consumers had transitioned to community living and Hali was not providing direct intervention, the "services" that provided therapeutic benefit were the meaningful work tasks engaged in at an organization created to help them resume appropriate life roles.

Principle 2B of the Code and Ethics Standards— "make every effort to ensure continuity of services or options for transition to appropriate services to avoid abandoning the service recipient" (AOTA, 2010a, p. S20)—despite being aimed at clients receiving direct therapy services, has some relevance to this situation. In this case, *services* refers to participation in worker roles in the office. Abrupt termination of these roles for consumers without an appropriate transition plan in place could be construed as a form of abandonment. Hali's refusal to participate in unethical actions and her resolve to protect the clients resulted in a positive outcome, the benefits of which were extended to many more participants through the transitional work program.

CONCLUSION

Occupational therapy services in the mental health arena are delivered in diverse practice settings to meet the needs of clients with a wide range of disorders and occupational performance deficits. Dilemmas and ethical issues can arise in any of these venues and challenge the occupational therapy practitioner. Ethical practice includes ensuring that client autonomy and confidentiality are maintained, even in relatively unstructured, community-based models. In more medically based settings, where group intervention and programs may be facilitated by staff from multiple disciplines in addition to occupational therapy, ethical issues often involve addressing competence and role delineation. In addition, other issues can arise as a result of simultaneous personal and therapeutic relationships and ineffective service delivery or staffing models. Although this chapter was dedicated to ethics in mental health practice, readers can easily draw parallels to practice in all areas.

With the AOTA *Centennial Vision* highlighting practice development in unique and community-based settings (AOTA, 2007; Baum, 2007; Christiansen, 2004), practitioners are ethically bound to monitor themselves and their workplace to ensure that high standards are met. Ethical principles and other ethics resources can guide practitioners in addressing these challenges in a professional manner while meeting the client's needs for safety, autonomy, and beneficial intervention. Knowledge and application of the Code and Ethics Standards and other relevant practice guidelines can help mental health occupational therapy practitioners provide care that protects and benefits clients.

REFERENCES

American Occupational Therapy Association. (2007). AOTA's *Centennial Vision* and executive summary. *American Journal of Occupational Therapy, 61,* 613–614. doi: 10.5014/ajot.61.6.613

American Occupational Therapy Association. (2008). Occupational therapy practice framework: Domain and process (2nd ed.). *American Journal of Occupational Therapy, 62,* 625–683. doi: 10.5014/ajot.62.6.625

American Occupational Therapy Association. (2009). Guidelines for supervision, roles, and responsibilities during the delivery of occupational therapy services. *American Journal of Occupational Therapy, 63,* 797–803. doi: 10.5014/ajot.63.6.797

American Occupational Therapy Association. (2010a). Occupational therapy code of ethics and ethics standards (2010). *American Journal of Occupational Therapy, 64*(6 Suppl.), S17–S26. doi: 10.5014/ajot.2010.64S17

American Occupational Therapy Association. (2010b). *2010 occupational therapy compensation and workforce study.* Bethesda, MD: AOTA Press.

American Occupational Therapy Association. (2010c). Standards of practice for occupational therapy. *American Journal of Occupational Therapy, 64*(6 Suppl.), S106–S111. doi: 10.5014/ajot.2010.64S106

Baum, M. C. (2007). Presidential Address—Centennial challenges, millennium opportunities. *American Journal of Occupational Therapy, 60,* 609–616. doi: 10.5014/ajot.60.6.609

Brown, C., Rempfer, M., & Hamera, E. (2009). *The Test of Grocery Shopping Skills.* Bethesda, MD: AOTA Press.

Castaneda, R. (2010). Therapeutic relationships in difficult contexts: Involuntary commitment, forensic settings, and violence. In M. K. Scheinholtz (Ed.), *Occupational therapy in mental health: Considerations for advanced practice* (pp. 199–214). Bethesda, MD: AOTA Press.

Christiansen, C. (2004, September 20). AOTA's *Centennial Vision:* A map for the future. *OT Practice, 9*(17), 10.

Haiman, S. (1995). Dilemmas in professional collaboration with consumers. *Psychiatric Services, 46,* 443–445.

Haiman, S. (2004, September). A parent/consumer-driven community program: Authentic occupational therapy. *Home and Community Health Special Interest Section Quarterly, 11,* 1–4.

International Center for Clubhouse Development. (2009). *What is a Clubhouse?* Retrieved from www.iccd.org/whatis.html

Lowenstein, D. A., Amigo, E., Duara, R., Guterman, A., Hurwitz, D., Berkowitz, N., . . . Eisdorfer, C. (1989). A new scale for the assessment of functional status in Alzheimer's disease and related disorders. *Journals of Gerontology, Series B: Psychological Sciences and Social Sciences, 44,* 114–121.

McLean Hospital. (2010). *Adult: Behavioral health partial hospital program—Services.* Retrieved from www.mclean.harvard.edu/patient/adult/bhphp.php

Newman, M. B., Barabási, A.-L., & Watts, D. J. (2006). *The structure and dynamics of networks.* Princeton, NJ: Princeton University Press.

Scheiber, S. C. (2004). The psychiatric interview, psychiatric history, and mental status examination. In R. E. Hales & S. C. Yudovsky (Eds.), *Essentials of clinical psychiatry* (2nd ed., pp. 33–66). Washington, DC: American Psychiatric Association Press.

Treatment Advocacy Center. (2009). *Severe shortage of psychiatric beds sounds alarm bell.* Re-

trieved from www.treatmentadvocacycenter.org/index.php?option=com_content&task=view&id=81&Itemid=247

U.S. Department of Health and Human Services. (1996). *The Health Insurance Portability and Accountability Act of 1996.* Retrieved from www.cms.gov/HIPAAGenInfo/Downloads/HIPAALaw.pdf

U.S. Psychiatric Rehabilitation Association. (2010). *CPRP exam application requirements.* Retrieved from netforum.avectra.com/eweb/DynamicPage.aspx?Site=USPRA&WebCode=cprpeligibility

Productive Aging

12

Janie B. Scott, MA, OT/L, FAOTA

What is productive aging? Dr. Ethel Percy Andrus first mentioned the construct in 1947 when advocating to insurance companies on behalf of older retired teachers. The organization, National Retired Teachers Association, later became AARP. Dr. Robert N. Butler, the founding director of the National Institute on Aging, also used the term *productive aging* in his early work and throughout his career. He emphasized exercise, nutrition, social engagement, and naps as important to living a healthy and productive life (Agnvall, 2010). *Productive aging* is the continued participation of older adults in self-care, work, volunteering, informal caregiving, civic participation, and engagement in leisure and social activities as they grow older.

People's engagement in their chosen occupations varies over time and is contingent on their health, interests, and abilities (see Figure 12.1). Occupational therapy practitioners consult for and intervene with the aging population by providing recommendations to improve energy conservation and community mobility and identifying strategies for time management, work simplification, coping, and social and leisure participation in response to changing needs and interests (Scott, 2009). This chapter illustrates how the *Occupational Therapy Code of Ethics and Ethics Standards (2010)* (referred to as the "Code and Ethics Standards"; American Occupational Therapy Association [AOTA], 2010b) provides

guidance for occupational therapy practitioners in ethical practice as they support older adults in aging productively.

OCCUPATIONAL THERAPY'S ROLE IN PRODUCTIVE AGING

Productive aging applies to both older adults who are well and those who are living with illness or disabilities. Occupational therapy can help them achieve their goals by "supporting health and participation in life through engagement in occupation" (AOTA, 2008, p. 626). AOTA, through the *Occupational Therapy Practice Framework: Domain and Process* (AOTA, 2008), articulated the profession's overall goal as facilitating clients' ability to maintain balance between different areas of occupation (e.g., activities of daily living [ADLs], rest and sleep, leisure, social participation) to enable them to have a productive life. It is imperative to consider the relationship of client factors (e.g., values, beliefs, spirituality) to a client's ability to maintain this balance in daily life, thereby achieving a productive and quality life. Through the occupational therapy process, practitioners can help facilitate the productive participation of older adults.

AOTA has recognized the importance of helping occupational therapy practitioners address the

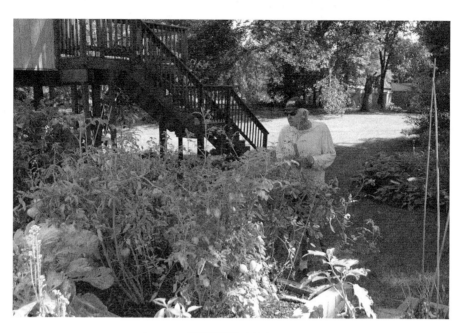

FIGURE 12.1

The demand for occupational therapy services will increase as the population ages. Occupational therapy practitioners provide interventions aimed at productive aging for clients with interests such as continuing to work, resuming functional activities after a disability, or gardening.

desire of older adults to remain productive. AOTA's Gerontology Special Interest Section and e-mail forum are important sources of information and continuing education to help prepare the profession to meet this portion of society's needs. When 2,000 members of AOTA participated in the development of the *Centennial Vision*, they included productive aging as one of the six practice areas of critical importance (Baum, 2006), reflecting both the number of occupational therapy practitioners who work with older adults and the anticipated increase in demand for services such as safety assessments, rehabilitation, and low vision services that older adults will need as they age.

An AOTA Ad Hoc Group on Aging/Gerontology was convened to examine "the future of aging and the challenges that confront the profession as a result of this longevity revolution" (Lysack et al., 2007, p. 1). The Ad Hoc Group delineated occupational therapy's opportunities with and contributions to older adults as follows:

- A holistic approach to working with the client to develop creative solutions to challenges in completing daily occupations

through our use of task analysis and adaptation within a framework attentive to the individual's personal, physical, and social context.

- A focus on creating a meaningful lifestyle.

- A focus on client values/client-centered care.

- A focus on performance of real-life activity.

- A focus on the value of habit and routine (normalcy) in everyday life.

- A focus on meaningful occupation as both the intervention and the outcome. (Lysack et al., 2007, p. 12)

The Ad Hoc Group presented several issues and recommendations to the AOTA Board of Directors. The list was long and inclusive and included suggestions such as

- Expanding the aging focus beyond rehabilitation to "a focus on healthy aging and

disability prevention and health promotion"
(Lysack et al., 2007, p. 2)

- Providing caregiver and consumer education
- Addressing mental health
- Developing innovative community-based practice models
- Advocating for reimbursement
- Engaging in lifelong learning
- Transferring research into best practices
- Promoting the use of assistive technologies and devices to support productive aging.

Occupational therapy professionals, the group noted, are ready to respond to the growing demand for services to promote productive aging:

The profession is uniquely trained to promote functional independence, quality of life and social participation in the face of chronic disease and disability. . . . Occupational therapists facilitate optimal occupational performance and community participation across the full spectrum of ability, from healthy adults actively engaged in their communities to those who are coping with serious physical and mental health conditions in more supported environments like assisted living facilities and nursing homes. (Lysack et al., 2007, p. 1)

DEMOGRAPHIC TRENDS IN PRODUCTIVE AGING

As McGuire, Lusk, and Bousfield (2010) noted, "The 'senior tsunami' is coming, and the need for occupational therapists to address the needs of older adults is growing" (p. 1). Two decades from now, an estimated 1 in 5 U.S. residents will be an older adult (Centers for Disease Control and Prevention [CDC] & Merck Company Foundation, 2007). Cities and states across the United States will need to examine and expand the range of services available to older adults, including medical, housing, transportation, and support services. Occupational therapy practitioners will have many opportunities to provide services to meet the needs of this increasingly diverse population in a culturally sensitive manner.

An emphasis on productive aging has implications both for housing and for the workforce. Many retirees want to age in place rather than move to warmer climates, retirement communities, or institutions (Agnvall, 2010), and "residing in one's preferred living arrangement and community mobility are two of the greatest challenges to maintaining occupational integrity" (Beitman, 2009, p. CE-1). Unless these two conditions are met, opportunities for productive aging are severely compromised.

A 2005 AARP report on older workers and employment projected a shortage of younger workers with experience to fill the gaps left by older, experienced workers, and health care is an area where shortages are expected. At the same time, partly because of economic necessity and partly out of a desire for continuing productivity, older adults may choose to work part-time or switch careers at traditional retirement age; according to the AARP (2005), "average retirement age may actually rise as the baby boomers approach retirement. Among the factors contributing to this shift are longer life expectancies and Americans' desire to stay involved and active in their later years" (p. 67). Changing expectations about retirement require that people plan strategies for retirement in advance (e.g., Fuscaldo, 2011).

The CDC and the Merck Company Foundation (2007) projected that "by 2030, the changing face of older adults in the United States will be evident" (p. 3): 72% of the U.S. population will be White, 11% will be Hispanic, 10% will be Black, and 5% will be Asian. Occupational therapy practitioners are committed to diversity and inclusion in their practice; as noted in the Code and Ethics Standards, "members of AOTA are committed to promoting inclusion, diversity, independence, and safety for all recipients in various stages of life, health, and illness and to empower all beneficiaries of occupational therapy" (AOTA, 2010b, p. S17).

Principle 3I of the Code and Ethics Standards obligates practitioners to "take appropriate steps to facilitate meaningful communication and comprehension in cases in which the recipient of service, student, or research participant has limited ability to communicate (e.g., aphasia or differences in language, literacy, culture)" (AOTA, 2010b, p. S21). Occupational therapy practitioners are also guided by Principle 4F to "provide services that reflect an understanding of how occupational therapy service delivery can be affected by factors such as economic status, age, ethnicity, race, geography, disability, marital status, sexual orientation, gender, gender identity, religion, culture, and political affiliation" (AOTA, 2010b, p. S22). Vignette 12.1 describes a situation in which an occupational therapist is challenged to provide culturally appropriate practice.

VIGNETTE 12.1. FACILITATING A TRANSITION TO RETIREMENT WITH CULTURAL COMPETENCE

Camila was a 59-year-old Hispanic woman recently admitted to a community behavioral health program following a 28-day admission to the behavioral health unit of a local hospital. Camila's treatment for bipolar illness was complicated because of a recent diagnosis of diabetes secondary to obesity. Medication management, new meal preparation guidelines, and Camila's difficulty in adhering to schedules complicated her psychiatric, medical, and occupational therapy care. During the course of her hospitalization, Camila decided that the stress of her maintenance job was too much and that she would retire in 6 months at age 60.

Camila's occupational therapist, **Elaine**, had recently obtained her certification. Elaine recognized that Camila had multiple occupational therapy needs (e.g., managing time, planning meals, expanding leisure interests, developing a retirement planning strategy); however, Elaine was uncomfortable working with Camila because of the cultural and language differences between them. Elaine discussed her feelings with **Nick**, her supervisor, who reminded her of her obligations under Principles 3I (facilitate open and collaborative dialogue with clients and their comprehension of services) and 4F (provide services that reflect an understanding of ethnicity and culture) of the Code and Ethics Standards, which underscore occupational therapy practitioners' obligation to take cultural orientation into account in service delivery. Cultural competence was important to Nick because of the community program's outreach to underserved populations. Practitioners were expected to locate translators when language barriers existed and to learn about sociocultural beliefs that may affect the therapeutic relationship with clients and their families.

To that end, Elaine and Nick agreed to the following plan to support the evolution of Elaine's cultural sensitivity and competence. Elaine would

- Locate resources to facilitate her communication with Camila (e.g., Thrash, 2006)
- Identify a process to obtain real-time language translation services
- Explore healthy and culturally sensitive food preferences that Camila could use
- Assist Camila, if she was interested, in reconnecting with her religious community
- Pursue further knowledge about the cultural habits and preferences of Camila and Elaine's other clients and use that knowledge to increase her *cultural interfacing,* which includes the verbal and nonverbal communications used in interactions between people of different cultures and languages (Bloomfield, 1994).

ETHICAL DILEMMAS IN SERVICE DELIVERY TO OLDER ADULTS

Occupational therapy practitioners who face ethical dilemmas in providing services to older adults need to consider whether to attempt to resolve the situation locally through direct communication with the supervisor or primary party involved, whether to file an ethical or legal complaint, or whether the best solution is to resign. This section discusses some of the ethical situations practitioners encounter during the delivery of occupational therapy services to older adults.

Aging in Place

Many older adult occupational therapy clients live independently or with supports in the community and desire to continue aging in place. Occupational therapy, with its focus on productive aging and aging in place, will be in high demand as such clients age. Many practitioners in this area primarily focus on making the home environment accessible to allow older adults and people with disabilities to continue living in their homes through home modifications. On a broader scale, occupational therapy with clients aging in place works to ensure livable communities through modifications to the home environment, community mobility, access to occupational therapy and other health care services, and access to employment (Fagan & Cabrera, 2008). Occupational therapy service delivery includes safety assessments of the home and community, recommendations and education to elderly clients and caregivers on environmental modifications, resources that connect elders to community services, and consultations to builders, organizations, and agencies.

Occupational therapy practitioners also support clients' desire to age in place by providing driver screening and evaluations, training seniors in the use of public transportation, providing sensitivity training to drivers, and enabling the use of adaptive equipment for driving, ADL performance, and employment productivity. Beitman (2009) observed that "occupational therapy intervention for older adults living in the community is most beneficial when it is client-centered and focused on health maintenance and successful adaptation to challenges associated with the aging process" (p. CE-6).

Entry-level education for occupational therapists addresses this area of practice through course content on universal design and environmental modifications. Practitioners can advance their knowledge in this practice area through AOTA continuing education and credentialing (e.g., Specialty Certification in Environmental Modification), the National Association of Home Builders Certified Aging in Place Specialist designation, and other academic and continuing education programs.

Public support for occupational therapy and other services to promote aging in place comes from legislation (see *Olmstead v. L.C.*, 1999) and initiatives through the Administration on Aging and aging advocacy organizations. The U.S. Department of Health and Human Services (DHHS; 2010), in the document *Healthy People 2020*, detailed the nation's health objectives for the next decade, among them to "improve the health, function, and quality of life of older adults" (DHHS, 2011b, para. 1). This document incorporates aging-in-place perspectives into many focus areas and objectives, such as fall prevention, engagement in leisure activities including exercise, and caregiver access to training and support, areas that are ideal for occupational

therapy intervention (DHHS, 2011a). As the DHHS (2011b) noted,

> Most older adults want to remain in their communities as long as possible. Unfortunately, when they acquire disabilities, there is often not enough support available to help them. States that invest in such services show lower rates of growth in long-term care expenditures. (para. 3)

In Case Study 12.1, an occupational therapist confronts competing priorities in her own efforts to age in place.

CASE STUDY 12.1. BALANCING ETHICAL OBLIGATIONS TO ENABLE AGING IN PLACE

Marcie, a 61-year-old wife, mother, and grandmother, was an occupational therapist working in a community-based senior center. Her duties included program evaluation and planning, group leadership, and client advocacy with community agencies. Her husband, **Stephen**, was 66 and became disabled after sustaining a left-sided stroke while playing tennis. Marcie was now the primary breadwinner for the family. Her position at the senior center required that she work a flexible schedule that included weekends when the center offered special events. Stephen began attending the center to be near his wife and to have mealtime supervision, opportunities for social engagement, and limited physical activity. The senior center context met both Marcie's and Stephen's needs.

After a few months, Stephen's dependence on Marcie began to have a negative impact on her work performance. Stephen wanted Marcie to have lunch with him each day, go with him on center outings, and help him perform some of his ADLs. If Marcie attended to all of Stephen's needs, she would not have time to fulfill her job responsibilities. Marcie was torn between the duties she owed in her position at the senior center and to her husband. She identified the following dilemmas:

- Stephen wanted Marcie to eat lunch with him every day. Before he attended the senior center, Marcie used her lunchtime to interact with center members or contact community agencies on clients' behalf to arrange for services. Did Marcie have a greater duty to attend to Stephen's needs or to continue to function in her position as she had previously? Was Marcie obligated to work through her lunch, or was she entitled to alter her behavioral patterns and choose to use her lunchtime to eat with her husband?

- Stephen wanted Marcie to go on center outings with him. Center staff often alternated in attending these events. If Marcie attended the ones that included Stephen, would she be able to attend to the needs of the other members? Would Marcie become more of a center member than staff? Did the center benefit from having Marcie so involved?
- Marcie was also conflicted about whether Stephen should be included in the groups she led. Would her attention be too directed to Stephen, to the detriment of the other group members' needs?

Some questions for Marcie to consider are the following:

- What are Marcie's duties and responsibilities in her position with the agency? Has she discussed her dilemmas with her supervisor? If she acquiesces to Stephen's requests, will she still be meeting the essential requirements of her job?
- Should Marcie have a frank conversation with Stephen about her conflicted feelings? She doesn't want to hurt his feelings, but she feels compelled to share her thoughts with him. If Marcie's income is a major concern, they need to decide what to do so as not to jeopardize Marcie's job.
- Are current center members harmed by the diversion of Marcie's attention?

Marcie considered the following possible courses of action:

- Have Stephen decrease his time at the senior center or switch to a different one. This action might give Marcie more space and time to do her job. Is it a good option, even though it might risk Stephen's physical and emotional health?
- Schedule Stephen into groups and activities that do not involve Marcie, giving each of them greater autonomy.

- Discontinue her current pattern of working through lunch and spend that time socializing with Stephen. If she chooses this option, she may have to realign her work duties in collaboration with her supervisor.

The responses to these questions will help Marcie analyze whom she owes the greatest duty to and how she decides between the two competing priorities. Once she more clearly understands the pros and cons of her dilemma, she can use an ethical decision-making model (see Chapter 10, this volume) to help crystallize her thinking before making recommendations to her husband and employer.

Case Study 12.2 describes an occupational therapist's efforts to balance ethical principles in ensuring adequate care for her home care clients.

CASE STUDY 12.2. ADDRESSING CLIENT AND CAREGIVER NEEDS IN HOME CARE

Deidre, 73, and her partner, **Alex**, 82, were retired. Alex had had a mild stroke 12 years previously, and 1½ years ago he had had quadruple bypass surgery. Deidre maintained an active schedule, exercising daily, snow skiing a few times a year, reading journal articles, and maintaining an active social life.

Deidre was diagnosed with Parkinson's disease 3 years ago and was feeling the consequences of the disease physically, cognitively, and emotionally. Deidre devoted a significant amount of her time to maintaining her own wellness and trying to stay actively and socially engaged with Alex and their friends, but Deidre's acceptance of her diagnosis was difficult. Alex and their occupational therapist, **Regina**, were working with Deidre to encourage her to consider her current and future needs relative to her ability to age in place.

Although Deidre was the primary focus of the occupational therapy intervention, Regina felt it was imperative to consider Alex's needs and level of function so that he could optimize his health and remain a supportive caregiver. Regina wanted to ensure that she would not be breaching the Code and Ethics Standards or Medicare policies by providing occupational therapy services to both Deidre and Alex. She reviewed several ethical decision-making models (e.g., those discussed in Chapter 10, this volume), the Code and Ethics Standards, and Medicare policies, specifically billing for caregiver education under Part A. She used the series of steps described in Chapter 10 to guide her decision making.

Regina sought first to gather the facts. Alex and Deidre could both benefit from occupational therapy intervention, but Medicare sets limits on reimbursement for people receiving home health services. Deidre needed evaluation and possible intervention regarding environment, safety, energy conservation, and executive functions. Alex would benefit from stress management techniques, transfer and home safety strategies, and methods to provide Deidre with emotional support. The key people involved were Deidre, Alex, Alex and Deidre's friends and family, and Medicare. Deidre and Alex had a long-term relationship, and support was available from family and friends.

Regina was a licensed occupational therapist in good standing with the state regulatory board and AOTA and within the community, and she wanted to provide high-quality occupational therapy services to this couple. Deidre and Alex would do whatever was necessary, including privately pay for services, to enable them both to age in place. Regina's dilemma was as follows: Could she ethically and legally provide occupational therapy services to both Alex and Deidre?

Regina listed the following possible courses of action:

- Evaluate and intervene only with Deidre, and offer caregiver training to Alex under the Medicare rules
- Accept private payment by the couple, and evaluate and provide recommendations as she and her clients saw fit
- Investigate and advocate for other sources of funding for the required services and environmental modifications
- In light of Deidre's potential cognitive deficits, provide caregiver instruction and environmental adaptation that may benefit the needs of both for energy conservation (Vance, Siebert, & O'Sullivan, 2006).

Regina's actions needed to be consistent with the following principles of the Code and Ethics Standards: Principle 1, Beneficence; Principle 2C (avoid relationships that exploit the client); and Principle 4, Social Justice, especially Principles 4A (uphold the profession's altruistic responsibilities) and 4E (advocate for clients to obtain needed services through available means).

In her research, Regina checked with the Centers for Medicare and Medicaid Services (n.d.) and found an online document, *Caregiving Education,* that noted the following:

> Medicare Part A covers home health services that include skilled nursing care and medical social services, both of which may involve caregiver education. For example, medically necessary training activities that require skilled nursing personnel to teach a patient and his caregiver how to manage treatment regimens can be considered a skilled nursing service covered under the home health benefit. (p. 2)

Regina also reviewed the original physician referral for occupational therapy evaluation and intervention, Medicare guidelines, Deidre's and Alex's priorities, and the Code and Ethics Standards.

Regina decided to set up a formal meeting with Deidre and Alex, and in the meeting she shared the results of her initial assessment and collaborated with them to develop an intervention plan. Regina agreed to provide the evaluation and services to Deidre in compliance with Medicare guidelines. At Regina's suggestion, Deidre agreed to contact the local Area Agency on Aging to see if grant funds or special programs were available to pay for environmental renovations. The three parties also agreed on a plan to reevaluate Deidra's and Alex's needs on a regular basis.

Institutional Care

In discussions on AOTA's *OTConnections,* an online discussion forum, occupational therapy practitioners often discuss ethical dilemmas they face. Among those they typically encounter in institutional settings are requests by supervisors to modify the results of evaluations, provide services to clients who in their professional opinion don't need services, document a client's care at levels that aren't accurate, pad the minutes billed to Medicare to reflect the facility's productivity standards, and document services when none were delivered (suspicions about Medicare fraud and abuse can be anonymously reported to the Medicare Hotline at 1-800-MEDICARE). Some participants consider leaving their employment rather than to compromise their ethics, be in noncompliance with state regulations, or participate in billing fraud. An occupational therapist's efforts to ensure that he is avoiding unethical practice in a skilled nursing facility are described in Vignette 12.2.

VIGNETTE 12.2. PROMOTING CLIENT WELL-BEING IN A SKILLED NURSING FACILITY

Amrit was an occupational therapist with several years of experience in acute care who was now working in long-term care. He was assigned to evaluate and work with a 93-year-old woman, **Zelda**, who was frail and had multiple chronic illnesses, including dementia. Zelda was recovering from a recent hip fracture and needed rehabilitative care. Amrit was concerned that Zelda was too old and frail to benefit from occupational therapy. He expressed his concerns to his supervisor, who instructed him to fulfill the referral because no other occupational therapist was available to evaluate and intervene. Amrit's dilemma existed because of his concern that he would devote valuable time to a person who was unlikely (in his professional opinion) to benefit from occupational therapy interventions while other patients needing occupational therapy services were unserved.

After thoughtful reflection and review of the Code and Ethics Standards and the AOTA advisory opinion on patient abandonment (Morris, 2011), Amrit realized that occupational therapy values and principles encouraged the advancement of Zelda's well-being through the administration of occupational therapy services. He considered Zelda's comprehensive needs and decided to focus her intervention on working with nursing staff to reduce her risk of falling, promoting her cognitive engagement, assessing her ability to summon help using the call button, and increasing her participation in dressing and feeding.

Discharge Planning

When the client's treatment in an institution comes to an end, occupational therapy practitioners have significant insights to contribute to the discharge planning process and need to embrace ethical principles to promote client safety and care. The Code and Ethics Standards obligate occupational therapy practitioners to terminate therapy in collaboration with the client when goals have been met (Principle 1H), to advocate for just and fair treatment for all clients (Principle 4D), and to advocate for clients to obtain needed services through available means (Principle 4E).

Atwal and Caldwell (2003) examined occupational therapy's role and participation in discharge planning and determined that occupational therapy practitioners unintentionally fail to uphold principles related to Autonomy and Confidentiality, Beneficence, Nonmaleficence, and Social Justice. Practitioners have an ethical obligation not only to contribute to the discharge planning process with interdisciplinary and multidisciplinary teams but also to participate on such teams equally and assertively. In Vignette 12.3, an occupational therapy student and her fieldwork supervisor struggle with their ethical obligation to participate assertively on a client's discharge planning team.

VIGNETTE 12.3. ADVOCATING FOR ADEQUATE DISCHARGE PLANNING

Selena was an occupational therapy student doing a Level II fieldwork assignment on a behavioral health inpatient unit of a community hospital. Her midterm evaluation was positive, with the comments focusing primarily on improving her communication skills, particularly her assertiveness during interactions with professional staff. Selena was reluctant to speak up at times (e.g., at team and discharge planning meetings). She was surprised to receive this feedback because her supervisor, **Marco**, rarely contributed in these settings.

Selena had been working with **Mrs. Boxer** following Marco's initial evaluation of her 2 weeks previously. Marco had identified several safety concerns in his assessment, and several of them remained unresolved, including short-term memory deficits, self-care, safety, and health. Selena voiced to Marco her concerns about Mrs. Boxer's plans to be discharged to her home. The day after their discussion, a discharge planning meeting was held involving the entire team, including family members. Team members mentioned some minor problems with short-term memory; however, all felt that Mrs. Boxer was safe to go home. Although Selena and Marco had information to the contrary, they were not asked for their input, and they did not offer their opinions.

Selena was distressed immediately after the meeting adjourned for a short break. She knew that the occupational therapy professionals had important information that should have been communicated to the team, and she expressed this to Marco. They realized that they had a duty to the patient and her family to share their knowledge and potentially protect Mrs. Boxer from a premature discharge that involved a high potential for injury. Although the team had moved on to the discussion of another patient, Selena and Marco returned to the subject of Mrs. Boxer and communicated their reports and recommendations. Privately, they both recognized the dangers that could result from silence and failure to advocate for their patients, and they established personal goals to overcome their lack of assertiveness and to consistently speak up on behalf of their patients in all future meetings.

Hospice and End-of-Life Care

Should conversations about productive aging include hospice and end-of-life care? Occupational therapists' ethical obligation to serve clients continues in the late stages of clients' lives. The Code and Ethics Standards remind us that "the concept of *freedom* and personal choice is paramount in a profession in which the desires of the client must guide our interventions" (AOTA, 2010a, p. S17). Support for clients' dignity, also a foundational value in occupational therapy, is critical in the end stages of life. Principle 1, Beneficence; Principle 3, Autonomy and Confidentiality; and Principle 4, Social Justice, establish occupational therapy practitioners' responsibility to provide services to all clients, even those with a terminal condition, and to avoid an authoritative or paternalistic attitude toward clients by listening to their wishes and engaging them collaboratively in the therapeutic process.

Although, as Benthall and Holmes (2011) noted, "outcomes for this population are not about permanent independence or rehabilitation" (p. 9), occupational therapy emphasizes occupational engagement for people throughout the life span, and

preparing to die and dying are part of that process. The role of occupational therapy continues to be to support the skills and activities that are important to clients and that contribute to their quality of life (Benthall & Holmes, 2011). Pizzi (2010) discussed the construct introduced in the palliative care literature of a "good death," which he believed could be achieved through the power of occupation: "Well-being and wellness can be goals for people with terminal illnesses" (p. 493).

Occupational therapy's role in end-of-life care includes strategies to enhance participation in meaningful occupations as well as specific ways to obtain reimbursement for these skilled services. Medicare, Medicaid, and other third-party payers supplement the cost of these needed services (Benthall & Holmes, 2011). Practitioners use their knowledge and experience in task analysis, energy conservation, psychosocial conditions, and the aging process to introduce new strategies, including use of assistive and adaptive devices, to facilitate engagement in meaningful activities important to the client. Vignette 12.4 demonstrates a violation of the Code and Ethics Standards in end-of-life care.

VIGNETTE 12.4. ADDRESSING A LACK OF VIGILANCE IN HOSPICE

Mandy was an occupational therapist and independent contractor with experience in the practice area of productive aging in a skilled nursing facility, a state behavioral health hospital unit, and an assistive living residence. She decided to expand her practice to include traditional home health services and hospice care to older adults living in their homes.

Mandy enjoyed working with clients in their homes. She felt that the care she delivered was more focused on each person's needs and priorities. Mandy developed close and rewarding relationships with some of her clients and their families. Occasionally her clients demonstrated their appreciation by taking her to lunch or giving her gift cards and other gifts. She enjoyed the attention and welcomed the gifts. Sometimes she used the gifts, and at other times she exchanged them for cash. Mandy found herself engaging in relationships with elderly clients at the end of their lives in order to deceptively attempt to obtain gifts and bequests, often by taking advantage of their diminished cognitive state. When a family member filed a complaint with the home health agency who contracted Mandy to provide occupational therapy services, the agency terminated her employment. The complaint alleged that Mandy exploited the complainant's parent by taking advantage of her poor judgment to obtain money and gifts from her.

David, the agency's vice president, filed a police report and reported Mandy to the state board regulating occupational therapy practice. He also filed a complaint with the AOTA Ethics Commission (see AOTA, 2010a) citing violation of Principle 2C (avoid relationships that exploit the client), Principle 2G (avoid situations in which one is unable to maintain clear professional boundaries), Principle 2J (avoid exploiting any relationship to further one's own interests at the expense of the best interests of the client), Principle 5 (comply with regulations applicable to the profession of occupational therapy), and Principle 5J (report all gifts and remuneration from clients and their families).

When a client or family member offers a gift to an occupational therapy practitioner, the practitioner should review the Code and Ethics Standards, the National Board for Certification in Occupational Therapy (NBCOT) *Candidate/Certificant Code of Conduct* (NBCOT, 2010), institutional policies, and federal regulations for relevant guidelines. AOTA, NBCOT, and some state regulatory boards advise the occupational therapy practitioners they govern or regulate to avoid harming the person under their care. For example, Principles 1, 2, and 3 of AOTA's Code and Ethics Standards (AOTA, 2010b); NBCOT Principle 6 (NBCOT, 2010); and one board of occupational therapy practice (Maryland) advise against permitting one's desire for financial gain to interfere with decisions made about client care (Department of Health and Mental Hygiene, 2008). Harm may occur when a patient or client tries to express his or her appreciation to the therapist through gift giving when the gesture may cause financial or emotional harm.

Regulations established to govern the receipt of gifts for federal employees can be complex. Under some circumstances, employees may accept coffee, a doughnut, plaques, certificates, or other gifts of less than $20 (Office of the General Counsel, 2010). These guidelines help protect practitioners from engaging in relationships leading to conflicts of interest. Additional information about the eth-

ics of receiving gifts is found in Chapter 21 of this volume.

CONCLUSION

Occupational therapy practitioners must have the knowledge, skills, and cultural competence to embrace AOTA's *Centennial Vision*: "We envision that occupational therapy is a powerful, widely recognized, science-driven, and evidence-based profession with a globally connected and diverse workforce meeting society's occupational needs" (Baum, 2006, p. 610). When working with older adults to maximize their productive aging, practitioners must incorporate evidence-based research into their practice, regardless of whether services are delivered in institutional settings or the community. Fulfilling the *Centennial Vision* will not only advance the profession but also build confidence and awareness among older adults who strive to age productively.

The construct of productive aging has been used for decades to promote an emphasis on occupational performance areas that are important to older adults. Occupational therapy has an important role in helping older adults develop, increase, or maintain ADLs and instrumental activities of daily living, work and volunteer roles, leisure pursuits, civic activities, and caregiving roles. The contexts for service provision include skilled nursing facilities, hospices, senior centers, private homes, employment settings, and community recreational programs, among other settings. Occupational therapy practitioners also work with older adults as they transition from one phase of life to another (e.g., from full-time work to retirement). The Code and Ethics Standards and other resources can help occupational therapy practitioners examine and resolve ethical dilemmas during service delivery.

REFERENCES

AARP. (2005). *The business case for workers age 50+: Planning for tomorrow's talent needs in today's competitive environment*. Retrieved from http://assets.aarp.org/rgcenter/econ/workers_fifty_plus.pdf

Agnvall, E. (2010, June 8). How to live a longer, happier life. *AARP Bulletin*. Retrieved from www.aarp.

org/health/longevity/info-06-2010/how_to_live_a_longer_happier_lifesubhed__longevity_expert_robert_butler_has_the_answers.html

American Occupational Therapy Association. (2008). Occupational therapy practice framework: Domain and process (2nd ed.). *American Journal of Occupational Therapy, 62,* 625–683. doi: 10.5014/ajot.62.6.625

American Occupational Therapy Association. (2010a). Enforcement procedures for the *Occupational Therapy Code of Ethics and Ethics Standards. American Journal of Occupational Therapy, 64*(6 Suppl.), S4–S16. doi: 10.5014/ajot.2010.64S4

American Occupational Therapy Association. (2010b). Occupational therapy code of ethics and ethics standards (2010). *American Journal of Occupational Therapy, 64*(6 Suppl.), S17–S26. doi: 10.5014/ajot.2010.64S17

Atwal, A., & Caldwell, K. (2003). Ethics, occupational therapy and discharge planning: Four broken principles. *Australian Occupational Therapy Journal, 50,* 244–251.

Baum, M. C. (2006). Presidential Address—Centennial challenges, millennium opportunities. *American Journal of Occupational Therapy, 60,* 609–616. doi: 10.5014/ajot.60.6.609

Beitman, C. L. (2009). Wellness interventions in community living for older adults. *OT Practice, 14*(3), CE-1–CE-8.

Benthall, D., & Holmes, T. (2011). End-of-life care. *OT Practice, 16*(9), 7–10.

Bloomfield, R. D. (1994). Cultural sensitivity and health care. *Journal of the National Medical Association, 86,* 819–820.

Centers for Disease Control and Prevention, & Merck Company Foundation. (2007). *The state of aging and health in America.* Whitehouse Station, NJ: Merck Company Foundation.

Centers for Medicare and Medicaid Services. (n.d.). *Caregiving education.* Retrieved from www.cms.gov/MLNProducts/downloads/MLN_CaregivingEducation.pdf

Department of Health and Mental Hygiene. (2008). Title 10, Subtitle 46. Board of Occupational Therapy Practice, chapter 2 *Code of Ethics.* Retrieved from http://dhmh.maryland.gov/botp/docs/comar/10.46.02.00.pdf

Fagan, L., & Cabrera, C. (2008). AOTA's societal statement on livable communities. *American Journal of Occupational Therapy, 63,* 847–848. doi: 10.5014/ajot.63.6.847

Fuscaldo, D. (2011). *10 steps to get you ready for retirement.* Retrieved from www.aarp.org/work/social-security/info-05-2011/10-steps-to-retire-everyday.1.html

Lysack, C., Fagan, L., Mallison, T., Peterson, M., Rogers, J., Toto, P., & Warren, M. (2007). *Ad Hoc Group on Aging/Gerontology report to the executive board.* Retrieved from www.aota.org/News/Centennial/Background/AdHoc/2006/40398.aspx?FT=.pdf

McGuire, M. J., Lusk, L. A., & Bousfield, C. K. (2010, March). Private practice occupational therapy serving older adults. *Gerontology Special Interest Section Quarterly, 33*(1), 1–4.

Morris, J. F. (2011). Patient abandonment. In D. Y. Slater (Ed.), *Reference guide to the Occupational Therapy Code of Ethics and Ethics Standards* (2010 ed., pp. 199–204). Bethesda, MD: AOTA Press.

National Board for Certification in Occupational Therapy. (2010). *NBCOT candidate/certificant code of conduct.* Retrieved from www.nbcot.org/pdf/Candidate-Certificant-Code-of-Conduct.pdf

Office of the General Counsel. (2010). *Ethics frequently asked questions.* Retrieved from www.nasa.gov/offices/ogc/general-law/ethicsfaq.html#gifts1

Olmstead v. L. C., 527 U.S. 581 (1999).

Pizzi, M. A. (2010). Promoting wellness in end-of-life-care. In M. E. Scaffa, S. M. Reitz, & M. A. Pizzi (Eds.), *Occupational therapy in the promotion of health and wellness* (pp. 493–511). Philadelphia: F. A. Davis.

Scott, J. B. (2009). Consultation. In E. B. Crepeau, E. S. Cohn, & B. A. B. Schell (Eds.), *Willard and Spackman's occupational therapy* (11th ed., pp. 964–972). Philadelphia: Lippincott Williams & Wilkins.

Thrash, J. (2006). *Common phrase translation: Spanish for English speakers for occupational therapy, physical therapy, and speech therapy.* Burbank, CA: Author.

U.S. Department of Health and Human Services. (2010). *Healthy People 2020.* Retrieved from www.healthypeople.gov/2020/TopicsObjectives2020/pdfs/HP2020_brochure.pdf

U.S. Department of Health and Human Services. (2011a). *Healthy People 2020 topics and objectives—Older adults, interventions and resources.* Available at healthypeople.gov/2020/topicsobjectives2020/ebr.aspx?topicId=31

U.S. Department of Health and Human Services. (2011b). *Healthy People 2020 topics and objectives—Older adults, overview.* Retrieved from healthypeople.gov/2020/topicsobjectives2020/overview.aspx?topicid=31

Vance, K., Siebert, C., & O'Sullivan, A. (2006). *Occupational therapy: Skills for the job of living for your patients, skills for achieving outcomes for your home health agency* [Fact sheet]. Retrieved from www.aota.org/Practitioners/PracticeAreas/Aging/Tools/38512.aspx?FT=pdf

Children and Youth: Ethics in Service Provision Across Contexts

13

Susanne Smith Roley, OTD, OTR/L, FAOTA, and Mary Alice Singer, MA, OTR/L

Societies place a high value on protecting children and youth, one of the most vulnerable populations. This vulnerability is reflected in the laws and guidelines societies enact to protect children and youth, such as child protective services, child custody, and institutional review boards. The public outcry against those who exploit the vulnerability of children and youth and fail to protect them is echoed in the media; for example, the cover of *Time* magazine's June 2010 issue presented the provocative title, "Why Being Pope Means Never Having to Say You're Sorry," a reference to the way the Catholic Church managed clergy who committed crimes against children in their care (*Time* Magazine, 2010).

Occupational therapy practitioners' concern for children addresses their need for food, love, and shelter (see Figure 13.1) but goes beyond these basic needs. Pediatric practices include children with a wide variety of presenting concerns and diagnoses (Smith Roley, Blanche, & Schaaf, 2001). Occupational therapy practitioners work with individuals, organizations, and populations related to children and youth from prenatal care to age 21 years. Depending on the area of pediatric practice, occupational therapy practitioners require different skill sets. Examples of types of practice that require distinct competencies include

- Counseling pregnant women
- Delivering school-based or private practice services

- Providing early identification of developmental risks in an Early Head Start program
- Providing interventions to premature infants and their parents in a neonatal intensive care unit
- Working in prevocational training centers, juvenile detention facilities, women's shelters, and community mental health centers.

Occupational therapy practitioners who work with children and youth also work with their caregivers in various family constellations, cultural contexts, environments, and communities. Clients' concerns are central to the provision of occupational therapy; thus, family-centered care is imperative. Because caregivers spend the most time with their children, know them the best, and have the largest impact on their development, they are the cornerstone of service provision to this population. Occupational therapy interventions often provide a critical source of support for development, remediation, education, and resilience in the lives of children who are at risk or who have disabilities and their families.

Occupational therapy practitioners are obligated to provide services in compliance with laws and professional standards. As such, practitioners are bound by the standards of care espoused by the occupational therapy profession to ensure that each client receives the services he or she needs to fully participate in society (American

149

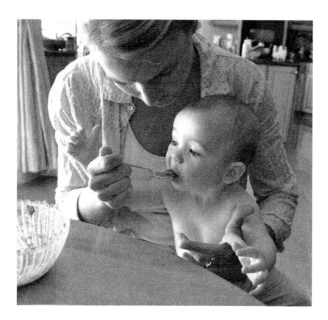

FIGURE 13.1

Practitioners often consult with parents on feeding techniques while on a home visit.

Occupational Therapy Association [AOTA], 2010a, 2010c). Principle 4B of the *Occupational Therapy Code of Ethics and Ethics Standards (2010)* (referred to as the "Code and Ethics Standards"; AOTA, 2010a) obligates occupational therapy practitioners to "take responsibility for educating the public and society about the value of occupational therapy services in promoting health and wellness and reducing the impact of disease and disability" (p. S22).

To provide evidence-based and value-driven services, occupational therapy practitioners rely on high-quality occupational therapy education, research, administration, and innovations in practice and depend on the utmost integrity of the people, programs, and systems that provide them. Authorities and mentors often set the bar for what to do and what not to do; when this is not the case, situations arise that require practitioners to make tough choices. They base their practice on promoting clients' engagement in occupation to support participation and health within the domain and process of occupational therapy (AOTA, 2008). The value of engagement in activities drives *what* the practitioner will do;

the values of altruism, equality, freedom, justice, dignity, truth, and prudence drive *how* the practitioner will do it (AOTA, 2010a).

Occupational therapy practitioners must be aware of potential conflicts of interest and must decline to engage in activities corrupted by motives of self-interest. Part of professional practice is ongoing vigilance for possible conflicts linked to personal gain such as salary, power, and position. In addition, practitioners need to act responsibly by discussing potential conflicts, requesting feedback from peers and authorities, and finding ways to approach conflicts so that the outcome is in the best interest of the client and the profession.

In this chapter, the seven principles of the Code and Ethics Standards are applied to occupational therapy practice with children and youth. It is trite, but true, that everybody makes mistakes; Table 13.1 provides examples of mistakes violating each of the seven principles in the Code and Ethics Standards. Ethical practitioners strive for best practice, recognize their mistakes, confront concerns affecting the lives of children and families, immediately take steps to report and repair errors, and make a firm conviction not to participate actively or passively in potentially harmful or dishonest situations.

PRINCIPLE 1: BENEFICENCE

Occupational therapy is a helping profession. Although multiple motivations bring someone to the profession, the desire to positively influence the lives of others is often the strongest driving force. Although they also may desire the other benefits, such as salaries, professional prestige, friendships, or standing in the local community, in the end occupational therapy practitioners working with children and youth should primarily wish to provide services that benefit this important segment of society. Clients in this area of practice necessarily include both children and youth and their primary caregivers (AOTA, 2008). Therefore, it is essential to provide services that respect the values and beliefs of families and other caregivers.

Occupational therapy practitioners gather essential information from families and caregivers to better understand the child and improve the

TABLE 13.1
Vignettes Describing Breaches of the Code and Ethics Standards in the Practice Area of Children and Youth

PRINCIPLE	VIGNETTE
1. Beneficence	**Michelle**, an occupational therapist, provided a thorough community-based evaluation of an adolescent, **Todd**, who was experiencing heightened anxiety and depression with suicidal thoughts. The evaluation provided an analysis of Todd's deficits but did not acknowledge his strengths. Michelle knew several immediate environmental modifications that would help Todd, but she did not share them with the family because she believed that this information involved remediation and wished to bill for the information. Michelle provided community-based suggestions over an 8-week period, rather than as part of the evaluation report, consuming Todd's annual allotment of insurance coverage for occupational therapy. Besides breaching Principle 1, Beneficence, Michelle also violated Principle 2, Nonmaleficence; Principle 5, Procedural Justice; and Principle 6, Veracity.
2. Nonmaleficence	**Michael**, an occupational therapist, was working with **Fred**, who was macrocephalic due to hydrocephalus, nonverbal, and blind and had cerebral palsy with contractures of the elbow and wrist. Michael decided that stretching the joints was necessary. The mother reported that Fred, who was typically good-natured and happy during therapy sessions, whined and cried throughout the stretching. Michael insisted that stretching was necessary and that Fred had to work through the pain. Later, a doctor discovered that Michael had torn Fred's biceps tendon. Michael violated Principle 2A, "Avoid inflicting harm or injury to recipients of occupational therapy services, students, research participants, or employees" (AOTA, 2010a, p. S20).
3. Autonomy and Confidentiality	**Carla** was an occupational therapist working in a private practice serving a variety of children with difficulties. Her desk was visible from the parent waiting room area. She turned from working on a report to talk with a child. While she and the child were talking, a parent walked by, read portions of the report open on her computer screen, and proceeded to discuss this private information with another parent in the waiting room. The mother of the child discussed in the report overheard the conversation and was mortified and angry. Carla violated Principle 3G, "Ensure that confidentiality and the right to privacy are respected and maintained regarding all information obtained about recipients of service, students, research participants, colleagues, or employees" (AOTA, 2010a, p. S21).
4. Social Justice	A **pediatric practice** in an urban area specialized in occupational therapy services for children with special needs, including an early intervention program. Several practitioners on the staff were aware of a growing non-English-speaking population in the neighborhood who were not seeking access to these services and thus were missing the opportunity for early identification of developmental disorders and autism. A practitioner with grant writing and oversight experience identified a federal grant that could expand the practice's early intervention services to non-English-speaking children and presented her idea to the practice's executive directors. The executive directors, however, did not want to "bother" with providing services to "immigrants."

(continued)

TABLE 13.1 (*cont.*)

PRINCIPLE	VIGNETTE
5. Procedural Justice	A **5-year-old child** experiencing learning and behavior difficulties at school was referred to **Shawna**, an occupational therapist. Shawna informed the parents of the child that there was a lengthy waiting list for evaluation and intervention. They were anxious for their child to receive services as quickly as possible, so **the child's father** offered to purchase and donate any piece of equipment needed for the practice, implying that he wished the child to be moved to the top of the waiting list. Shawna rechecked the schedule and "found" an unexpected opening, ignoring the waiting list. She scheduled the child and provided the parents her wish list of equipment for the gym.
6. Veracity	**Kenan**, an adolescent receiving inpatient intervention for cancer, was provided occupational therapy services. The administrator insisted that the occupational therapist, **Akeia**, continue to see Kenan until discharge. Following reevaluation using the Canadian Occupational Performance Measure (Law et al., 2005) and other assessments, however, Akeia determined that Kenan had achieved all appropriate goals. The administrator also directed Akeia to use billing codes that did not reflect her intervention but had been preapproved by the insurance company.
7. Fidelity	A nonprofit organization providing specialized services for children invited **Cassandra**, an occupational therapist, to be a member of the board of directors. Cassandra accepted the position, even though her ownership of a for-profit business providing products and programs similar to those of the nonprofit organization constituted a conflict of interest. During the following year, she successfully lobbied for several of her business affiliates to fill vacant board positions; she intended to close two departments of the nonprofit and change key staff in the other departments and needed the additional votes to do so. With the new board members in place, Cassandra moved to the board chair position and proceeded to fire long-standing staff, replacing them with staff members loyal to her.

Note. AOTA = American Occupational Therapy Association.

co-occupations they engage in—that is, activities that are intrinsically shared (e.g., parenting and being parented, family dining). Vignette 13.1 describes a situation in which occupational therapists promoted Beneficence in an early intervention setting.

VIGNETTE 13.1. PROMOTING BENEFICENCE IN SERVICES TO FAMILIES

A group of occupational therapy practitioners provided services as part of an early intervention program focusing on children with autism and their families. Several families traveled more than 60 miles each way to come to the weekly program. The practitioners were aware that the program director took on clients who could be receiving services closer to their homes to prevent a competing program from receiving the business. The program director refrained from sharing information about geographically closer services with the families. The practitioners identified the following options to address this dilemma:

- Tell the families in private about other options for services.
- Meet with the director to discuss their discomfort with the situation.
- Solicit more clients within a reasonable geographic region.

- Set up meetings with other similar agencies to discuss the referral process to better meet the needs of families.
- Suggest providing unique and sophisticated intervention options that warrant the extra effort by families to attend that early intervention program.

After reviewing all of the possible plans of action, the practitioners developed a plan for soliciting more clients in the surrounding area. They also met with the therapy team at an agency closer to the families in question to create a referral plan to better serve the families. The final step was a meeting with the director of the program to update him on the networking and to suggest ways that the children and families would be better served. The proposal of a plan for attracting new clients allowed the meeting to go smoothly.

PRINCIPLE 2: NONMALEFICENCE

Primum non nocere means "First, do no harm." This phrase, commonly used in medicine, reminds practitioners to humbly consider whether to intervene would be worse than to do nothing. When working with vulnerable children and youth, occupational therapy practitioners must commit to updating their knowledge and skills to ensure that their clients are receiving the best possible services. This commitment is necessary both when entering practice with children and youth and when changing focus within this practice area. Practitioners must obtain specialized knowledge and skills, particularly in settings (e.g., a neonatal intensive care unit) or situations (e.g., difficulty with eating, feeding, and swallowing) in which clients are the most vulnerable. Entry-level skills and abilities can be honed through practice and mentorship, but when the client needs expertise beyond the practitioner's skill level, the practitioner must find resources such as a mentor or a competent practitioner to assist in the intervention.

The more educated the occupational therapy practitioner, the better he or she is able to communicate with parents or guardians, caregivers, and professionals, who rely on practitioners to provide expertise that supports their efforts to care for their children under stressful conditions.

Caregivers are critical to a child's well-being; therefore, their input must be included in intervention planning, intervention, and follow-up programs. If practitioners educate parents and other caregivers regarding the purpose and methods used during intervention, parents and other caregivers are more likely to carry this learning over into the settings where children spend most of their time. Parent education begins with evaluation results, which must be written in language that parents understand. Collaboration between practitioners and parents or caregivers is paramount in creating a support system for children at home and in the community. In Vignette 13.2, a practitioner confronts a dilemma involving the duty to do no harm.

VIGNETTE 13.2. ENSURING THE AVOIDANCE OF HARM

While diapering a child with Down syndrome during an early intervention program, the occupational therapist noticed bruises on the child's legs. The nanny had mentioned to the therapist that she was frustrated with the child's hyperactivity and lack of compliance when told to do something. Both parents were away on a business trip. The therapist suspected that the nanny had used corporal punishment on the child. The various responsibilities of the occupational therapist in this situation are as follows:

- Prevent further harm from happening to the child.
- Report suspected abuse to child protective services.
- Notify the child's parents about her suspicions and be aware of any future incidents.
- Inform the administration of the early intervention program about the suspected abuse.
- Consult with the nanny on positive behavioral approaches.
- Provide the nanny with contact information for the social worker on staff for assistance if needed.

The first step the therapist took to prevent further harm to the child was to notify the child's parents and the program's administrator of her suspicions. The therapist provided the nanny with written information on positive behavioral approaches and opened a dialogue with the nanny about intervention strategies specific to the behavior she was finding difficult to manage. She gave the nanny a referral to a local respite program to add support. The child's parents returned home and, after meeting with the nanny, decided to hire additional help for the nanny when they were both going to be out of town at the same time.

PRINCIPLE 3: AUTONOMY AND CONFIDENTIALITY

Infants and children often do not have a voice in decision making related to their care, so the adults responsible for their well-being must be very sensitive to their best interests. Occupational therapy practitioners require finesse to understand the primary needs of infants, children, and youth and advocate for their best interests while traversing cultural differences in caregiving, parenting styles, and families' hopes and dreams, as well as limitations in funding streams and service delivery models.

Occupational therapy practitioners often have access to sensitive information about their clients when providing services, including not only health and educational records but also family dynamics and financial status. The obligation to sustain confidentiality is expressly stated in laws such as the Health Insurance Portability and Accountability Act (U.S. Department of Health and Human Services, 1996). Protecting the privacy of clients' written records is easy, however, compared with sustaining their privacy when collaborating with other parents or professionals and when addressing a history of child abuse or neglect. Vignette 13.3 describes the efforts of an occupational therapist to resolve an ethical dilemma involving confidentiality.

VIGNETTE 13.3. WEIGHING CONFIDENTIALITY AGAINST NONMALEFICENCE

As part of a nonpublic agency (NPA) service, **Juanita**, an occupational therapist, provided twice-weekly direct services to **Megan**, a student, as indicated on

Megan's individualized education program (IEP). On 3 out of 4 occasions over a 2-week period, Megan had had a grand mal seizure on the day Juanita was to provide therapy. The seizures had lasted about 20 minutes each, and the teacher told Juanita not to worry because she had handled it by wrapping the child in a blanket in the corner of the classroom until the seizure subsided. On the fourth therapy day, Juanita happened to be at the school when Megan's mother picked her up, and Juanita told her about the seizure activity and suggested that she call the physician and have Megan's blood checked for medication levels. The mother told her that because the physician did not expect to draw blood for another 4 months, she hadn't thought to request it earlier.

The physician determined that because Megan had grown, the prescription was too weak. When the prescription was modified, the seizure activity was eliminated. Later that week, Juanita received a call from the teacher reprimanding her for speaking directly to Megan's mother and undermining the teacher's authority. Juanita consulted the Code and Ethics Standards and found that Principle 2, Nonmaleficence, and Principle 3J—"Make every effort to facilitate open and collaborative dialogue with clients and/or responsible parties to facilitate comprehension of services and their potential risks/benefits" (AOTA, 2010a, p. S21)—applied in this case. She considered the following courses of action:

- Review the school district's policy related to health management specific to seizures.
- Request an emergency IEP team meeting, including the parents, and invite members of the child's medical team.
- Approach the district about the need to revise the line of supervision for NPA-related services.
- Cease providing services to this district because of the conflict between their policies and Juanita's legal and moral obligations.

After reviewing the school district's policy regarding seizures, Juanita determined that Megan's teacher had neglected to follow established procedures and alert both the school principal and Megan's parents of the increase in her seizure activity. She requested an emergency IEP team meeting, at which Megan's parents, teacher, and other therapy providers agreed on immediate notification of her parents regarding changes in the frequency of seizures or Megan's overall behavior. Juanita scheduled a meeting with the principal of the school to clarify the line of supervision for NPA-related services and arranged ongoing direct contact with the principal instead of the classroom teacher. Juanita felt she could continue to provide therapy services to this district with the new accommodations to ensure Megan's health and safety.

PRINCIPLE 4: SOCIAL JUSTICE

The occupations of children and youth may differ from those of other age groups, but the overarching goal of occupational therapy practice is still engagement in occupation to support health and participation, regardless of the age, disability, economic status, culture, or ethnicity of the client (see Figure 13.2). Access to and engagement in needed and desired activities are intrinsic to the health and well-being of children and youth and to their eventual participation as contributing members of society. Provision of occupational therapy services allows the child to be an active family and community member to the best of his or her ability. Practitioners strive to provide needed services to individuals, populations,

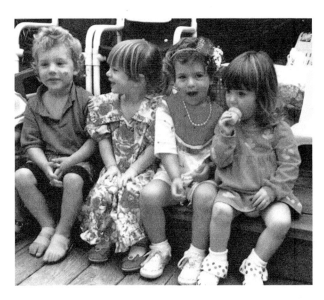

FIGURE 13.2

Consideration of the social needs of children within their communities is important in promoting child development and well-being.

and organizations without economic, ethnic, or cultural bias. Occupational therapy services are not limited by cultural or political boundaries and are provided with the aim of enhancing health and participation in the lives of youth and children. The occupational therapist in Vignette 13.4 faces a dilemma regarding a family's ability to pay for services.

VIGNETTE 13.4. PROMOTING ACCESS TO SERVICES FOR ALL

Trisha, a private practitioner, provided an independent occupational therapy evaluation to a family referred by a child advocacy group. On completing the evaluation, the father paid for the evaluation in cash, proudly stating that he had saved for 1 year to provide this evaluation for their child. Trisha realized that the father was a day laborer and did not have a bank account. She realized that her fees were a significant drain on the family's resources, but she had already committed to further services at a mutually agreed-on fee, including creating goals and objectives, consulting with the child's school district, and attending the IEP meeting. Trisha identified the following potential options to address this dilemma:

- Continue with the services as previously negotiated.
- Return the money for the evaluation to the father.
- Take the money and purchase something for the family.
- Provide the remainder of the agreed-on services with no further charge.

Trisha considered the ethical issues in this case and came to the following conclusions: She was providing a service to the family, and they needed to reimburse her, but the fees that she charged should not put undue financial strain on a family already stressed by a child with serious health issues. Trisha made the decision to establish a sliding scale for her services and charged the family a reduced fee for the overall evaluation, recommendations, and attendance at the IEP. This reduction in fees allowed the family to purchase equipment Trisha recommended to enhance the health and well-being of their child.

PRINCIPLE 5: PROCEDURAL JUSTICE

Procedural Justice includes ensuring high standards of adherence to laws, rules, and regulations and continuing competence. Regardless of the type of services provided, occupational therapy practitioners must adhere to the Code and Ethics Standards and apply them to their work with children and youth (Figure 13.3). Practitioners must provide appropriate supervision and mentoring for staff therapists, particularly those new to an area of practice. Regardless of whether the payer is a family, school district, employer, insurance company, or state or federal agency, fees for services should be fair and commensurate with the services provided.

Organizations often have guidelines for gifts and contributions made by clients, but if the family pays the provider directly, it is especially important to limit the type and value of gifts. It is critical for practitioners to understand cultural differences related to gift giving and the implications of giving or receiving any gifts, large or small; significant gifts from the client may be construed as bribes for better attention or extended services or as extortion on the part of a practitioner taking

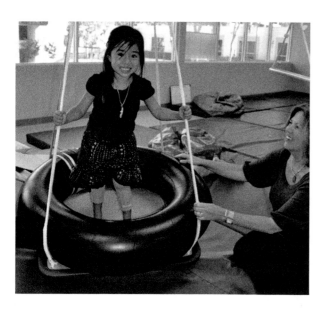

FIGURE 13.3

Practitioners are obligated to update their professional skills and use research-based practice techniques.

advantage of a desperate family's desire to help their child. In Vignette 13.5, the occupational therapist must decide how best to adhere to laws, rules, and regulations in response to pressure by a parent to disregard a custody agreement.

VIGNETTE 13.5. ENSURING ADHERENCE TO LEGAL OBLIGATIONS

Derek, a school-age child, attended a social skills training class led by **Bianca**, an occupational therapist, at a clinic. Derek's parents were in the process of a contentious divorce and custody settlement agreement, and each had independently requested that Bianca testify as a witness during Derek's custody hearing. In the meantime, the noncustodial parent under the current custody agreement tried to pick Derek up following therapy during days that were assigned to the custodial parent. No social workers or attorneys were available for consultation at the clinic. Bianca identified the following options to address this dilemma:

- Consult with the AOTA Ethics Commission and the state regulatory board.
- Insist that the custodial parent be the only person transporting the child to therapy.
- Suggest that the parents go to mediation.
- Decline to provide testimony during the hearing.
- Meet with Derek's parents, and if they are unable to agree on who will transport Derek to and from therapy, discharge the child from the caseload.

Bianca scheduled a meeting with both of Derek's parents and explained that testifying in court for either parent compromised her neutrality and impaired her ability to provide therapy for Derek that was child centered. She gave the parents a referral to a family therapist who was experienced in conflict resolution and suggested that to support Derek, both parents needed to focus on behavior that put his needs first. She explained that conflict over who was transporting Derek was impairing the therapeutic environment she was attempting to create for Derek and stated that she would not release him to the noncustodial parent. Bianca made it clear that these conditions were not negotiable and that the parents were free to choose another therapist if they did not feel they could agree to them. Derek's parents agreed to her stipulations and attended mediation to work out their issues.

PRINCIPLE 6: VERACITY

Accurate and reliable information provided to consumers of occupational therapy services and collaborators in the professional community is fundamental to the integrity of occupational therapy services. Occupational therapy practitioners are often the ones who work most closely with clients and their families to ameliorate the effects of challenges to their ability to carry out activities of daily living. Clients and their caregivers deserve the most accurate information in a format that enables them to best understand and apply that information. Practitioners must present information in a way that enhances understanding and avoids impairing family dynamics. In Vignette 13.6, an occupational therapist must repair the damage caused by a colleague who violated the ethical principle of Veracity.

VIGNETTE 13.6. RECTIFYING A BREACH OF VERACITY

The parents of **Eileen**, a 5-year-old child who was having difficulty in school, requested a second-opinion evaluation by **Agnes**, an occupational therapist. Eileen had a history of developmental delays and extreme sensory sensitivities for which she had received intervention. Another occupational therapist from the same practice, **Roger**, had recently evaluated Eileen. The parents complained that they had spent a lot of money for a report that was confusing and did not address their concerns. Roger had reported findings from prior assessments completed by other therapists but based his recommendations solely on observations in his office. Roger's evaluation report was written haphazardly, emphasized erroneous theories about neurology that lacked support in the literature, and claimed that with extensive intervention in his clinic, Eileen would be completely cured. Not only was the information incorrect; it was impossible to pick out the salient information about Eileen that would be used to guide intervention.

Agnes communicated her concerns about Roger's report to her supervisor and set up a team meeting with the family. In the meeting, she described for the family how services were provided and intervention decisions made in their facility but avoided making disparaging remarks about Roger. Agnes also considered the following steps:

- Discuss her concerns with Eileen's parents regarding the need for additional testing and evidence-based review of information about Eileen's occupational performance and her needed and desired engagement in activities and, with the parents' permission, provide a complete evaluation and report on Eileen.
- Provide a suggested reading list for parents to read over time.
- Write a concise and easily understood evaluation report with recommendations.
- Give the parents handouts that explain home and community activities that will benefit Eileen.
- Discuss the situation with the state regulatory board, the National Board for Certification in Occupational Therapy (if Roger is certified), and AOTA's Ethics Commission (if Roger is an AOTA member), supplying facts and documentation as necessary.
- If Eileen's parents provide consent, provide a copy of her current report and recommendations to Roger, the original therapist.
- Demonstrate intervention strategies within the sessions and explain how Eileen's parents can adapt them during the week to support her progress toward therapy goals.
- Provide Eileen's parents a home program for follow-up to therapy; update the program periodically as Eileen progresses.

Agnes scheduled a meeting with Eileen's parents and explained the need for further evaluation with standardized tests to determine her level of occupational performance in comparison to her same-age peers. After Eileen's parents agreed to further evaluation, Agnes provided an evaluation with a clear explanation of Eileen's functional levels with goals and recommendations for community and home activities that would help Eileen achieve her goals. Eileen's parents observed her therapy sessions and were provided with explanations of therapy approaches and ways to adapt them for home follow-up. Agnes recommended reading for Eileen's parents about her challenges and ways to support her at home, school, and the community. Agnes determined that Roger was not a member of AOTA but was licensed through the National Board for Certification in Occupational Therapy. She reported him to the state regulatory board, and they began an investigation into his practice.

PRINCIPLE 7: FIDELITY

The principle of Fidelity requires practitioners to practice reliably and faithfully and to make and keep commitments to others. Colleagues who are trusted implicitly are the ones who do what they say and say what they do; they are trustworthy and follow through on their commitments or responsibilities. Being reliable ensures that clients can trust the information and interventions provided. To ensure this level of reliability, practitioners must be honest about their knowledge base and the limitations of their expertise. They also must avoid unnecessary disruptions to their personal and professional lives because of negligence, difficulty prioritizing, or lack of attention to essential duties and the needs of others. Vignette 13.7 describes the issues an occupational therapist faced in protecting the competencies of her own and other professionals.

VIGNETTE 13.7. ENSURING FIDELITY TO SCOPE OF PRACTICE

Mariko, an occupational therapist providing rural home health services for homebound, medically fragile children, was asked by her employer to provide speech, nursing, and physical therapy to clients after being given cross-training in each of the other disciplines. Mariko saw that sufficient professionals were not available to meet the needs of these children. She knew the professional community in the area and wished to maintain and develop her relationships with colleagues and organizations in the area. But she also knew that if she refused, she

would lose her job, and this high-needs population might not be served. Mariko considered the following courses of action:

- Seek consultation and mentorship with experienced home health therapists and administrators.
- Provide the administrator with relevant sections from licensure laws and the Code and Ethics Standards.
- Attend as much continuing education as possible to cover the needs of these children and families.
- Review scope of practice documents (e.g., AOTA, 2010b).
- Consult frequently with other disciplines on issues relevant to the cases.
- Limit the caseload to force the agency to hire more therapists.
- Refuse to offer services outside of those covered by licensure laws.

Mariko decided to meet with the administrator and provide him with both the scope of practice standards and relevant sections of the licensure laws. She discussed her hesitancy to provide therapeutic intervention outside of her area of expertise. The administrator agreed to provide her with continuing education for this population of clients. Mariko sought out mentorship from home health therapists in her area who understood the client population she was dealing with. She established monthly meetings with other therapists in her area for support and mentorship.

CONCLUSION

When working with children and youth, their best interest is the ultimate goal of occupational therapy. This goal influences the ways in which occupational therapy practitioners make decisions about what to do and how to do it. It is not enough to follow the example of others; it is essential to examine the ways in which actions or nonactions potentially influence others. Sometimes ethical practice requires going against the status quo. Practitioners who are uncertain about the right thing to do will benefit from seeking the advice of those who are knowledgeable about professional ethics and wise in their implementation.

REFERENCES

American Occupational Therapy Association. (2008). Occupational therapy practice framework: Domain and process (2nd ed.). *American Journal of Occupational Therapy, 62,* 625–683. doi: 10.5014/ajot.62.6.625

American Occupational Therapy Association. (2010a). Occupational therapy code of ethics and ethics standards (2010). *American Journal of Occupational Therapy, 64*(6 Suppl.), S17–S26. doi: 10.5014/ajot.2010.64S17

American Occupational Therapy Association. (2010b). Scope of practice. *American Journal of Occupational Therapy, 64*(6 Suppl.), S70–S77. doi: 10.5014/ajot.2010.64S70

American Occupational Therapy Association. (2010c). Standards of practice for occupational therapy. *American Journal of Occupational Therapy, 64*(6 Suppl.), S106–S111. doi: 10.5014/ajot.2010.64S106

Law, M., Baptiste, S., Carswell, A., McColl, M. A., Polatajko, H., & Pollock, N. (2005). *The Canadian Occupational Performance Measure* (4th ed.). Ottawa, Ontario: CAOT Publications.

Smith Roley, S., Blanche, E. I., & Schaaf, R. (Eds.). (2001). *Understanding the nature of sensory integration with diverse populations.* San Antonio, TX: Pro-Ed.

Time Magazine. (2010, June 7). *Why being Pope means never having to say you're sorry* [Cover illustration by T. O'Brien based on photograph by Andreas Solaro/AFB/Getty Images]. Retrieved from www.time.com/time/covers/0,16641,20100607,00.html

U.S. Department of Health and Human Services. (1996). *Health Insurance Portability and Accountability Act of 1996.* Retrieved from www.cms.gov/HIPAAGenInfo/Downloads/HIPAALaw.pdf

Ethics in Health Promotion and Wellness

14

S. Maggie Reitz, PhD, OTR/L, FAOTA

Health promotion includes efforts to ensure access by members of the public to the knowledge, information, and strategies they need to minimize threats to health and maximize well-being. Occupational therapy practitioners have long been involved in the promotion of health and well-being among individuals and have the potential for greater involvement with communities and populations (Reitz, 2010; Reitz & Scaffa, 2010). The number of occupational therapy practitioners engaging in this type of practice has been small (American Occupational Therapy Association [AOTA], 2010b). Although many of the same skill sets are used in this practice area as in other areas, practitioners may need to acquire additional skills, knowledge, and experience to provide interventions in an ethical manner.

Each of the principles in the *Occupational Therapy Code of Ethics and Ethics Standards (2010)* (referred to as the "Code and Ethics Standards"; AOTA, 2010a) applies to occupational therapy practice that promotes health and well-being. The relationships between the seven principles of the Code and Ethics Standards and health promotion practice are discussed in this chapter. A recurring theme in the vignettes and case studies presented is the importance of obtaining current and relevant knowledge and competencies surrounding health promotion before engaging in this type of practice.

PRINCIPLE 1: BENEFICENCE

Occupational therapy health promotion services are interventions designed to enhance the pursuit of wellness in individuals, families, institutions, and populations. The intended outcome of these efforts is optimal quality life, health, and wellness (AOTA, 2008). Outcomes are facilitated through customized initiatives that facilitate clients' abilities to make positive, self-directed choices about occupational engagement in their pursuit of wellness. Clients, whether individuals, families, or communities, determine their own definition of wellness on the basis of values shaped by culture, age, ethnicity, geography, and other unique factors. Practitioners support the principle of Beneficence, which focuses on ensuring that clients receive a benefit from services, by respecting clients' values and their right to self-determination.

Educating occupational therapy students in a manner that supports their development of knowledge and skills to provide health promotion services through the various levels of care provision (e.g., individuals, groups, families, communities, populations) is supported by this principle. Preparation of occupational therapy students for this practice area is the subject of Case Study 14.1.

CASE STUDY 14.1. PROMOTING COMPETENCY FOR COMMUNITY PRACTICE

Yael was hired as the third faculty member in a new occupational therapy department at a small liberal arts college that recently began offering graduate programs. She was excited to move from a health promotion–focused, community-based practice working with older adults, caregivers, and various agencies to an academic position. Yael had taught for 10 years before taking time off to care for her mother. She wanted to return to academia to get students excited about working in community- and population-based programming because she saw the potential for the profession to influence more lives. Once she took a closer look at the curriculum, however, she realized there was no coursework to prepare students for community-based practice. When she questioned **Martha**, the program director, she was told that the students were going to be well trained in the use of an occupational profile across diagnostic groups and that they would be able to easily generalize this process to families and communities.

Yael considered her next step. She remembered attending an ethics presentation at the state occupational therapy association's conference and reviewed her notes from the presentation. She also identified relevant principles from the Code and Ethics Standards. Yael was concerned that the students' ability to benefit from their occupational therapy education might be limited by the current curriculum design, and thus the program would be in violation of Principle 1, Beneficence. The students' preparedness to address issues surrounding social justice (i.e., Principle 5) also could be limited.

Next, Yael reviewed the current accreditation standards for entry-level master's-degree programs (Accreditation Council for Occupational Therapy Education [ACOTE], 2012). She was simultaneously pleased and dismayed when she identified 10 ACOTE standards directly related to health promotion and community-based practice (see Table 14.1). Although she was pleased that this much attention was directed to a practice area she loved, she was dismayed because the proposed curriculum at her college could be out of compliance with many, if not all, of these standards.

Yael requested a formal meeting with Martha to review the curriculum and ACOTE standards and to formulate a plan to cover the material called for in the standards. The plan Yael developed included the addition of a community-based class, which she volunteered to develop and teach, as well as earlier infusion of additional content on family theory and community practice. Martha was embarrassed about her lack of knowledge about these standards and thanked Yael for her efforts to ensure that the program and curriculum would meet or exceed the standards.

PRINCIPLE 2: NONMALEFICENCE

Occupational therapy practitioners are reminded of the importance of preventing harm by Principle 2, Nonmaleficence. The potential to do harm is very real in health promotion practice. Examples of well-meaning health promotion interventions with the potential to result in physical or fiscal harm to a community include the following:

- Using a boilerplate process to replicate a fitness program in all the senior centers in a county or local jurisdiction without customizing the program to meet the interests, health needs, and values of each center's membership
- Replicating programs with no formal evaluation process in place, thereby failing to include a mechanism to uncover and address unforeseen negative effects
- Supporting or assisting programs that use or promote fear to change behavior in adolescents and young adults without an understanding of the complex role of fear in health decision making; research evidence has shown that fear is ineffective in changing the desired health behavior and in some cases can encourage the opposite, unhealthy engagement, in this age group (Prevention First, 2008)
- Establishing a health promotion program in an at-risk community with no plans to sustain the program once funding ends.

Failure to consider potential harm when developing health promotion programs can result in negative ripples of influence that travel through a

TABLE 14.1
ACOTE Standards Related to Health Promotion and Community-Based Practice

No.	STANDARD
B.2.4	Articulate the importance of balancing areas of occupation with the achievement of health and wellness for the clients.
B.2.5	Explain the role of occupation in the promotion of health and the prevention of disease and disability for the individual, family, and society.
B.2.6	Analyze the effects of heritable diseases, genetic conditions, disability, trauma, and injury to the physical and mental health and occupational performance of the individual.
B.2.9	Express support for the quality of life, well-being, and occupation of the individual, group, or population to promote physical and mental health and prevention of injury and disease considering the context (e.g., cultural, personal, temporal, virtual) and environment.
B.5.17	Develop and promote the use of appropriate home and community programming to support performance in the client's natural environment and participation in all contexts relevant to the client.
B.5.18	Demonstrate an understanding of health literacy and the ability to educate and train the client, caregiver, family and significant others, and communities to facilitate skills in areas of occupation as well as prevention, health maintenance, health promotion, and safety.
B.5.19	Apply the principles of the teaching–learning process using educational methods to design experiences to address the needs of the client, family, significant others, communities, colleagues, other health providers, and the public.
B.5.26	Demonstrate use of the consultative process with groups, programs, organizations, or communities.
B.6.1	Evaluate and address the various contexts of health care, education, community, political, and social systems as they relate to the practice of occupational therapy.
B.6.5	Analyze the trends in models of service delivery, including, but not limited to, medical, educational, community, and social models, as their potential effect on the practice of occupational therapy.

Note. ACOTE = Accreditation Council for Occupational Therapy Education.
Source. ACOTE (2012).

community or population, compromising future efforts to gain access to the community.

Blatant abuse of a community's trust to meet personal needs or goals as a researcher or student or to collect data for a publication, grant, or course without concern for the long-term welfare of the community is unethical and in direct violation of Principles 1, 2A (avoid inflicting harm or injury on clients), and 2C (avoid relationships that exploit clients). To ensure a win–win outcome in community-based health promotion programming and research, plans must address the sustainability of services or the program at the outset of negotiations. Fail-

ure to do so will undermine access to the community by future students, researchers, or others seeking research participants. The Tuskegee experiment (1932–1972), in which researchers studied the long-term effects of syphilis among a group of African-American men without notifying participants of their diagnosis or offering treatment for them or their partners, should be a warning to all who engage in public health or health promotion research without concern for the impact on the population. The legacy of this experiment is lingering mistrust of government public health officials and researchers (Jones, 1981; Thomas & Quinn, 1991).

PRINCIPLE 3: AUTONOMY, CONFIDENTIALITY

The pursuit of wellness is a self-directed activity of individuals, communities, populations, or a society. One cannot impose wellness on a person or community; it must be initiated by the client. Although health promotion programs are developed to encourage health behavior change and the adoption of a wellness philosophy, deciding how to use the delivered information or experience rests solely with the client. When decisions are made regarding what programs are needed in a community, care should be taken to include community members and leaders in the needs assessment and decision-making process (Fazio, 2010).

The principle of Autonomy should be upheld while assessing needs, developing programs, and evaluating outcomes with communities as well as individuals. As shown in Case Study 14.2, knowledge of health behavior literature and support from other disciplines can enhance occupational therapy practitioners' work and success as well as their adherence to the Code and Ethics Standards.

CASE STUDY 14.2. FOSTERING AUTONOMY IN PROGRAM PLANNING

Veranda enjoyed living and working in the city. She loved commuting to her job as an occupational therapist at the city hospital via mass transit. Having grown up in a quiet rural area on a farm, she thrived on the hustle and bustle of city life. The hospital had recently received a grant to promote the health and well-being of families in the surrounding area. Staff could apply for funds to develop programs in support of the hospital's initiative. Veranda decided that the best way to improve the families' health and well-being was to provide basic parenting training. She was successful in obtaining funding to provide an evening parenting tips program. Because she had observed that the parents who brought their children for outpatient occupational therapy always seemed rushed, she decided that time management would be the focus of the first session, and on the basis of the attention that the obesity epidemic was receiving in the media, she selected healthy eating habits as the second topic for the evening.

Veranda was in a hurry as she prepared for the parenting class. The night before, she remembered that 5 years previously, a professor in her university health class had provided materials on the two topics she planned to discuss. Veranda located her class notebook, removed the professor's name and copied the material onto hospital letterhead, and made copies for the parenting class.

The night of the first session, she was happy to see 10 people in attendance. The program started off well, as Veranda was a friendly, outgoing person who could put people at ease. Veranda sensed a growing tension as she distributed the materials on time management and healthy eating she had copied. Nevertheless, she proceeded to review the time management information, and when she sensed that the information was not being well received, she announced a break. During the break, one of the transport aides, **Teddy**, who was attending the class, told her that there were people in the room who could read only at about a 9th-grade level, and they were embarrassed and frustrated with the materials. Teddy further explained that he knew about the SMOG readability assessment (National Cancer Institute [NCI], 2001) from his health education graduate studies. Veranda thanked Teddy for the information.

After the break, Veranda switched to discuss the importance of serving fresh fruits and vegetables as part of a healthy diet. These materials contained more visuals and less text, so Veranda thought she was back on track. However, one attendee stood up and said, "Honey, I know you mean well, but where am I supposed to get these fresh fruits and vegetables?" Veranda was speechless and said, "I don't understand." The person calmly explained that the closest grocery store was 10 miles away and that although some convenience stores in the area carried fruits and vegetables, the selection was limited, the quality was poor, and the cost was high. Veranda asked if there were any farmers' markets in the area and was told there were none on that side of the river.

Veranda thought quickly on her feet; she needed to do something to reconnect with the group. She used her occupational therapy problem-solving skills and knowledge of occupational therapy theory, specifically the Ecology of Human Performance (Dunn, Brown, & McGuigan, 1994), to develop a potential plan for the next session. After thanking people for coming, she asked, "What do you think about spending next week's session having you introduce me to the local neighborhood and then brainstorm ideas to get a farmers' market on this side of the river?" Teddy said, "Now, that is much more like what we need!"

Teddy stayed after the others left. He gently asked Veranda if she had ever studied any health behavior frameworks or theories. She replied that she had not. Teddy suggested she start by reading two free sources that were easily available online. The first was *Theory at a Glance* (NCI, 2005), and the second was known in health education and behaviors circles as the "pink book" (NCI, 2001). Veranda spent time the following weekend reviewing the materials. She became excited about blending health behavior theories with occupational therapy theories to support the development of a farmers' market. She also asked Teddy if he would be co-facilitator for the project. Veranda was happy that the group's effort could be far more meaningful than she first imagined. Instead of merely affecting the 10 people who had attended the group, the group's combined efforts to obtain a farmers' market could benefit the entire community.

PRINCIPLE 4: SOCIAL JUSTICE

Health promotion, especially at the community and population levels, can help address the disparities in health seen in the United States (U.S. Department of Health and Human Services, 2010). The presence of the principle of Social Justice in the Code and Ethics Standards and the fact that health and wellness is one of the focus areas of AOTA's *Centennial Vision* (Baum, 2006) support the need for continued focus on health promotion and community health in occupational therapy practice.

Although the *Centennial Vision* and ACOTE standards reflect an appreciation and acknowledgment of the important role of occupational therapy practitioners in health promotion (see Table 14.1), the latest AOTA workforce survey indicated that only 3% of occupational therapy practitioners work in the community. Because this number includes practitioners who work not only in health promotion but also in assisted living, group homes, and other community settings, the proportion of practitioners who have health promotion as their primary work focus is very small indeed (AOTA, 2010b). Not included in these figures, however, are the health promotion efforts of

occupational therapy practitioners working in other areas such as hospitals or schools; the professional literature provides little or no evidence of the impact of this work. The profession as a whole has a shared responsibility to determine the next best steps to take to ensure that Principle 4B (educate the public about the value of occupational therapy in promoting health and wellness) and Principle 4C (promote activities that benefit the health status of the community) are upheld.

PRINCIPLE 5: PROCEDURAL JUSTICE

Principle 5, Procedural Justice, obligates occupational therapy practitioners to "comply with institutional rules, local, state, federal, and international laws and AOTA documents applicable to the profession of occupational therapy" (AOTA, 2010a, p. S22). In Case Study 14.2, Veranda failed to uphold this principle in her parenting program because she did not have the full complement of skills necessary to provide a parenting class, as required by Principle 5F (maintain continuing competence and improve knowledge and skills). She had no knowledge of the health behavior change literature. In addition, Veranda presented healthy eating information using the food pyramid (Figure 14.1; U.S. Department of Agriculture [USDA], 2005) instead of the updated "My Plate" tool (Figure 14.2; USDA, 2011),

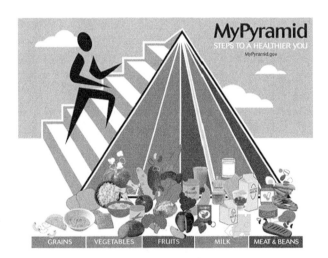

FIGURE 14.1

MyPyramid: Food guidance system recommended by the U.S. Department of Agriculture, 2005–2011.

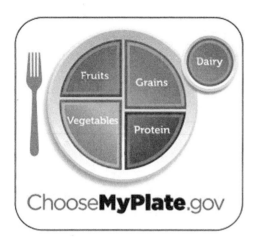

FIGURE 14.2

MyPlate: Food guidance system recommended by the U.S. Department of Agriculture since 2011.

which is much easier to understand (Vastag, 2011). Occupational therapy practitioners must remain current on the available knowledge and evidence to deliver health promotion services ethically.

PRINCIPLE 6: VERACITY

Health promotion practice, like any other area of practice, requires practitioners to be truthful in their work. Veranda failed to uphold Principles 6I (give credit when using the work of others) and 6J (do not plagiarize). As Teddy and Veranda talked about the source of the material she distributed, they realized that she had plagiarized and failed to recognize the work of her professor. At a minimum, Veranda needed to try and contact her professor to apologize and ask what actions she would like Veranda to take. She also needed to alert her supervisor to her mistake and follow supervisor and hospital guidance as long as the advice was in alignment with the Code and Ethics Standards.

PRINCIPLE 7: FIDELITY

Principle 7 requires occupational therapy practitioners to "treat colleagues and other professionals with respect, fairness, discretion, and integrity" (AOTA, 2010a, p. S24). As has been

seen throughout this chapter, health promotion frequently intersects with other areas of practice, settings, and disciplines. For these initiatives to be successful, practitioners need to take care to nurture respectful and professional relationships. Positive partnerships both enhance client health promotion services and support the principle of Fidelity. Failure to uphold this principle can negatively affect service delivery, as shown in Vignettes 14.1 and 14.2, and can even place one's license or livelihood at risk. Vignette 14.2 ends with questions to give readers the opportunity to analyze the ethical dilemmas themselves.

VIGNETTE 14.1. MAINTAINING FIDELITY IN PROGRAM DEVELOPMENT

Colleagues **Lilly** and **Irene** developed a fall prevention program while working for a private hospital. They both spent a lot of time working on the project and were very proud of the program, including the title, TREAD (*Trip Reduction Education, Analysis, Demonstration*) Safely. Irene left the facility to develop a private practice. While grocery shopping, Lilly noticed a set of flyers advertising a fall prevention program with Irene's picture. The title and program description appeared to be exactly the same as those they had developed at the hospital. Lilly was shocked that Irene had stolen and replicated the program because it belonged to the hospital.

Lilly, knowing that one should handle ethical issues locally before escalating to a complaint, contacted Irene and shared her concerns. At first, Irene shrugged it off, but when she saw how upset Lilly was, she offered to pay Lilly a percentage of the profit from the program. Lilly declined this solution and told Irene that she would contact the hospital administration and state board of practice to report Irene's unethical behaviors unless she cancelled the program and refunded any payments received.

VIGNETTE 14.2. OBSERVING FIDELITY IN ASSISTING COLLEAGUES

Dean had a background in private practice with children and youth in a bustling mid-Atlantic metropolitan area. He was hired as an assistant professor at a private faith-based university 45 miles east of the city in a rural farming community at the foot of the Appalachian Mountains. The chair of the occupational therapy department, **Kate**, met with Dean to share the mission of the university and the guidelines for promotion and receipt of tenure. In the ensuing discussion, Kate encouraged Dean to become involved in health promotion service learning within the community to position himself for success at the university.

Being pragmatic, Dean thought he would provide an evaluation service embedded in a class he was scheduled to teach the following fall semester. Dean spent the next 9 months securing resources (e.g., a meeting place at the library) for a weekly evaluation clinic for young children. He anticipated community interest in the free evaluation service and expected the students to gain useful hands-on practice experience.

The first 2 weeks went by with no one showing up for the free evaluation service. He was perplexed and concerned. Dean sought guidance from **Sam**, a health science faculty member who had been teaching at the university for 20 years. Sam asked questions about Dean's background knowledge of health promotion and Appalachian culture. Dean acknowledged that he had very little. Sam provided him with resources about Appalachian culture and suggested he visit a local museum. Sam also suggested that he become familiar with health behavior models and frameworks, which would help him better plan and implement programs once he became known to and knowledgeable about the community he sought to assist.

Using the four-step decision-making model introduced in Chapter 10, analyze the situation. Be sure to identify the ethical principles Dean violated. Consider Kate's responsibility in the situation; did her behavior violate any of the principles? What should Dean do to address the situation in its totality?

CONCLUSION

Occupational therapy practitioners are trained to provide health promotion services to clients that directly relate to the completion of activities of daily living and instrumental activities of daily living with individuals. However, there is a need for occupational therapy practitioners to become involved in prevention and health promotion activities beyond the scope of the individual client. According to AOTA,

There are three critical roles for occupational therapy practitioners in health promotion and disease or disability prevention: to promote healthy lifestyles; to emphasize occupation as an essential element of health promotion strategies; and to provide interventions, not only with individuals but also with populations. It is important that occupational therapy practitioners promote a healthy lifestyle for all individuals and their families, including people with physical, mental, or cognitive impairments. (AOTA, 2008, p. 696)

Occupational therapy practitioners who wish to provide services at the community or population level should remain current on the literature on health behavior, health education, and public health and should consider partnering with experts in these areas to jointly provide services.

REFERENCES

Accreditation Council for Occupational Therapy Education. (2012). 2011 Accreditation Council for Occupational Therapy Education (ACOTE®) standards. *American Journal of Occupational Therapy, 66*(6 Suppl.), S6–S74. doi: 10.5014/ajot.2012.66S6

American Occupational Therapy Association. (2008). Occupational therapy in the promotion of health and the prevention of disease or disability. *American Journal of Occupational Therapy, 62,* 694–703. doi: 10.5014/ajot.62.6.694

American Occupational Therapy Association. (2010a). Occupational therapy code of ethics and ethics standards (2010). *American Journal of Occupational Therapy, 64*(6 Suppl.), S17–S26. doi: 10.5014/ajot.2010.64S17

American Occupational Therapy Association. (2010b). *2010 occupational therapy compensation and workforce study.* Bethesda, MD: AOTA Press.

Baum, M. C. (2006). Presidential Address—Centennial challenges, millennium opportunities. *American Journal of Occupational Therapy, 60,* 609–616. doi: 10.5014/ajot.60.6.609

Dunn, W., Brown, C., & McGuigan, A. (1994). The ecology of human performance: A framework for considering the effect of context. *American Journal of Occupational Therapy, 48,* 595–607. doi: 10.5014/ajot.48.7.595

Fazio, L. S. (2010). Health promotion program development. In M. E. Scaffa, S. M. Reitz, & M. A. Pizzi (Eds.), *Occupational therapy in the promotion of health and wellness* (pp. 195–207). Philadelphia: F. A. Davis.

Jones, J. H. (1981). *Bad blood: The Tuskegee syphilis experiment—A tragedy of race and medicine.* New York: Free Press.

National Cancer Institute. (2001). *Making health communication programs work: A planner's guide.* Bethesda, MD: National Institutes of Health. Retrieved from www.cancer.gov/cancertopics/cancerlibrary/pinkbook/page1

National Cancer Institute. (2005). *Theory at a glance: A guide for health promotion practice* (2nd ed.). Bethesda, MD: National Institutes of Health. Retrieved from www.cancer.gov/theory.pdf

Prevention First. (2008). *Ineffectiveness of fear appeals in youth alcohol, tobacco and other drug (ATOD) prevention.* Springfield, IL: Prevention First. Retrieved from www.prevention.org/Professionals/ProfDev/documents/IneffectivenessofFearAppealsinYouthATODPrevention-FINAL.pdf

Reitz, S. M. (2010). Historical and philosophical perspectives of occupational therapy's role in health promotion. In M. E. Scaffa, S. M. Reitz, & M. A. Pizzi (Eds.), *Occupational therapy in the promotion of health and wellness* (pp. 1–21). Philadelphia: F. A. Davis.

Reitz, S. M., & Scaffa, M. E. (2010). Public health principles, approaches, and initiatives. In M. E. Scaffa, S. M. Reitz, & M. A. Pizzi (Eds.), *Occupational therapy in the promotion of health and wellness* (pp. 70–95). Philadelphia: F. A. Davis.

Thomas, S. B., & Quinn, S. C. (1991). The Tuskegee syphilis study, 1932 to 1972: Implications for HIV education and AIDS risk education programs in the Black community. *American Journal of Public Health, 81,* 1498–1505.

U.S. Department of Agriculture. (2005). *My Pyramid tracker.* Retrieved from www.fns.usda.gov/eatsmartplayhardhealthylifestyle/Tools/mypyramidtracker.htm

U.S. Department of Agriculture. (2011). *My Plate.* Retrieved from www.choosemyplate.gov/food-groups/

U.S. Department of Health and Human Services. (2010). *Healthy People 2020* [Brochure]. Retrieved from www.healthypeople.gov/2020/TopicsObjectives2020/pdfs/HP2020_brochure.pdf

Vastag, B. (2011, June 3). Moving from pyramid to plate. *Washington Post,* p. A4.

15

Work and Industry: Ethical Considerations in Designing an Injury Prevention Program

Jeff Snodgrass, PhD, MPH, OTR/L

Work and industry is a well-established area of practice for occupational therapy practitioners. Because the profession has always been strongly grounded in work as a central occupation, occupational therapy practitioners are found in a variety of settings where they intervene with people who have acquired a work-related injury. Traditional venues include outpatient settings, either hospital based or freestanding, and inpatient rehabilitation centers, as well as clients' homes and work sites (Kaskutas & Snodgrass, 2009).

This chapter describes a case study (Case Study 15.1) that poses several ethical dilemmas in an industrial work site setting. The occupational therapist in the scenario works as an independent contractor providing on-site services in a variety of work sites, including work reconditioning, preplacement tasks and job simulation for return to work, post–job offer screenings, ergonomic services (including activity and environmental modifications), and injury prevention programs. Relevant principles of the *Occupational Therapy Code of Ethics and Ethics Standards (2010)* (referred to as the "Code and Ethics Standards"; American Occupational Therapy Association [AOTA], 2010) are identified and used to help frame the ethical problems. After considering the ethical dilemmas and associated ethical tensions, the best options for addressing the dilemmas and the possible outcomes of the decisions are explored.

CASE STUDY 15.1. CONFRONTING ETHICAL DILEMMAS IN A WORK SITE PROGRAM

Susan, an occupational therapist working as an independent contractor, established a limited liability corporation (LLC) 5 years ago when she decided to leave her longtime employer to provide occupational therapy services at work sites in her region. Her contracting service was called Occupational Rehabilitation Consulting Services, LLC.

Susan enjoyed relative success with several companies by establishing comprehensive injury prevention and ergonomic programs. She presented her positive outcomes at a regional occupational safety and health symposium that was well attended by local and state health safety officials, plant managers and supervisors, and health care providers. After her presentation, she was approached by the human resources (HR) director of a midsize company in the local area that produced small engine parts for a large automobile manufacturer. The HR director was very interested in discussing Susan's recent successes with designing and implementing injury prevention programs and invited her to visit the company's facility to meet with management and safety professionals.

On her arrival at the facility, Susan was given a tour and saw firsthand the operations and production areas. Following the walkthrough of the facility,

Susan sat down with the company's president, HR director, safety and health manager, and senior production supervisor. The president expressed his concern about the company's rising work-related injury rates and resultant increase in workers' compensation claims and costs. The HR director went on to explain that over the past several years, their workers' compensation costs had skyrocketed because of coverage of medical treatment and benefits paid while their injured workers were recuperating away from work. Through their discussion, Susan determined that this company was indeed committed to reducing injuries and improving the overall quality of the work environment.

At the conclusion of this first meeting, Susan was asked if she would be willing to work with the company to design and implement a comprehensive injury prevention program. Susan replied that she would certainly consider the opportunity, but she would first need to conduct a preliminary needs assessment to determine the magnitude of the problem. Both parties (Susan and the company) agreed to draw up an initial letter of agreement (see Figure 15.1) to establish a working relationship between the manufacturing company and Susan's company.

Once the letter of agreement was signed, Susan began her work in earnest as a consultant. She requested access to their Occupational Safety and Health Administration (OSHA) Log of Work-Related Injuries and Illnesses (Form 300) for the past 3 years and overall workers' compensation costs for the same period. OSHA Form 300 logs are used to classify work-related injuries and illnesses and to note the extent and severity of each case (OSHA, 2004b). The company president initially expressed concern about revealing this information, but Susan reassured him that all information would be treated with strict confidentiality. The HR director suggested that she sign a disclosure statement to protect the company's private and sensitive information and any proprietary information she might be privy to during her needs assessment. Susan signed the disclosure statement and began reviewing the company's OSHA Form 300 logs.

Before presenting her final needs assessment analysis, Susan reviewed the latest U.S. Bureau of Labor Statistics (2010) data for cases requiring days away from work for musculoskeletal disorders by nature of injury and part of body. Susan used the national data as a means for benchmarking and comparing the company's rate of injury with the national standard.

Following the preliminary needs assessment, Susan concluded that the company had indeed had a significant number of OSHA-recordable work-related injuries over the past 3 years. In fact, she had been provided with 5 years of data from the company's workers' compensation insurance carrier, and she discovered that the company's OSHA-recordable work-related injuries amounted to hundreds of thousands of dollars in compensable workers' compensation claims. Susan's comparison of the company's injury rates with the national data from the U.S. Bureau of Labor Statistics (2010) indicated that the company's average days away from work due to musculoskeletal injuries was 8 days longer than the national average. Most of the company's OSHA-recordable injuries were related to overexertion and repetitive work. The most common injuries were to the low back (e.g., low back strains, sciatica) and upper extremities (e.g., rotator cuff tears, lateral epicondylitis, carpal tunnel syndrome). From a thorough review of the records, Susan found that the company had received several OSHA citations under the OSHA General Duty Clause (OSHA, 2004c) related to poor work station designs, excessive exposures to awkward postures and forceful exertions (e.g., lifting, pushing, pulling, and carrying), and repetitive motions.

The HR director scheduled a meeting with Susan and the safety and health manager to discuss the results of her preliminary needs assessment. This meeting revealed that the company had not addressed most of the OSHA citations. The HR director pulled Susan aside after the meeting and informed her, "You need to report all of your findings directly to me rather than sharing them with the president and other managers." He explained that it was important to first report the findings to him to create a "proper flow of information."

Susan began to design a comprehensive injury management and prevention program. She conducted a series of roundtable discussions and focus interviews with senior administration, middle management, frontline supervisors, and rank-and-file employees. From these roundtable discussions, Susan noted several emerging themes, including an organizational culture that lacked transparency and a general distrust of management among the rank-and-file employees. However, a strong theme

Susan Therapist
Occupational Rehabilitation Consulting Services, LLC

Dear President and CEO:

Thank you for the opportunity to provide my consulting services to Premier Auto Parts Manufacturing. This letter summarizes our conversation on August 15 regarding this project and will serve as the agreement between us.

I agree to perform the following services for Premier Auto Parts Manufacturing:

- Conduct preliminary analyses of injury rates through interviews with employees, a review of injury record logs, and a walkthrough of your facility.
- Form a committee comprising management representatives and frontline employees with myself as chair to guide and advise the process.
- Perform comprehensive ergonomics evaluations on workstations identified as potential or known problem areas.
- Develop a series of recommendations to minimize or prevent work-related musculoskeletal disorders.
- Perform additional related tasks as mutually agreed on by the president and me.

In consideration for my performance of these services, you agree to pay me at the rate of $85.00 per hour. I will be paid the amount of $1,000.00 on September 1, after which date I will begin work on the project. Upon completion of the project, I will submit an invoice that totals my hours on this project, multiplies them by my hourly rate of $85.00, and subtracts the amount advanced on September 1 from the total. The total remaining amount will be due within 30 business days after the date on the invoice.

If this agreement accurately summarizes the terms of our earlier conversation, please sign below on this and the attached copy. Retain one copy for your records and return one to me.

Best regards,

Susan Therapist, MS, OTR/L
Occupational Rehabilitation Consulting Services, LLC

Agreed to by:

Premier Auto Parts Manufacturing

FIGURE 15.1

Sample letter of agreement between a work site occupational therapy consultant and an auto parts manufacturing company.

that reverberated during these discussions was acknowledgment that the status quo was no longer acceptable and assurance by all stakeholders that they were willing to make the commitment to reimagine their company as a leader in workplace safety and as an employee-supportive work environment.

Following the roundtable discussions and focus interviews, Susan formed a Safety and Health for Injury Prevention (SHIP) committee. All levels of the organization were represented on the SHIP commit-

tee, and Susan was chair. Ground rules established for committee meetings included the following:

- All ideas are worthy.
- Critical debate on the issues at hand should be seen as important and necessary.
- Personal attacks and insults are forbidden.
- Everyone must contribute to the process and allow his or her voice to be heard.
- Inaction is unacceptable. Recommendations to reduce, if not ameliorate, the company's

work-related injury rates is the goal of the committee.

The initial, rollout phase of the program involved management and select employees, as agreed on by the SHIP committee. The committee targeted one part of the manufacturing area, which included two shift supervisors and 12 employees. Working directly with the supervisors and employees, Susan conducted ergonomic evaluations on each of the four small-parts assembly workstations. Following the evaluations, she first presented the findings to the HR director. Although he expressed concern regarding her findings, he agreed that she should present her findings to the SHIP committee, discuss issues and concerns, and then begin problem solving and implementing solutions with the employees.

The full phase-in of the program began once the initial phase was successfully completed. At this stage Susan started experiencing significant resistance from the HR director and safety and health manager, both of whom were members of the SHIP committee. Their resistance mostly came in the form of expressions of concern regarding her findings. The HR director and safety and health manager were concerned that Susan's findings were too critical of the company's current work practices and that her findings would create potential OSHA violations that could lead to citations. At first, Susan believed the resistance she encountered was merely the typical resistance to change she had seen in many other companies where she implemented similar programs. Susan had learned that change does not come easy in most instances, and part of her job was to cultivate and facilitate a culture of change to enable her programs to be successful.

One day, however, Susan was invited to a meeting with the HR director and safety and health manager to "discuss progress to date." During the meeting, they informed Susan that the company was concerned because her program had identified several deficiencies (excessive repetitive motions, forceful exertions, and awkward postures involving the upper extremities) on their small-parts assembly line that might be "red flags" to OSHA and the state's occupational and safety health administration. In addition, since the initial implementation of the program, the company had experienced a significant increase in employees reporting musculoskeletal discomfort and other OSHA-recordable injuries, and they worried that this increase would trigger an inspection by a state health compliance officer to investigate the increase. The HR director and safety and health manager asked Susan to refocus her program to encourage employees to "work through the pain and discomfort" rather than report their injuries so the company could meet the production schedule and minimize the number of recordable injuries while implementing the program.

Susan realized that she faced a dilemma that was beginning to cause significant ethical tension. She decided to address the ethical tensions by applying a process for making ethical decisions.

ETHICAL DECISION MAKING

Ethical decision making is akin to decision making with a client; it includes evaluation, development of an intervention plan, and assessment of outcomes (AOTA, 2008). Most ethical decision-making frameworks or models follow similar steps (see Chapter 10, this volume). The process for analyzing ethical problems used in this chapter combines Purtilo and Doherty's (2011) and Thomas's (2004) frameworks into the following six-step process:

1. Gather relevant information, and identify key issues.
2. Identify the type of ethical problem, and clarify the facts.
3. Analyze the problems, and identify the stakeholders.
4. Explore the practical alternatives and possible courses of action.
5. Select and complete the best course of action.
6. Evaluate the process and outcomes.

Susan's situation is not unique for health care professionals; occupational therapy practitioners face ethical dilemmas on a daily basis. When faced with a dilemma, one must take care not to allow emotions to overrule an objective examination of the situation at hand. To adequately and appropriately address the ethical tensions described in the case study, Susan applied the six-step process to help her remain objective and exercise sound judgment.

Gather Relevant Information and Identify Key Issues

Susan faced several possible issues that she felt compelled to address before moving forward with her program. Susan reflected on the situation and identified three essential issues.

First, Susan determined that failing to inform the company's senior administration about the risk factors she identified was a problem. She recalled the HR director's directive to report all findings directly to him rather than sharing them with the president and other managers. She now wondered if this process of reporting was typical procedure or reflected a culture of silence and lack of transparency. She believed that the SHIP committee was the place to address and discuss her findings, which in turn were reported to the president via meeting minutes and reports.

Second, Susan considered the company's history of OSHA violations that had gone unresolved. Susan recognized her responsibility to confront the key stakeholders in the company because of her belief that the company had a duty and legal obligation to address OSHA citations. Susan also knew that this discussion might be unpleasant and could have negative consequences.

Finally, Susan was concerned about the HR director's request that she refocus her program to encourage employees to "work through pain and discomfort" rather than reporting their injuries in order to maintain the production schedule and minimize reports of recordable injuries. Susan understood from her educational background and practice experience that it's common for workers in labor-intensive jobs to experience a certain amount of pain and discomfort. However, she also understood that workers who experience significant pain and discomfort are at much greater risk for developing a work-related musculoskeletal disorder (Zuccarello, 2010). In fact, she knew that epidemiological studies have found a strong correlation between exposures to work-related risk factors (e.g., forceful exertions and repetitive motions) and musculoskeletal injuries (e.g., Kaskutas & Snodgrass, 2009).

Identify the Type of Ethical Problem and Clarify the Facts

As a member of AOTA, Susan was bound by the Code and Ethics Standards, which had been adopted by her state regulatory board. She used the Code and Ethics Standards as a resource and guide to help identify the ethical problems she encountered. Susan determined that the following ethical principles had been or might be violated: Principle 1, Beneficence; Principle 5, Procedural Justice; and Principle 6, Veracity.

Principle 1: Beneficence

Susan was especially concerned that the company had received numerous citations from the state's occupational safety and health administration and OSHA that had gone unresolved. Thus, she believed that segments of the company were acting unethically. This belief stemmed from Principle 1M of the Code and Ethics Standards, which states the need to "report to appropriate authorities any acts in practice, education, and research that appear unethical or illegal" (AOTA, 2010, p. S19). In addition, the HR director's request that she advise workers to work through pain and discomfort violated Principle 1B, which obligates practitioners to "provide appropriate evaluation and a plan of intervention for all recipients of occupational therapy services specific to their needs" (AOTA, 2010, p. S19). Susan feared that asking employees to work through their pain was similar to asking them to ignore what could be a sign of a significant problem, especially in light of the evidence of a connection between exposure to work-related risk factors, reported discomfort, and the development of musculoskeletal injuries.

Principle 5: Procedural Justice

Susan's conversations with the HR director and safety and health manager led her to fear that the company was failing to follow both state and federal rules. In addition, she believed that not reporting her concerns to the company's president compromised her integrity and the ethical principle of Procedural Justice. After reviewing the Code and Ethics Standards, Susan believed she risked violating Principle 5B—"be familiar with and seek to understand and abide by institutional rules, and when those rules conflict with ethical practice, take steps to resolve the conflict" (AOTA, 2010, p. S22)—and Principle 5N—"actively participate with employers in the formulation of policies and procedures to ensure legal, regulatory, and ethical compliance" (p. S23). Therefore, Susan felt compelled to highlight to senior administration where the potential violation of rules existed and encourage the formulation of appropriate policies and procedures to ameliorate the violations.

Principle 6: Veracity

The lack of truthfulness was Susan's most significant concern. She believed that on several occasions she had been asked to hide her findings by sharing them with only a select few and to discourage employees from reporting problems. Susan realized that she would violate Principle 6B if she complied with these requests; Principle 6B of the Code and Ethics Standards obligates practitioners to "refrain from using or participating in the use of any form of communication that contains false, fraudulent, deceptive, misleading, or unfair statements or claims" (AOTA, 2010, p. S24).

Analyze the Problems and Identify the Stakeholders

Susan identified the key stakeholders in this situation as herself, the HR director, the safety and health manager, members of the SHIP committee, frontline employees, and the president. Susan used two perspectives on ethics—human rights and utilitarianism—to provide insight into the situation and help resolve her ethical tension (Thomas, 2004). Weighing these two perspectives helped Susan gain a clearer picture of the situation and decide on her best course of action.

From the human rights perspective, Susan recognized the importance of maintaining the dignity of all of those involved and her obligation to protect those most vulnerable to work-related injuries (i.e., the frontline workers) if it all possible. Susan believed that being asked to "work through the pain" compromised the frontline workers' dignity by discouraging them from reporting their symptoms and discomfort.

Using the utilitarian perspective, Susan looked at the potential consequences of her action (and inaction) and how each action would affect the entire company. She determined that the overall benefits of implementing her program far outweighed the potential costs of ignoring workers' reported symptoms and suppressing findings from the president. In fact, Susan had presented this cost–benefit analysis to the key stakeholders when she initially presented her program. She cited numerous empirical studies that found a significant return on investment when companies implemented comprehensive injury prevention programs.

Susan also considered the laws, rules, and regulations that govern workplace safety. Susan was very familiar with the federal Occupational Safety and Health Act of 1970, which requires that employers provide their employees with working conditions that are free of known dangers (OSHA, 2004a). Workers have the right to a safe work environment that is free from conditions that pose a risk of serious harm. Thus, Susan knew that the company was bound by federal law to provide workers with a safe work environment and to address any known issues.

In addition to incorporating ethical perspectives and considering issues of jurisprudence, Susan also found it helpful to draw on prior experiences from her own work and the work of trusted colleagues in the field. This action is a recommended strategy when facing ethical challenges (Thomas, 2004). After doing some background investigation and networking with several colleagues and recognized experts in the field of industrial rehabilitation, Susan found an emerging theme of resistance by employers to acknowledge and address identified risk factors shared by others who had faced similar dilemmas.

Explore the Practical Alternatives and Possible Courses of Action

After much critical thought and deliberation, Susan developed a list of possible courses of action she could take to address the identified ethical issues:

- Do nothing; simply continue to implement the program and keep her concerns to herself.
- Confront the HR director about his insistence on keeping information from the president.
- Raise her concerns and identified issues in a SHIP committee meeting and perhaps together devise a plan of action to deal with the issues at hand.

- Work with frontline employees on program implementation despite the lack of support from the HR director and safety and health manager.
- Meet with the president and share her concerns about the suppression of information and lack of support for the program.
- Report the company's violations directly to OSHA and the state regulatory agency.

Select and Complete the Best Course of Action

Susan spent the better part of a weekend considering the key issues, identifying and analyzing the ethical problems, and detailing possible courses of action. She decided to schedule a one-on-one meeting with the company president to share her concerns. During the meeting, Susan was able to objectively present the key issues, the identified ethical issues, and what she believed were the best strategies to address her concerns in order to continue with her program's implementation. The president expressed concern about the suppression of findings and the lack of transparency in the organization. He informed Susan that he wished to meet with her and the SHIP committee to establish an open and honest dialogue regarding the issues and solutions.

After meeting with the president, Susan called a meeting of the SHIP committee and president. The meeting was very difficult for Susan to lead and facilitate, but in the end she was able to establish an open and honest dialogue between the key stakeholders concerning the ongoing implementation of the program. Following this meeting, members of the SHIP committee reached a consensus, and Susan felt confident that the implementation of her program would proceed as planned.

Evaluate the Process and Outcomes

Susan spent time reflecting on and evaluating the process she used to resolve her ethical dilemma. Susan compared and contrasted the ethical issues with this company with her past experience in similar situations. She scheduled a lunch meeting with her mentor to further discuss and consider how she handled the situation and what, if anything, she should have done differently. She and her mentor came to the re-

alization that Susan did indeed handle the situation appropriately by addressing the issue directly with the company's president. However, her mentor provided one suggestion for consideration should she be faced with this type of ethical dilemma in the future. Susan's mentor suggested that Susan always include in her initial meetings with prospective clients the need for transparency and veracity of reporting when discussing any and all ergonomic assessment findings and recommendations. Her mentor noted that the potential for ethical dilemmas is always present, but using strong communication skills is critical to successful resolution of dilemmas.

CONCLUSION

Susan arrived at a satisfactory conclusion following a formal process of ethical decision making. The process involved gathering relevant information, identifying the ethical problems, applying ethical perspectives to analyze the problems, identifying stakeholders, exploring alternatives, selecting the best course of action, and evaluating the outcomes. This systematic process for ethical problem solving can help occupational therapy practitioners practicing in work site (and other) settings address and resolve ethical issues.

REFERENCES

American Occupational Therapy Association. (2008). Occupational therapy practice framework: Domain and process (2nd ed.). *American Journal of Occupational Therapy, 62,* 625–683. doi: 10.5014/ajot.62.6.625

American Occupational Therapy Association. (2010). Occupational therapy code of ethics and ethics standards (2010). *American Journal of Occupational Therapy, 64*(6 Suppl.), S17–S26. doi: 10.5014/ajot.2010.64S17

Kaskutas, V., & Snodgrass, J. (2009). *Occupational therapy practice guidelines for individuals with work-related injuries and illnesses.* Bethesda, MD: AOTA Press.

Occupational Safety and Health Administration. (2004a). *Occupational Safety and Health Act of 1970.* Retrieved from www.osha.gov/pls/oshaweb/owasrch.search_form?p_doc_type=OSHACT&p_toc_level=0&p_keyvalue=&p_status=CURRENT

Occupational Safety and Health Administration. (2004b). *OSHA forms for recording work-related injuries and illnesses.* Retrieved from www.osha.gov/record keeping/new-osha300form1-1-04.pdf

Occupational Safety and Health Administration. (2004c). *Sec. 5, Duties.* Retrieved from www.osha. gov/pls/oshaweb/owadisp.show_document?p_ table=OSHACT&p_id=3359

Purtilo, R., & Doherty, R. F. (2011). *Ethical dimensions in the health professions* (5th ed.). Philadelphia: Elsevier.

Thomas, J. C. (2004). *Public health ethics modules.* Retrieved from http://oce.sph.unc.edu/phethics/index.htm

U.S. Bureau of Labor Statistics. (2010). *Case and demographic characteristics for work-related injuries and illnesses involving days away from work.* Retrieved from www.bls.gov/iif/oshcdnew.htm

Zuccarello, V. (2010, September). The use of ergonomic analysis in medical causation cases to support or debunk compensability claims for musculoskeletal disorders. *Work and Industry Special Interest Section Quarterly, 24*(3), 1–4.

Participation, Disability, and Rehabilitation

16

Barbara L. Kornblau, JD, OTR, FAOTA

Ethical issues that may arise during the practice of occupational therapy in the rehabilitation context are discussed in this chapter. Occupational therapy practitioners do not "therapitize" their clients. Rather, occupational therapy is an interactive, client-centered process. This belief is clearly articulated in Principle 3 of the *Occupational Therapy Code of Ethics and Ethics Standards (2010)* (referred to as the "Code and Ethics Standards"; American Occupational Therapy Association [AOTA], 2010). It is the ethical responsibility of occupational therapy practitioners to "respect the right of the individual to self-determination" (AOTA, 2010, p. S20).

This responsibility is accomplished through a collaborative process involving jointly proposed interventions by the occupational therapy practitioner and the client that are occupation based (AOTA, 2008, 2010). As an interactive process, occupational therapy in the rehabilitation context involves a dynamic balance among the rights, responsibilities, and duties of both the occupational therapy practitioner and the recipient of services.

In this chapter, this dynamic balance is explored through a series of case studies after relevant terms are defined and potential ethical issues are identified. The case studies involve typical scenarios that occur in occupational therapy practice, as well as potential future situations that may result from changes in health and disability policy, such as the Patient Protection and Affordable Care Act (ACA; 2010) and the Americans With Disabilities Act (ADA) amendments (Americans With Disabilities Act of 1990, as amended; ADA).

RELEVANT TERMINOLOGY

Three terms crucial to the discussion of client-centered care in rehabilitation are defined to help establish the foundation for the case studies. These terms are *participation, disability,* and *rehabilitation*. The discussion of the term *disability* is the most extensive of the three and includes a review of different philosophical models as well as a discussion of issues resulting from the multiple definitions of the term.

Participation

The World Health Organization (WHO; 2002) defines *participation* as "involvement in a life situation" (p. 10). The *Occupational Therapy Practice Framework: Domain and Process* (AOTA, 2008) incorporates principles found in the WHO's (2001) *International Classification of Functioning, Disability and Health* (ICF) and uses some *ICF* definitions, such as the definition of *participation* (AOTA, 2008, p. 660). The World

Bank defines *activities* as "basic deliberate actions undertaken in order to accomplish a task, such as getting dressed or feeding oneself" (Mont, 2007, p. 3) and *participation* as "activities that are integral to economic and social life and the social roles that accomplish that life, such as being able to attend school or hold a job" (pp. 3–4).

The outcome of client-centered occupational therapy intervention is increased participation in activities or occupations considered by the client to be important or meaningful (AOTA, 2010). Occupational therapy researchers often study client outcomes for specific conditions in terms of participation (Kim & Colantonio, 2010).

Disability

Disability is a more complicated term, and definitions vary. Many definitions exist, and the definition used in a given instance depends on attitudes, context, or policy.

Some view disability through an internally focused lens, which looks at people with a disability as the root cause of their own functional limitations, whereas others focus on external factors in society that place barriers in the way of people with disabilities and their ability to function. Historically, several categorical definitions of disability have come from several models, including the moral model, the tragedy/charity model, the medical model, the rehabilitation model, the disability or empowerment model, the social model, the occupational therapy model, and the rights model.

Moral Model and Tragedy/Charity Models

One example of an older, outdated model still followed in some cultures is the *moral* model, which associates disability with sin, shame, and guilt (Kaplan, 2010). According to this philosophy, a person has a disabling condition as the result of a moral transgression committed by that person or a family member. A related model, called either the *tragedy* or *charity* model, assumes that people with disabilities need to be taken care of, require charity, and deserve to be pitied (Disabled World, 2010b; Landmine Survivors Network [LSN], 2007).

Both models connote a negative view of the person. Neither model considers the competence

of people with a disability, instead taking a paternalistic view of them. People seen in this light are perceived as being unable to do anything for themselves. A contemporary example of an organization using this view of disability is Jerry's Kids. The treatment of children on the muscular dystrophy telethon reflects a focus on encouraging pity to raise money for the children's care.

Medical Model

Proponents of the *medical* model provide another disempowering definition of disability focusing on the person (Disabled World, 2010c; Kaplan, 2010; LSN, 2007). Advocates of the medical model view disability as a health issue arising from and residing in the person and resulting in his or her inability to function (Mont, 2007). This perspective stems from a view that illness needs to be cured or fixed. The emphasis is on the belief that a physician or other health care provider is empowered to "correct" the disability without regard for the societal barriers people with disabilities face (Disabled World, 2010b; Kaplan, 2010; LSN, 2007).

Use of the medical model, like use of the charity and moral models, tends to isolate these people. Those who use the medical model treat people with disabilities as sick and encourage care in hospital and institutional environments rather than empowering them to participate in the community (LSN, 2007).

Rehabilitation Model

Like those who ascribe to the medical model definition of disability, the proponents of the *rehabilitation* model, also called the *expert* or *professional* model, define a person with a disability as one who needs interventions from a rehabilitation professional to make up for "deficiency" caused by the disability (Kaplan, 2010; LSN, 2007). As in previously discussed definitions, the person with a disability is seen through a lens focused on the person's deficits.

Rehabilitation professionals who follow this approach believe that they know what a person needs solely on the basis of an assessment of the person's impairment. The expert acts for the passive client, creating a rehabilitation system that may be authoritative or paternalistic in nature and may fail to consider the principle of self-determination. Today's vocational rehabilitation system is an example of this model in action (Disabled World, 2010b; Kaplan, 2010).

Disability or Empowerment Model

Proponents of the *disability* or *empowerment* model view disability as a "normal aspect of life" as opposed to a defective or deviant aspect of life (Kaplan, 2010). Those using this model view disability as a result of factors external to the person. Disability is a function of inadequate support services; "attitudinal, architectural, sensory, cognitive, and economic barriers" (Kaplan, 2010, para. 6); and the stigma born of the tendency of those without disabilities to generalize about those who have disabilities in spite of the spectrum of variations within the disability community (Kaplan, 2010).

Service providers who ascribe to this model, such as occupational therapy practitioners, empower people with disabilities to make their own decisions about the intervention and services they want. Service providers act in a consultative role to provide guidance to empower a person with a disability to achieve his or her own goals in spite of the external barriers imposed by society (Disabled World, 2010b).

Social Model

The *social* model of disability is the model most closely related to an occupational therapy perspective on disability. The social model defines disability in a broader context and integrates the internal and external foci. A condition may cause an impairment that limits a person's ability to function and participate in everyday life, but society causes the disability by placing barriers in the way (Disabled World, 2010c). Disability comprises a complex set of factors that arise from the social environment, such as physical barriers in the environment, that intentionally or unintentionally exclude people with disabilities (Disabled World, 2010a).

Within the social model, disability is viewed as "arising from the interaction of a person's functional status with the physical, cultural, and policy environments" (Mont, 2007, p. 2). The concept of disability as an outcome of the interaction between a person and the environment is prominent in this model (Mont, 2007). Whereas the medical model is person specific and the disability model is heavily focused on the environment, the social model "is neither person nor environment specific" (Mont, 2007, p. 3).

Occupational Therapy Model

The *occupational therapy* model of disability that has evolved since the profession's inception involves application and expansion of the social model. Occupational therapy professionals look at disability in terms of function and participation as defined by the WHO (2010a; see also AOTA, 2008). The WHO has defined *disability* as

> an umbrella term, covering impairments, activity limitations, and participation restrictions. An impairment is a problem in body function or structure; an activity limitation is a difficulty encountered by an individual in executing a task or action; while a participation restriction is a problem experienced by an individual in involvement in life situations. (WHO, 2010a, para. 1)

The WHO views disability as "a complex phenomenon, reflecting an interaction between features of a person's body and features of the society in which he or she lives" (WHO, 2010a, para. 2). Disability, according to occupational therapy theory, is a result of the dynamic interaction among the person, the environment, and the tasks the person wants to perform or goals for greater societal participation (AOTA, 2008; Law et al., 1996).

Rights Model

The *rights* model of disability put forth by the United Nations is an extension of the social model. The disability rights movement advocates for equality for people with disabilities in many areas, including housing, education, employment, full inclusion in society, and other social and political contexts. In the United States, this movement resulted in the passage of the ADA in 1990, the

Individuals With Disabilities Education Act (IDEA; 1990), and the Fair Housing Act Amendments (1988), among other laws and policies. On an international level, the disability community facilitated the development of the Universal Declaration of Human Rights, which set a baseline standard for human rights recognizing the "inherent dignity and . . . the equal and inalienable rights of all members of the human family" (United Nations, 1948, para. 1) and advocating for people with disabilities to have these same rights. In 2006, the United Nations formally adopted the Convention on the Rights of Persons with Disabilities (CRPD), an international treaty to give all people with and without disabilities the same rights (United Nations, n.d.).

The United Nations also defines disability in terms of participation in society, but it adds the concept of *participation* on an equal basis. In the CRPD, *disability* is described as "an evolving concept" that "results from the interaction between persons with impairments and attitudinal and environmental barriers that hinder their full and effective participation in society on an equal basis with others" (United Nations, n.d., para. 5).

Proponents of the rights model view a person with a disability as a "rights holder" entitled to determine the course of his or her own life like other members of society (LSN, 2007). Barriers such as architectural or attitudinal barriers that society places in the way of people with disabilities—whether intentionally or unintentionally—are viewed as violations of basic human rights, thereby transforming the *needs* of people with disabilities into *rights* to which they are entitled (LSN, 2007).

Ethics Issues Presented by Definitions of Disability

The various models of disability present different definitions of disability, each of which raises ethical concerns. Although the moral and charity models are outdated and are not embraced by the occupational therapy profession, some practitioners may have been raised with these values or may live in cultures that still subscribe to them. Even though occupational therapy education attempts to change students' view of disability to one of empowerment and respect for the right of people to self-determination (see Principle 3 of the

Code and Ethics Standards), sometimes ingrained values still influence practitioners' actions.

Occupational therapy practitioners may find themselves tempted to function in a medical model, viewing themselves in the role of "fixer" instead of showing respect for the client's right to self-determination and decision making as indicated by Principle 3 of the Code and Ethics Standards. The medical model is antithetical to the emphasis in the Code and Ethics Standards on autonomy and self-determination, as is the rehabilitation model, which also promotes paternalistic views of decision making for the client or clients rather than self-determination.

Impact of Multiple Definitions of Disability

In the world of health and disability policy, multiple definitions of disability make the development of policy difficult and confusing. The federal government has a plethora of definitions of disability depending on the funding source or federal program (Adler, 1991). For example, Social Security determines disability benefits on the basis of a strict definition of whether or not a person can work (Social Security Administration, 2010). Within the IDEA, disability is defined using a list of specific impairments. If a child has one of those impairments (e.g., autism, orthopedic impairment) and requires special education and related services, then the child is considered a "child with a disability" (IDEA, 1990, §602(3)).

This conceptualization differs greatly from that used in the ADA (1990), which provides a much broader definition that takes into account a person's ability to participate in major life activities:

(1) Disability. The term "disability" means, with respect to an individual—
  (A) a physical or mental impairment that substantially limits one or more major life activities of such individual;
  (B) a record of such an impairment; or
  (C) being regarded as having such an impairment. (§3)

Multiple definitions of disability present unique issues for occupational therapy researchers, service providers, and educators. Researchers who study the impact of disability or the effect of an occupational therapy intervention on a group must select a definition of disability to apply to potential participants. Those who seek to perform a meta-analysis, a systematic review, or comparative effectiveness research on the same topic must be aware that previous investigators may have used different definitions of disability; definitions may have changed over time; and multiple, different definitions may be in use at any one time (Adler, 1991; Mont, 2007; U.S. Census Bureau, 2009).

Students may find keeping track of multiple definitions of disability daunting. For example, a pediatrics professor may teach one definition of disability according to the IDEA, a class on physical disabilities may use a different definition, classes on environmental modifications may use another, and classes on job analysis may use the Social Security definition.

The multiple definitions of disability affect how occupational therapy practitioners view people with disabilities and, consequently, how they behave around and treat people with disabilities. For example, those who view people with disabilities under the moral or charity model of disability will likely treat clients, research participants, and students with disabilities paternalistically because these models disempower or limit people with disabilities. Attitudes of family members toward people with disabilities may influence how occupational therapy direct service providers, researchers, and educators treat those people as their clients, research participants, or students.

The policy-related definitions also affect occupational therapy clinical service delivery. Who qualifies for occupational therapy services? What definition of disability qualifies a person for benefits, and for which benefits? Researchers must use care in deciding on the definition they use to determine whether people qualify as participants. How can educators make reasonable accommodations to their programs for students with disabilities if they are not sure which students qualify as individuals with disabilities? Which definitions do they teach to students for which practice areas?

Rehabilitation

The WHO has described rehabilitation as an important process that facilitates participation and promotes the right to self-determination for people with disabilities. The WHO stated that "rehabilitation of people with disabilities is a process aimed at enabling them to reach and maintain their optimal physical, sensory, intellectual, psychological and social functional levels" (WHO, 2010b, para. 1). Rehabilitation provides people with disabilities "with the tools they need to attain independence and self-determination" (WHO, 2010b, para. 1).

According to the WHO, the United Nations, and other international organizations, "rehabilitation is now viewed as a process in which people with disabilities or their advocates make decisions about what services they need to enhance participation," and in addition, "rehabilitation services should no longer be imposed without the consent and participation of people who are using the services" (International Labour Organization [ILO]; United Nations Educational, Scientific and Cultural Organization [UNESCO]; & WHO, 2004, p. 3). This empowerment model reminds us that "professionals who provide rehabilitation services have the responsibility to provide relevant information to people with disabilities so that they can make informed decisions regarding what is appropriate for them" (ILO, UNESCO, & WHO, 2004, p. 4).

The WHO's definition and viewpoint are represented in Principle 3 of the Code and Ethics Standards. Principle 3 states that "occupational therapy personnel shall respect the right of the individual to self-determination" (AOTA, 2010, p. S20). Self-determination is a key principle of rehabilitation. People with disabilities should have the right to enter into a collaborative relationship with occupational therapy practitioners, as described in Principle 3A. Proposed interventions must be shared with clients or their advocates so they can make informed decisions about what they see as appropriate for them to reach their own goals.

CHANGING HEALTH AND DISABILITY POLICIES

Federal, state, and local laws and policies affect the practice of occupational therapy. Laws cover many aspects of occupational therapy practice and patient care, including privacy, reimbursement, and even the size of the sign one can display outside a practice or clinic. Principle 5 of the Code and Ethics Standards states that "occupational therapy personnel shall comply with institutional rules, local, state, federal, and international laws and AOTA documents applicable to the profession of occupational therapy" (AOTA, 2010, p. S22). In practice, this means that occupational therapy practitioners have an ethical obligation to familiarize themselves with changes in laws that affect occupational therapy service delivery, education, and research.

For example, the ADA was amended in 2008 to make up for limitations the Supreme Court had placed on the impact of the ADA. In 1999, the Supreme Court had decided three cases in one day that severely restricted the employment rights of people with disabilities under the ADA by narrowing the definition of who could be considered an individual with a disability (*Albertsons, Inc., v. Kirkingburg,* 1999, 527 U.S. 55; *Murphy v. United Parcel Service, Inc.,* 1999, 527 U.S. 516; *Sutton v. United Air Lines, Inc.,* 1999, 527 U.S. 472). The 2008 ADA amendments afforded protection to more people with disabilities, increasing their ability to participate in work and other meaningful activities. The changes broadened the reach of the ADA to include more people under the definition of individuals with disabilities and, in particular, those whom Congress originally intended to be covered by the act (ADA Amendments Act of 2008).

The ACA (2010), the U.S. health care reform law, also will affect people with disabilities and occupational therapy practice. People with disabilities who previously could not purchase insurance will be able to do so on the exchanges and will no longer face discrimination in employer-based insurance (see §1201 *et seq.*). The essential benefits package for insurance plans sold on the exchanges includes rehabilitation and habilitation. Before the ACA, many insurance plans did not cover habilitation. With an expectation that 30 million more people will be covered and that rehabilitation and habilitation will be included in the basic benefits package, occupational therapy practitioners will likely see more demand for services.

The ACA also calls for teaching cultural competence to health professionals at all levels and, for the first time, specifically includes disabilities

awareness under the umbrella of cultural competence (see §5307). Occupational therapy educators and practitioners, in concert with their patients and clients with disabilities, can play a role in developing new curricula to address this need.

The U.S. government will promulgate more rules and regulations required by the ACA that will affect occupational therapy practice. Principle 4 of the Code and Ethics Standards, Social Justice, speaks to the ethical obligation to advocate for just and fair treatment of clients. Occupational therapy practitioners are also encouraged to look beyond touching the lives of individual clients or families by engaging in education that promotes the health and well-being of the broader community. In addition, Principle 4E clearly supports practitioners' advocacy role in giving input and feedback as new government regulations are developed.

The preceding discussion provides merely a few examples of contemporary policy changes that affect occupational therapy practice. A respected, nonpartisan source for learning more about changes in health care policy and law is the Henry J. Kaiser Family Foundation (2011), an independent source from Kaiser Permanente; resources are available at www.kff.org.

CASE STUDIES

Work in rehabilitation often presents occupational therapy practitioners with ethical dilemmas, especially in a world where health care and disability policy are constantly changing. Four typical examples of how ethical dilemmas may arise in practice and how occupational therapists can address the issues are presented in this section (Case Studies 16.1–16.4).

CASE STUDY 16.1. ADVOCATING FOR CLIENT AUTONOMY

Mrs. Washington, a 72-year-old woman, was recovering from a stroke. She was able to participate in more meaningful and necessary occupations and was looking forward to returning to live in her own home. She and her occupational therapist, **Olive**, discussed the tasks she needed to be able to do to live at home, and they practiced those activities with assistive technology as part of her rehabilitation program. They planned to do a home visit, but Mrs. Washington's adult daughter did not agree with the plan because she preferred that her mother live in a nursing home, where she would be safer. She didn't want her mother to return to her own home because she was worried her mother might "fall or something." Mrs. Washington's daughter appealed to Olive: "Please, help me convince my mother that she is not safe living at home. I want her in a nursing home or assisted living facility where she will be supervised."

This situation raised many concerns for the occupational therapist. Olive knew that Mrs. Washington could live alone, but pursuant to Principle 1, Beneficence, of the Code and Ethics Standards, she was concerned for Mrs. Washington's well-being and safety. She planned a home assessment collaboratively with Mrs. Washington; together, they set short-term goals to meet the ultimate goal of returning home. Mrs. Washington could complete the tasks she needed to in order to live independently and demonstrated this in the simulated clinic apartment. On the basis of her assessment, Olive was confident that Mrs. Washington would not be in any danger if she returned to her own home, but she wanted to do the actual home assessment to be absolutely sure that Mrs. Washington would be safe. This action comports with Principle 1, Beneficence, of the Code and Ethics Standards, which provides an ethical obligation to demonstrate "a concern for the well-being and safety of the recipients" of services (AOTA, 2010, p. S18). Moreover, Principle 1B (appropriate evaluation and plan of intervention) supports an occupational therapist in performing a home assessment to meet a client's specific needs.

Mrs. Washington's daughter's request, although it reflected what she believed was best for her mother, may have been an unconscious attempt to interfere with her mother's autonomy and replace her mother's wishes with her own. Principle 3, Autonomy, Confidentiality, asserts the occupational therapist's ethical obligation to respect a service recipient's right to self-determination. Mrs. Washington was the recipient of service to whom Olive's ethical obligations applied, not her daughter. Although it would be an uncomfortable conversation, Olive was obligated to inform Mrs. Washington's daughter that she could not encourage Mrs. Washington to

change her wishes without medical reason because Mrs. Washington had a right to self-determination. Olive's responsibility was to see that Mrs. Washington could exercise that right.

CASE STUDY 16.2. ADDRESSING CONFLICT OF INTEREST AND CONFLICT OF COMMITMENT

Ahmed was a 35-year-old man who had survived a serious hit-and-run car accident that left him with a spinal cord injury and quadriplegia at the C-7 level. He had lived in a nursing home since his accident 5 years previously because his aging mother could not care for him at home. The lone young adult in a nursing home filled with elders, Ahmed wanted to work and live in the community like other people his age. He believed that to enable him to live in the community, all he needed was some assistance, such as personal assistant services, after he relearned some basic instrumental activities of daily living.

Ahmed's wishes were closer to reality under the ACA, which provides incentives for states to provide services to people in the community through the Community First Choice Option (see §2401). This option enables state Medicaid plans to choose home- and community-based services and supports as the rule rather than the exception. This option applies to Medicaid-eligible people with disabilities with incomes up to 150% of the federal poverty level who would otherwise require institutional or nursing home care. As an incentive to states to choose this option, states that opt in receive an additional 6% of the federal government's share of Medicaid costs (referred to as the Federal Matching Assistance Percentage) for 5 years (Isaacs, Morris, & Kornblau, 2011). Ahmed's state had announced plans to participate in the Community First Choice Option.

Ahmed consulted with **Alyssa**, the nursing home's occupational therapist. He wanted her to assist him in becoming more independent in many of the skills he had learned during his rehabilitation program 5 years ago but that he had not had an opportunity to use in the nursing home, such as meal preparation. He wanted Alyssa to work with him to prepare him for community living. He spoke to his physician and obtained the necessary occupational therapy referral.

This situation presented an ethical dilemma for Alyssa. She identified a potential conflict of commitment between her client's interest in preparing to live in the community and her employer's interest in his remaining in the nursing home. Her employer, the nursing home owner, was in business to make money and made that money by keeping beds filled. In fact, the owner of the facility had lobbied Congress against the Community First Choice Option part of ACA. It was not in the employer's best interest for Ahmed to move out of the facility and into the community; therefore, occupational therapy intervention was contrary to the employer's interests.

However, Ahmed had a right to live in the community (*Olmstead v. L.C.,* 1999, 527 U.S. 581), and the ACA gave him some tools for self-empowerment. In a collaborative relationship, Alyssa could provide Ahmed with the remaining tools he needed to realize his goal of living in the community. Principle 3 of the Code and Ethics Standards instilled in Alyssa the duty to respect Ahmed's right to autonomy and self-determination. Moreover, under Principle 1A, Alyssa had a duty to respond to Ahmed's referral for occupational therapy services in a timely manner because Ahmed had a right to intervention. Occupational therapy practitioners also have an ethical obligation or duty to look out for the well-being of service recipients, so Alyssa had an obligation to Ahmed.

In contrast, Principle 7E, Fidelity, of the Code and Ethics Standards imposes an ethical obligation to avoid conflicts of interest or commitment in employment. Alyssa's duty to work with Ahmed so he could live in the community was in direct conflict with her employer's wishes. At the same time, Principle 4, Social Justice, imposes an ethical duty on occupational therapy practitioners to advocate for fair and just treatment for all clients and to encourage employers to abide by the highest standards of social justice. This principle translated into an obligation for Alyssa to advocate for Ahmed with her employer to help him meet his goal of community living.

CASE STUDY 16.3. HELPING OR HARMING A RECIPIENT OF SERVICES

Robin was a 39-year-old woman with rheumatoid arthritis in numerous joints in both her lower and upper extremities. She took several medications, including a biologic, which seemed to keep her pain and symptoms under control most of the time, enabling her to work as a preschool teacher. Robin saw an occupational therapist, **Danilo**, for hand splints and activities of daily living training, which, in concert with her medications, improved her level of participation. She also worked with Danilo on ways to decrease future deformities and implement work simplification and energy conservation techniques.

Robin began to experience pain with exertion and left her job because she could no longer chase preschool children around the classroom. After 6 months, she asked Danilo for help so she could get Social Security disability benefits. As with most potential beneficiaries, her initial application had been denied. Robin had engaged an attorney, and a hearing date approached. She asked Danilo to testify at her hearing about her current functional limitations.

Danilo believed that Robin could work at something, in spite of her functional limitations, even though he knew that Social Security would probably approve Robin's application for benefits. He knew that the diagnosis of inflammatory arthritis in multiple joints with some functional limitations would meet Social Security's criteria for a person with a disability. Danilo was not sure he felt comfortable testifying because he believed that everyone should have to work and that benefits should be reserved for people with serious disabilities.

This situation presented the occupational therapist with a choice. Danilo could choose not to testify at all if he believed the testimony would harm the client. Principle 2 of the Code and Ethics Standards, Nonmaleficence, imposes an ethical obligation to refrain from actions that cause harm; the harm need not be physical in nature. Providing damaging testimony in Robin's case for benefits could be considered harm.

In contrast, Principle 1, Beneficence, imposes an ethical obligation to demonstrate concern for the well-being and safety of recipients of service. If the client meets the definition of a person with a disability under the Social Security criteria on the basis of an occupational therapist's factual, truthful testimony, then testifying may be considered responding to a request for occupational therapy services under Principle 1. Providing the testimony also is supported by Principle 4, Social Justice. Testifying would promote social justice for Robin by reflecting Danilo's "understanding of how occupational therapy service delivery can be affected by factors such as . . . disability" under Principle 4F (AOTA, 2010, p. S22).

Danilo needed to ensure, if he did provide the requested testimony, that it was accurate and objective pursuant to Principle 6, Veracity, of the Code and Ethics Standards. If Danilo could not testify truthfully in a manner that would help Robin as supported by Principle 1, Beneficence, he needed to explain that the testimony would probably cause Robin harm and, therefore, that Robin would probably not want him to testify. This disclosure would be an attempt to avoid violating Principle 2, Nonmaleficence.

In general, Danilo needed to reflect on his feelings and beliefs regarding work by people with disabilities. His beliefs may reflect outdated paternalistic models of disability that blame the person with the disability. His personal beliefs should not interfere with those of Robin or any of his clients. Principles 2E and 2G of the Code and Ethics Standards ascribe an ethical obligation to take appropriate actions to remedy personal limitations that might cause harm to Robin and to avoid situations in which the therapist "is unable to maintain clear professional boundaries or objectivity to ensure" Robin's well-being (AOTA, 2010, p. S20). Consequently, self-reflection should lead Danilo to separate his own personal beliefs about people with disabilities from Robin's case, look at the situation objectively, and focus on what is in his client's best interest.

CASE STUDY 16.4. PROMOTING CONFIDENTIALITY AND SOCIAL JUSTICE

Joaquin worked for a local manufacturing company. A veteran of Operation Iraqi Freedom, Joaquin sustained a below-knee limb loss, a traumatic brain injury (TBI), and posttraumatic stress disorder (PTSD) during his service. Under the ACA, Joaquin's employer applied for and received a grant to put a comprehensive workplace wellness program in place at the plant (ACA, 2010, see §10408). After acquiring the ACA grant, Joaquin's employer could give employees who participated in the wellness program substantial discounts on their health insurance premiums. Because of his disabilities, Joaquin was unable to participate in the workplace wellness program at the plant with his coworkers.

Joaquin called in an occupational therapist, **Maile**, as a consultant to help find some reasonable accommodations to enable him to participate in the comprehensive wellness program. He wanted to quit smoking, lower his stress level, and increase his activity level—all aspects of the program.

Obtaining a referral was not an issue because his state's licensure law allowed direct access to occupational therapy services, and Joaquin planned to pay Maile himself. Although he sought Maile's assistance, he was very concerned about disclosing his PTSD to his employer. He had heard his employer, a Vietnam War veteran, make disparaging comments about PTSD being a "whiner's syndrome." These comments made Joaquin feel very uncomfortable.

Maile accepted the assignment. She met with Joaquin and performed an assessment. Maile then contacted the employer to make an appointment to perform an assessment of the comprehensive workplace wellness program. She explained what occupational therapists do to modify the physical environment to enable people to participate in everyday tasks. Next, Maile interviewed the program director, took the appropriate measurements of the equipment, and observed the program in action. Afterward, she made an appointment to return to meet with the employer to make recommendations for reasonable accommodations to enable Joaquin to participate in the program.

At the meeting, the boss expressed his willingness to make the accommodations to the program, but he wanted to know specific information regarding Joaquin's disabilities and medical conditions. Maile informed the employer about Joaquin's limb loss and his TBI but not his PTSD, according to Joaquin's wishes. The employer agreed to make the accommodations.

Maile felt uncomfortable about revealing only part of Joaquin's story. A review of Principle 3, Autonomy, Confidentiality, of the Code and Ethics Standards showed her that, pursuant to Principles 3G and 3H, Maile had a duty to respect Joaquin's confidentiality and right to privacy and to maintain confidentiality of all communications. Joaquin gave Maile his permission to disclose his limb loss and TBI; she was ethically bound to keep the PTSD confidential. Maile was also bound by the Health Insurance Portability and Accountability Act (HIPAA) privacy regulations, which forbade her to disclose information for which she lacked Joaquin's express permission—in this case, the PTSD diagnosis (HIPAA Privacy Rules, 2007).

Maile's actions also fell within Principle 4, Social Justice, of the Code and Ethics Standards. Maile was ensuring the public good by supporting the right of a veteran with disabilities to participate in a workplace wellness program. She educated the public—Joaquin's employer—about the value of occupational therapy. Through her advocacy, she promoted activities that would benefit the health status of the community. She acted as an advocate for the fair treatment of Joaquin and assisted him in obtaining needed wellness services.

Although Maile felt uncomfortable because she revealed only part of Joaquin's diagnosis, she found comfort in Code and Ethics Standards in Principle 6, Veracity. This principle clarifies that "concepts of veracity must be carefully balanced with other potentially competing ethical principles" (AOTA, 2010, pp. S23–S24). "Veracity ultimately is valued as a means to establish trust and strengthen professional relationships. Therefore, adherence to the Principle also requires thoughtful analysis of how full disclosure of information may impact outcomes" (p. S24). In the context of this case study, had Maile disclosed information that competing sections of the Code and Ethics Standards required be kept private and confidential, she could potentially have caused Joaquin harm. Maile acted within the boundaries of the Code and Ethics Standards when viewed in its entirety.

CONCLUSION

The existence of multiple definitions of disability raises ethical and policy-related issues for occupational therapy practitioners in service delivery, education, and research. Occupational therapy practitioners need to stay current with changes in health and disability policy so that they can abide by the Code and Ethics Standards and provide quality care that facilitates self-determination in a collaborative manner.

As shown in the four ethical case studies in this chapter, occupational therapy practitioners must apply the principles of the Code and Ethics Standards in rehabilitation settings within the context of an ever-changing health and disability system. Changes in health and disability policy,

such as health care reform, will continue to affect occupational therapy service delivery, education, and research in the future.

REFERENCES

ADA Amendments Act of 2008, Congressional Debate, 110 Cong. Rec. H8286–8298 (daily ed. Sept. 17, 2008).

Adler, M. (1991). *Programmatic definitions of disability: Policy implications.* Washington, DC: U.S. Department of Health and Human Services, Office of Family Community and Long-Term Care Policy [now Office of Disability, Aging, and Long-Term Care Policy]. Retrieved from http://aspe.hhs.gov/daltcp/reports/prodefes.htm

Albertsons, Inc., v. Kirkingburg, 527 U.S. 555 (1999).

American Occupational Therapy Association. (2008). Occupational therapy practice framework: Domain and process (2nd ed.). *American Journal of Occupational Therapy, 62,* 625–683. doi: 10.5014/ajot.62.6.625

American Occupational Therapy Association. (2010). Occupational therapy code of ethics and ethics standards (2010). *American Journal of Occupational Therapy, 64*(6 Suppl.), S17–S26. doi: 10.5014/ajot.2010.64S17

Americans With Disabilities Act of 1990, as amended, Pub. L. 110–325, 42 U.S.C. 12101 *et seq.* (2008).

Disabled World. (2010a, December 20). *Definition of disabilities.* Retrieved from www.disabled-world.com/disability/types

Disabled World. (2010b, September 10). *Definitions of the models of disability.* Retrieved from www.disabled-world.com/definitions/disability-models.php

Disabled World. (2010c, December 20). *Disability information: Benefits, facts and resources for persons with disabilities.* Retrieved from www.disabled-world.com/disability

Fair Housing Act Amendments Act of 1988, Pub. L. 100–430, 42 U.S.C. §3601 *et seq.* (1988).

Health Insurance Portability and Accountability Act Privacy Rules, 45 C.F.R. § 164.102 *et seq.* (2007).

Henry J. Kaiser Family Foundation. (2011). *About the Kaiser Family Foundation.* Retrieved from http://kff.org/about/index2.cfm

Individuals With Disabilities Education Act of 1990, Pub. L. 101–476, 20 U.S.C. § 1400 *et seq.*

International Labour Organization; United Nations Educational, Scientific and Cultural Organization; & World Health Organization. (2004). *CBR: A strategy for rehabilitation, equalization of opportunities, poverty reduction and social inclusion of people with disabilities.* Retrieved from http://whqlibdoc. who.int/publications/2004/9241592389_eng.pdf

Isaacs, J., Morris, A., & Kornblau, B. L. (2011, April). *Answers to 20 often asked questions raised by those with disabilities about the one-year-old health reform law.* East Elmhurst, NY: United Spinal Association. Retrieved from www.unitedspinal. org/2011/04/18/answers-to-20-often-asked-questions-on-the-health-reform-law/

Kaplan, D. (2010). *The definition of disability.* San Diego, CA: Center for an Accesible Society. Retrieved from www.accessiblesociety.org/topics/demographics-identity/dkaplanpaper.htm

Kim, H., & Colantonio, A. (2010). Effectiveness of rehabilitation in enhancing community integration after acute traumatic brain injury: A systematic review. *American Journal of Occupational Therapy, 64,* 709–719. doi: 10.5014/ajot.2010.09188

Landmine Survivors Network. (2007). *Disability rights advocacy workbook* (2nd ed.). Retrieved from www. handicap-international.fr/kit-pedagogique/documents/ressourcesdocumentaires/apadoption/DisabilityRightsAdvocacyWorkbook2007.pdf

Law, M., Cooper, B., Strong, S., Stewart, D., Rigby, P., & Letts, L. (1996). Person–environment–occupation model: A transactive approach to occupational performance. *Canadian Journal of Occupational Therapy, 63,* 9–23.

Mont, D. (2007, March 1). *Measuring disability prevalence.* Washington, DC: World Bank. Retrieved from http://go.worldbank.org/VV2FGMBXU0

Murphy v. United Parcel Service, Inc., 527 U.S. 516 (1999).

Olmstead v. L.C., 527 U.S. 581 (1999).

Patient Protection and Affordable Care Act, Pub. L. 111–148, § 3502, 124 Stat. 119, 124 (2010).

Social Security Administration. (2010). *Disability planner: What we mean by disability.* Retrieved from www.ssa.gov/dibplan/dqualify4.htm

Sutton v. United Air Lines, Inc., 527 U.S. 472 (1999).

United Nations. (1948, December 10). *Universal Declaration of Human Rights.* Retrieved from www. udhr.org/udhr/default.htm

United Nations. (n.d.). *Convention on the Rights of Persons with Disabilities and optional protocol.* Retrieved from www.un.org/disabilities/documents/convention/convoptprot-e.pdf

U.S. Census Bureau. (2009, September 21). *Disability overview.* Retrieved from www.census.gov/hhes/www/disability/overview.html

World Health Organization. (2001). *International classification of functioning, disability and health.* Geneva: Author.

World Health Organization. (2002). *Towards a common language for functioning, disability and health.* Retrieved from www.who.int/classifications/icf/training/icfbeginnersguide.pdf

World Health Organization. (2010a). *Health topics: Disabilities.* Retrieved from www.who.int/topics/disabilities/en/

World Health Organization. (2010b). *Health topics: Rehabilitation.* Retrieved from www.who.int/topics/rehabilitation/en/

Administration and
Private Practice

17

Tammy Richmond, MS, OTR/L, FAOTA

Ethics "is a systematic study of and reflection on morality" (Purtilo & Doherty, 2011, p. 16). *Morals* or *morality* guides relationships between people, including stakeholders, to promote a high-quality and ethical life for people or for the community as a whole (Purtilo & Doherty, 2011). Stakeholders in a typical health care practice can include clients and potential clients, families, caregivers, referring professionals, staff, paying entities, suppliers, other colleagues, competitors, and health care oversight agencies. Private practice practitioners face an additional layer of stakeholders (i.e., federal and state oversight agencies, third-party payers) and challenges in that they operate not only as a practice but also as a business entity. They are in a unique position of balancing their duty to be the client's advocate with their desire to earn a financial profit. Professional and organizational morality is further complicated by current internal and external environmental factors such as

- Business laws and regulations being merged with health care laws and regulations
- Changes in managed care and health care reform, including reimbursement
- Increases in regulation and stronger ethical oversight
- Shifts in societal morality
- Shortages of clinicians and resources
- Differences in value or belief systems between stakeholders and the organization.

During economic turmoil and uncertainty, these already pressing issues and challenges loom even larger. Moreover, many private practice businesses do not have the luxury of having their own ethics committees, human resource departments, or legal teams of advisors. Business owners and managers are often left to sort out challenging ethical issues through their own initiatives. Management has the responsibility to ensure that ethical integrity exists throughout the organization and for all stakeholders. Practitioners have multiple obligations to fulfill and a careful balance to achieve between social and economic responsibilities in order to meet organizational objectives and achieve efficacy in service delivery (Nosse, Friberg, & Kovacek, 1999). In a survey of practitioners conducted by the American Occupational Therapy Association (AOTA) Ethics Commission (Slater & Brandt, 2009), the most commonly reported ethical concerns in practice included the following:

- Conflict with organizational policies
- Excessive pressure to meet productivity standards
- Lack of administrative support
- Reimbursement constraints.

Addressing ethics in the private practice workplace involves developing a systematic strategy to best satisfy all the stakeholders. The goal of ethical decision making, in the best of all possible worlds, . . . is a resolution to the dilemmas that is in the best interests of all involved parties—person receiving services, therapist, and third-party payer, along with management, family, and others depending on the particular situation. Sometimes it is a win–win, and sometimes it is choosing the least worst of several possible resolutions. (R. Hansen, personal communication, July 18, 2010)

In this chapter, the *Occupational Therapy Code of Ethics and Ethics Standards (2010)* (referred to as the "Code and Ethics Standards"; AOTA, 2010) is applied to private practice operations. The critical link among personal, professional, and organizational morals and behavior and the ways these contribute to ethical decision making in private practice are discussed. Legal and regulatory issues and their impact on an understanding of the factors contributing to dilemmas are explored. Approaches to selecting a framework for ethical decision making are discussed, and management strategies to prevent ethical tensions are provided.

The words *administration, management,* and *organization* are used in this chapter to refer to the role of occupational therapy practitioners in private practice who function as owners, partners, or business managers and who have the job tasks of commanding, planning, managing, or controlling both practice and business operations. Private practice owners are practitioners who are self-employed, including independent contractors. Although supervision is a common function of clinical management that carries additional ethical issues and overarching legal and regulatory concerns, this topic is beyond the scope of the chapter; ethical issues in supervision are addressed in many of the case studies and vignettes in this book.

Legal and regulatory guidelines are discussed as they apply to both the business and the health care provision aspects of private practice. The legal information provided is general; this chapter should not be used in place of legal counsel. Readers should seek expert counsel and opinion when appropriate. In addition, it is strongly recommended that readers routinely set aside time to stay abreast of current content on ethics and ethics in management sources, including the Web sites of AOTA, the National Board for Certification in Occupa-

tional Therapy, and the appropriate state regulatory boards. Texts such as *Ethical Dimensions in the Health Professions* (Purtilo & Doherty, 2011) and *Ethics in Rehabilitation: A Clinical Perspective* (Kornblau & Burkhardt, 2012) are recommended resources.

BEHAVIORAL GUIDANCE FOR ETHICS IN PRIVATE PRACTICE

A moral compass is essential in operating an ethical practice and performing as an ethical professional. One must understand that fulfilling one's duty to clients comes first. It is essential to disengage from personal values when providing quality care and certainly when resolving issues of ethics. This disengagement becomes more challenging in private practice, in which the need to care for both the client and the business can create ethical distress or dilemmas. Meeting the needs of both starts with reflection on the behavior involved in the main roles of the private practitioner.

Morality consists of the values, interests, attitudes, duties, virtues, and behaviors of people, communities, and societies as a whole. In the most basic sense, morality is about right and wrong conduct. Kohlberg identified four elements of moral behavior (cited in Gibbons, 1998, p. 2):

- *Moral sensitivity:* the ability to identify a dilemma and consider others' views
- *Moral judgment:* the ability to make ethical decisions by weighing principles and others' preferences and opinions
- *Moral motivation:* the ability to integrate a value system and sort through conflicts
- *Moral character:* the ability to carry out the decisions one knows to be moral.

Purtilo and Doherty (2011) viewed personal, societal, and group morality as overlapping subgroups of moral values. Likewise, ethics in management and business is predicated on the construct of a "trilevel" (Nosse et al., 1999) relationship among personal, professional, and organizational behaviors. In other words, morality relates to establishing an overall ethical culture for an organization. These overarching moral belief systems provide the framework for sound ethical decision making in private practice. Discussions of personal morality, professional morality, and organizational morality (see Figure 17.1) related to private practice and administration follow.

Personal Morality

By the time a typical health care practitioner is completing his or her education and starting a professional career, he or she has already internally synthesized a set of values or morals. Personal values and morals are developed throughout one's lifetime and are influenced by numerous factors, such as parental practices, cultural background, societal norms, education, personal experiences, and religious beliefs. Responses to moral issues are shaped by a personal process of ethical decision making, although one may not be consciously aware of it.

Nosse et al. (1999) called this concept *personal guidance*. This model of personal guidance or personal morality consists of a personal self-view influenced by one's inherent or selected values, attitudes, and interests (Nosse et al., 1999). As people evolve, personally embedded values, attitudes, and interests shape moral reasoning

and eventually become a personal moral compass or set of ethical principles used to resolve ethical tensions. Identification of one's personal morality prospectively influences one's professional ethical behavior and ethical decision making (see Table 17.1). In Vignette 17.1, an occupational therapist experiences an ethical dilemma in which a potential solution to a business problem conflicts with her personal morality.

VIGNETTE 17.1. ADDRESSING A CHALLENGE TO PERSONAL MORALITY

Jill was starting up a new private practice in occupational therapy. She knew a physician who would refer clients if Jill opened up a practice in his building. The physician gave Jill a printed list of the major insurance carriers with whom his office had contracts. She eagerly made several phones calls to the first few carriers and found out that she needed to set up her company as a corporation. In addition, the insurance carriers told Jill that if she wanted to get a contract to be "in network," she would need to join and be accredited by a medical or provider network. Jill contacted the provider network that serviced her geographic area to apply for membership and credentialing. The network sent her a membership

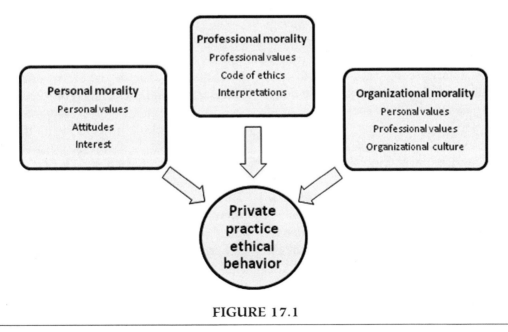

FIGURE 17.1

Overlapping subgroups of ethical behavior.

Source. From *Managerial and Supervisory Principles for Physical Therapists* (p. 37), by L. J. Nosse, D. G. Friberg, and P. R. Kovacek, 1999, Philadelphia: Lippincott Williams & Wilkins. Copyright © 1999 by Lippincott Williams & Wilkins. Adapted with permission.

TABLE 17.1
Ethical Principles Reflected in Personal Values, Attitudes, and Interests

Ethical Principle	Values	Attitudes	Interests
Beneficence	Kindness, safety	Empathy, protectiveness	Helping humanity
Nonmaleficence	Prudence, security	Obligation, duty	Due process
Autonomy, Confidentiality	Freedom, privacy	Self-determination, rights	Collaboration
Social Justice	Balance, equality	Altruism, appropriateness	Advocacy, promotion
Procedural Justice	Fairness, quality	Competence, compliance	High moral standards
Veracity	Truthfulness, honesty	Trustworthiness, worthiness	Expertise, recognition
Fidelity	Respect, integrity	Commitment, fairness	Mediation, negotiation

contract that stated she would be required to hire a physical therapist to meet the credentialing standards and the terms of the contractual relationship. Jill had not planned on hiring anyone and could not afford to hire a physical therapist.

The next day, she called her friend **Shaun**, with whom she had worked at the local hospital a few years previously and occasionally still went biking. She told Shaun of the opportunity with the physician and new startup practice. Shaun, who was a physical therapist and liked Jill, said he was willing to sign any paperwork to help her get the credentialing she needed to satisfy the provider network and the insurance carriers but that he could not work for her. Jill wasn't sure what she should do.

Jill's moral character was influenced by her personal values of integrity and honesty and her attitudes toward obligation and compliance with rules and laws. The need to meet the requirements of the provider network challenged Jill's moral character when matched with her desire to open a private practice and to meet the expectations of the referring physician. She needed to identify alternative options and weigh them against what was legal, ethical, and within her capabilities.

Professional Morality

As a member of a health care profession subject to state licensure, a practitioner's code of conduct and values are governed by certain standards de-signed to protect the public and to direct ethical actions. Practitioners have a *duty*, a social contract, to their clients to act as moral agents on the clients' behalf with all stakeholders involved in their medical care. They also have the duty to abide by the ethics of professional organizations and to follow federal and state laws. Practitioners' self-view is influenced by their professional values and interpretations of the Code and Ethics Standards, which then provide guidance for their professional behavior (Nosse et al., 1999). Values required at the professional level are grounded in the core values and attitudes of occupational therapy: altruism, equality, freedom, justice, dignity, truth, and prudence (AOTA, 2010, p. S17).

Interpretations of core values are shaped by the official documents available from AOTA and by a state's regulations, practice act, and code of ethics. State regulatory boards take core values and the code of ethics and create legally binding requirements for professional behavior that, if not followed, can result in serious penalties and disciplinary actions. Therefore, professional morality should align with the behavioral guidance to protect the public, advocate for the profession, and facilitate *self-regulation*, or the monitoring of one's own behaviors, activities, and adherence to professional, legal, and ethical standards. An ethical dilemma brought on by decreases in reimbursement is described in Case Study 17.1.

CASE STUDY 17.1. ADDRESSING A CHALLENGE TO PROFESSIONAL MORALITY

Ron was an occupational therapist who had owned his practice for over 10 years. He had two full-time practitioners who worked for him—an occupational therapist and a physical therapist—as well as a therapy aide. Ron worked with clients only part-time so he could devote the rest of his schedule to the business end of his practice. He performed all the financial management tasks, including the billing. Ron prided himself on recognizing emerging practice trends and was dedicated to his professional duty to promote best standards of care. The practice serviced patients with all types of diagnoses, including upper and lower orthopedic injuries, back and spine injuries, neurological disorders, and general chronic disorders (e.g., diabetes). The practice setting had a large gym area with equipment for therapeutic exercise and three private rooms for one-to-one intervention. Ron liked the idea of all of the staff feeling as if they were "part of the business family," so the practice was always full of conversation and handshakes. Ron regularly invited the staff to his house for dinners and holidays. **Marge**, the full-time occupational therapist, happened to be his sister-in-law.

Because of a recent decrease in reimbursement by most insurance carriers, including Medicare, Ron had been looking over the billing and accounting to see where he could cut costs so he wouldn't have to decrease employee benefits or staff. Ron mentioned his concerns about the clinic to Marge at the Friday night family dinner. Marge mentioned she had noticed that most physician referrals request therapy two or three times weekly and suggested that Ron consider scheduling clients three times weekly to take advantage of the physicians' referrals; she also shared her feeling that many of the clients probably could not handle therapy that often.

Ron pondered the idea all night and wondered if Marge was right; maybe their clients could be seen three times a week. He would have to schedule the first 30 minutes with a therapist and then have the therapy aide finish the session in order to schedule all their current clients. This action would bring in more profit but could also jeopardize quality of care, maybe even harm some clients, and create billing issues.

What is unique about professional morality in private practice is that the practitioner is the controller of self-regulation and has a wider range of discretion in applying the actions of duty in professional behavioral guidance and making professional decisions. Inversely, the employee of an organization may have duty and self-regulation imposed on him or her by policies and procedures.

Generally, no external oversight of behavior and decision making exists in private practice. For example, Ron was an owner, practitioner, and business administrator. He held the responsibility to decide what was right or wrong. Fewer checks and balances are typically in place in private practice, so implementing a personal professional code of ethics requires guidance. When this guidance is not present, ethical dilemmas often result from a flawed interpretation of professional duty and self-regulation within the complicated network of health care regulation and small business law (see Table 17.2).

Ron's understanding of the physicians' prescriptions reflected his interpretation of duty as it related to best standards of practice for his clients and his own core values of altruism, justice, and prudence. Moreover, Ron had a legal obligation not to unintentionally harm clients and an ethical responsibility not to promote employee behaviors that could create issues related to Principle 2, Nonmaleficence. In addition, he needed to ensure that he and his colleagues were faithful to Principle 1, Beneficence, as well as Principles 4, Social Justice, and 5, Procedural Justice, of the Code and Ethics Standards. Additionally, Ron's use of the therapy aide would depend on his state's scope of practice, insurance carriers' regulations, and acceptable billing practices. His decision could potentially open Ron and his practice to both legal and ethical infractions.

Ron's situation highlights the importance of private practitioners' ongoing commitment to training and maintaining their professional morality by understanding and using the Code and Ethics Standards to guide interactions with all stakeholders. The goal in professional morality is to create a professional foundation of expected moral conduct and moral reasoning; thereafter, "the burden is on practitioners to ensure that they are making clinical decisions that

TABLE 17.2
Professional Morality in Private Practice

Expectation	Possible Dilemma	Core Values[a]	Principles[a]
Level of competence	No recognized standards in place	Altruism, truth, prudence	Beneficence Procedural Justice Veracity
Informed consent	No written policy in place	All core values	Autonomy, Confidentiality
Scope of practice	Subjective definition of terms	Altruism, justice, prudence	Beneficence Nonmaleficence
Professional boundaries	Infringement on client Informal relationships	Equality, justice, dignity, prudence	Nonmaleficence Social Justice Fidelity
Promotion activities	Pro bono services to a special subgroup	Justice, truth, equality	Social Justice Beneficence
Duty	No policies or guidelines in place	All core values	All principles
Privacy	Discussion of work issues on social networks	Altruism, dignity, justice	Autonomy, Confidentiality Fidelity
Accurate reporting	Improper documentation	Justice, truth	Veracity Procedural Justice

[a]*Source.* American Occupational Therapy Association (2010).

are in compliance with the core ethical principles related to benefitting the consumer" (AOTA Ethics Commission, 2009, p. 1).

Organizational Morality

Maintaining an ethical and profitable professional practice in an age of decreasing reimbursement, higher costs of conducting business, and increasing competition can be a challenge (Kimberg, 2006). Two major factors contribute to organizational morality in private practice: One is the management of the practice as a health care organization, and the other is the management of the practice as a small business entity. The practitioner–owner needs to comply legally and ethically with both types of management duties. The goal of a private practice owner striving for organizational morality is to provide a positive organizational culture, an environment where ethical and legal behavior is role-modeled and consistently demonstrated. It is the responsibility of the practitioner–owner to

establish ethical guidelines for the organization's operations and employees. A lack of ethical operations and behavioral guidance can jeopardize the livelihood and success of the practice.

According to Nosse et al. (1999), the model of organizational self-view (i.e., organizational culture) is influenced by the mission, vision, and value statements of the private practice business. These fundamental administrative documents represent the organization's purpose, values, and beliefs about moral conduct within society, and they set the tone for workplace morality for employees. As a health care entity, the administration of a private practice has several managerial functions with respect to ethics (Opacich, 2003):

- Committing to follow the tenets, principles, and standards of the profession provided through official documents of the discipline and all applicable laws and regulations governing health care and business

- Ensuring the integrity of individual practitioners through establishing a culture of introspection, self-review, and staff development
- Implementing ethical clinical and organizational decision making
- Preserving the integrity of the professional community by obtaining necessary qualifications, certifications, licensure, and accreditations for services and delivery of services.

In Case Study 17.2, the new owner of a private practice must bring policies and procedures more into line with ethical practice.

CASE STUDY 17.2: ADDRESSING A CHALLENGE TO ORGANIZATIONAL MORALITY

Abigail was an occupational therapist who had advanced credentialing as a Certified Hand Therapist (CHT) and was a new business owner of a hand therapy practice. She recently bought an occupational therapy hand practice from another CHT, **Rhonda**, who had the reputation of being "the best" hand therapist in town. Several hand surgeons referred to the practice, so Abigail was convinced that she had invested well and would be able to continue to provide the reputable hand therapy services previously established.

Three therapists were already working at the clinic: a physical therapist named **Tom**; an occupational therapist, **Kathy**, who was working toward her advanced certification in modalities and hand therapy; and another CHT, **Brenda**, who had many years of experience. The clients were mainly field workers of Hispanic origin from the nearby agricultural farms who had sustained severe hand injuries requiring complex customized hand splints. The office administrator, **Claire**, had worked there for several years and seemed to handle all the business operations singlehandedly. Abigail was relieved to hear Claire state that she planned on continuing to work there until she retired in 5 years as long as Abigail continued to provide the benefits Rhonda had established.

Rhonda agreed to mentor Abigail for the first two weeks of ownership to help acclimate her to the ins and outs of the business. During her first week without Rhonda there, Abigail decided to go back to the office after hours to spend more time looking through the front office files and drawers to become better acquainted with the details of the business. When she arrived, she saw Brenda, the CHT, making a hand splint for a client sitting next to her. Abigail was surprised and decided to sit at the front desk and quietly look through files until Brenda was done and the client had left.

After the client departed, Abigail found Brenda and asked if they could discuss what had just happened. Brenda told Abigail that Dr. Alvarez routinely operated after hours and called Brenda to come in to fabricate hand splints needed postsurgery. Brenda also told Abigail that Rhonda had also come in as needed. Brenda went on to say that in exchange for her willingness to work after hours and overtime, Rhonda allowed her extra days off, paid her way to conferences, and gave her an end-of-the-year bonus. In fact, Brenda stated that she and her husband were celebrating their 20th anniversary and wanted to take three weeks off to meet some friends in Italy the next month. Abigail replied that she appreciated the information and would get back to Brenda about her time off.

After Brenda left, Abigail went to the filing cabinet to find Brenda's personnel file and see what was in Rhonda's employee agreement. Abigail read through the agreement but did not see any mention of extra days off or any of the other benefits Brenda discussed. She looked through the other employees' personnel files and found that none of them contained any mention of benefits, either. Abigail wondered how to comply with legal standards in employee contracts and benefits without losing her experienced professionals, thus potentially damaging the reputation of the practice.

In this case, the previous owner had established an organizational culture of informal professional boundaries and risky business practices built on bartering and undocumented negotiations. Several other contributing factors related to the organizational culture of private practices could lead to other ethical dilemmas for Abigail. These include

- Contractual relationships that facilitate over- or underutilization of services
- Difficulty confronting referral sources who intentionally or unintentionally promote unethical demands for services
- False sense of ethical compliance because owners assume that occupational therapy

practitioners are naturally ethical and have values that align with the profession

- Increasing numbers of people with chronic illnesses and an aging population in areas where access and quality-of-care issues are prevalent and services are restricted or limited
- Lack of formal ethics programs in private practices
- Limited formal ethical training
- Limited availability to owners and employees of knowledge, policies and procedures, and guidelines regarding health care and small business laws and regulations, including codes of ethics
- Need to make a profit versus obligation to advocate for clients and maximize their functional potential
- Sense that third-party payers place greater value on money than clients
- Tendency to implement informal standards
- Use of lower-cost personnel when state laws that define the use of aides and assistants are open for interpretation by the owner.

In summary, organizational morality incorporates management compliance with ethical practices, implementation of core values and minimum ethical standards, and education of employees on the code of conduct acceptable to the organizational culture of the business.

LEGAL AND REGULATORY ISSUES

Often the first question asked in solving ethical dilemmas is, "Is it legal?" There is an inevitable overlap between an organization's ethical and legal responsibilities in both practice and administration. Objective measures of ethics are defined by laws. For example, obtaining informed consent and a signed privacy statement is a prerequisite to intervention. The signed privacy statement is required by the Health Insurance Portability and Accountability Act of 1996 (HIPAA). As a business entity, the administration of a private practice must have a working knowledge of the state and federal legal requirements, laws, and regulations (e.g., tax laws and corporate or business laws) that affect ethics in private practice (see Table 17.3). During the ethical decision-making process,

legal and regulatory information can assist with systematically unraveling an ethical dilemma.

The current legal system is divided into two main sections: (1) criminal law and (2) civil law. *Criminal law*, both state and federal, covers any act committed against people or property, such as assault, embezzlement, robbery, perjury, and perverting the course of justice. A staff employee stealing supplies from a clinic can be charged with robbery. *Civil law* deals with wrongful acts (called *torts*) between individuals and organizations, and compensation or other remedies are allowed. An example of civil law malpractice is a practitioner who provides an intervention that negligently causes damage to the client, such as aggressive manual therapy to an osteoporotic limb that causes a fracture.

The primary difference between the two common law categories is intent: Criminal law involves malicious intent, whereas in civil law, malicious intent is missing. A case in which a practitioner intentionally harms a client by providing an intervention that leads to a serious injury is covered by criminal law, whereas a claim following an incident in which the client fell off a stool while practicing dressing with the therapist present and providing proper supervision would be argued under civil law.

Administrative functions of a private practitioner, such as billing and documentation, fall under another subdivision of civil law, called *administration law*, which governs activities of administrative agencies of federal and state governments (e.g., state health care licensing boards, Medicare). Management deals with many types of contracts: employee contracts, agency contracts, and provider contracts, which are regulated by contract laws.

Other general business laws that apply to private practice include employment regulation, environmental protection, facilities regulation, and financial management, as well as food, drug, and medical equipment manufacture, labeling, handling, sale and use, and quality. Decisions related to supplies and equipment can have serious consequences; for example, attempting to save money by cancelling the weekly pickup service for disposable hypodermic needles used for dispensing topical agents might expose the public to unsafe agents that could cause harm.

Legal and regulatory compliance with health care and business laws and regulations is a duty of occupational therapy practitioners and private

TABLE 17.3
Legal and Regulatory Categories That Affect Private Practice

CATEGORY	EXAMPLES
Access[a]	Public access and direct access
Employment law	Human resources Pay practices Employee health and safety
Environmental protection[a]	Cleaning of equipment
Financial management[a]	Medical records Fraud and abuse
Food, drug, and medical equipment manufacture, sale, and use[a]	Sale of products or topical medications Use of atypical physical agents
Civil law	Negligence Malpractice Informed consent
Criminal law	Embezzlement Robbery
Administrative law	State licensing Falsification of billing Government oversight
Contract law	Service contracts Provider contracts
U.S. Department of Health and Human Services	Medicare Medicaid State Children's Health Insurance Programs Health Insurance Portability and Accountability Act

Source. [a]From *Managerial and Supervisory Principles for Physical Therapists*, 3rd ed. (p. 185), by L. J. Nosse and D. G. Friberg, 2009, Philadelphia: Lippincott Williams & Wilkins. Copyright © 2009 by Lippincott Williams & Wilkins. Adapted with permission.

practice organizations. A majority of the federal health care laws and regulations that affect practitioners fall under the U.S. Department of Health and Human Services, including Medicare, Medicaid, State Children's Health Insurance Programs, and HIPAA. Common ethical and legal infractions involve the sharing of medical information about a client with others.

State health care laws and regulations consist of state occupational therapy licensing regulations and federally funded programs administered through corresponding state agencies such as the Individuals With Disabilities Education Act (1990) funded by the state department of education, which in turn has contracts with private practitioners or practices for specific services.

Health care and business laws and regulations can offer clarification in ethical and legal decision making. Experts can assist in resolving ethical dilemmas when legal and regulatory issues are at play.

RECOGNIZING COMMON SOURCES OF ETHICAL TENSION AND DILEMMAS

Key ethical issues in private practice can be found in each of the seven Code and Ethics Standards principles, which guide professional and organizational morality and approaches to ethical decision making. Ethical distress and dilemmas in private practice have familiar themes: lack of resources, motivation to make a profit, mandates or impositions from outside payers or referring entities, and varied interpretations of professional and organizational self-governance and duty. Common sources of ethical tension and dilemmas in private practice related to each of the seven principles are described in the sections that follow.

Principle 1: Beneficence

According to Principle 1 of the Code and Ethics Standards, "Occupational therapy personnel shall demonstrate a concern for the well-being and safety of the recipients of their services" (AOTA, 2010, p. S18; see also Chapter 3, this volume). Common dilemmas arise in the areas of level of competence (Principles 1E and 1G), evidence-based practice (Principle 1F), and termination of services (Principle 1H).

In the author's experience, termination of services is the most prevalent source of ethical tensions in private practice for at least two major reasons. First, terminating a client means ending financial profit for the practice. Second, clients, families, and even referral sources may push for continued services beyond the realistic functional potential of the client; this pressure is most evident among practitioners working in pediatrics and those subcontracting in skilled nursing facilities.

Maintaining competence also is a source of ethical tensions. Staff development may be decreased because of limited financial resources, so additional skills training is left up to the individual practitioner, who may have no intrinsic motivation to improve skills. Inadequate self-regulation in meeting the level of competence needed to provide skilled interventions can lead to services that unintentionally harm the client. In addition, a consistent referral source may encourage offering a type of service that falls outside the scope of the practitioners or organization. This disconnect facilitates possible tensions between physicians and providers, and practitioners face a reluctance to refer inappropriate clients elsewhere because of the potential for loss of income and loss of referral. Additionally, professionals who practice in isolation may be unmotivated to self-regulate their competence or may even deem it unnecessary.

Ethical tensions also arise in the area of providing evidence-based practice. Lack of financial

resources or appropriately skilled practitioners to meet quality of care standards in intervention (e.g., duration, number, or frequency of sessions) may result in services that fall outside of intervention protocols or scope of practice. In Case Study 17.1, Ron's organizational culture emphasized following evidence-based practices, but in his desire to bring in more profit, albeit for the sake of maintaining his staff and benefits, he considered promoting care outside of quality of care standards, thus potentially causing harm.

Principle 2: Nonmaleficence

Principle 2 reads, "Occupational therapy personnel shall intentionally refrain from actions that cause harm" (AOTA, 2010, p. S19; see also Chapter 4, this volume). Because of the autonomy of a private practice, two common examples of nonmaleficence are (1) maintaining clear professional boundaries with all stakeholders (Principles 2C, 2D, 2G, 2I, and 2J) and (2) avoiding client abandonment (Principle 2B).

As stated earlier, an informal organizational culture can result in more personal relationships forming throughout the operations. Owners, occupational therapy practitioners, and referral sources share more communication and responsibility for service outcomes, which leads to the formation of social bonds that can interfere with professional judgment, quality of care, or business operations, as seen in Case Study 17.2. This informality results in insensitivity or lack of awareness regarding whether or not the stakeholders are being harmed until legal negligence becomes apparent. Then what may have been a simple ethical dilemma at the outset becomes a complex legal issue, such as malpractice or labor law infringement.

Abandonment of clients is more subtle but happens regularly, mainly because of reimbursement limitations or restrictions. Practitioners may be less intrinsically motivated to extend the visits of clients who have insurance carriers, such as health maintenance organizations, that provide lower reimbursement rates.

Another factor commonly contributing to client abandonment is challenging family dynamics. For example, clients with complicated or chronic medical conditions and their family caregivers who have unrealistic or unfulfilled expectations of therapy outcomes may become disgruntled when therapy ends, creating a reluctance in the practitioner to appeal for additional therapy visits. In addition, productivity demands and financial pressures from owners can drive practitioners to schedule clients every 20 to 30 minutes with little consideration of the risks of rushing through clients.

Principle 3: Autonomy, Confidentiality

According to Principle 3, "Occupational therapy personnel shall respect the right of the individual to self-determination" (AOTA, 2010, p. S20; see also Chapter 5, this volume). Two important ethical and legal issues fall under this principle for private practice owners. The first is informed consent, which is legally required before an intervention can begin (Principles 3A, 3B, 3C, and 3J). The second is the HIPAA privacy statement that must be provided to each client, which must specify how to notify a privacy officer and provide space where the client can designate restrictions regarding sharing medical information (Principles 3G and 3H).

The informed consent is a legal document that contains specific elements for disclosure. Occupational therapy practitioners are supposed to discuss four main issues to ensure that the client has full knowledge and understanding of the following (Scott, 1997):

1. Recommended intervention ordered by the referral source
2. Potential risks of serious harm or complications so the client can accept or reject the intervention
3. Expected benefits and goals
4. Reasonable alternatives, if any, to the proposed intervention.

Ethical conflicts occur when the practitioner fails to tell the client about all the risks and complications and alternatives to the intervention plan. In fact, too many practitioners hand clients the informed consent without any explanation and expect them to read and sign it on their own cognizance.

The HIPAA privacy statement is standard documentation addressed during the intake or initial evaluation session, so it can easily be inadvertently omitted from the documentation or handed out but never signed and returned. Ethical infractions occur when a client's personal medical information is shared inappropriately, most often by being overheard by another client or therapist or by a family member. For example, a client in the waiting room may overhear the office administrator at the intake desk converse about another client or office matters openly and loud enough for others to hear. How these ethical breaches are handled is important; making a timely apology is the first step, followed by training practitioners, updating procedures, and reviewing and changing policies as needed to prevent further occurrences.

Principle 4: Social Justice

Principle 4 specifies that "Occupational therapy personnel shall provide services in a fair and equitable manner" (AOTA, 2010, p. S21; see also Chapter 6, this volume). Generally, the law allows practitioners to deny therapy services to clients who can't pay for them, but ethics requires practitioners not to deny or restrict services to certain subgroups of society. This issue is sizable for health care providers because insurance policies and care are typically available only to consumers who can afford them. This situation may change with health care reform, but discrepancies will remain to some degree because access to care will continue to be problematic. For example, clients living in a remote area of a state, where specialists and occupational therapy practitioners are not available, will be unable to receive the care they need even if they are eligible to receive those services under their insurance coverage. Inequity also arises when clients are provided inferior services or denied intervention on the basis of their religion, sexuality, or other discriminatory element.

Principle 5: Procedural Justice

In line with Principle 5, "Occupational therapy personnel shall comply with institutional rules, local, state, federal and international laws and AOTA documents applicable to the profession of occupational therapy" (AOTA, 2010, p. S22; see also Chapter 7, this volume). Here lies the important obligation of the practitioner–owner and the private organization to know, comply with, and implement both ethical and legal standards and the guidelines and regulations of the profession and of the business. Furthermore, if a practitioner is brought before an ethics committee or legal proceeding, ignorance does not exclude him or her from professional and business responsibilities to meet legal and ethical standards.

Procedural Justice was involved in the vignette and both case studies. Jill faced ethical distress in deciding whether to engage in unethical and illegal behavior to comply with the provider network's contract requirements. Ron reflected on his interpretation of intervention guidelines and reimbursement methodologies. Abigail was faced with legal contract and labor law issues along with unethical professional behaviors.

Principle 6: Veracity

According to Principle 6, "Occupational therapy personnel shall provide comprehensive, accurate, and objective information when representing the profession" (AOTA, 2010, p. S23; see also Chapter 8, this volume). Proper documentation for reimbursement purposes is a common ethical issue for private practice owners. This is a payer-driven dilemma when a payer

- Demands use of specific procedural codes encouraging unethical behavior through improper documentation
- Denies access to care without specific documentation or language
- Denies care or payment for care if documentation cannot support medical necessity, challenging the therapist to document unethically
- Restricts, limits, or denies authorization or payment without certain documentation or language.

Making changes to a medical record is illegal. Documenting accurate information is required legally and ethically. Nonetheless, a service provider contract is also a legal document, so coding and billing to meet the contract provisions of the payer may mean that the billing procedure does not accurately describe the intervention given. For example, if the fee schedule of the third-party payer does not include the service codes that accurately reflect the types of intervention appropri-

ate for the impairment the practitioner is treating, the practitioner may be forced to code or treat outside standards of care or treatment protocol.

In the case study of Ron, adding a third visit would have to be a justified medical necessity regardless of what the prescription indicated. Furthermore, federal law regarding billing of federal insurance (e.g., Medicare) clearly states that only "skilled" services can be billed, so does billing for intervention given by the therapy aide qualify? Ron could risk engaging in fraudulent billing.

Principle 7: Fidelity

Principle 7 states, "Occupational therapy personnel shall treat colleagues and other professionals with respect, fairness, discretion, and integrity" (AOTA, 2010, p. S24; see also Chapter 9, this volume). Competition for clients and referrals is a constant in private practice. A private practice business cannot survive without referrals, so professional relationships and the duty to show respect for other colleagues can be challenged. Furthermore, the encroachment of other professionals or paraprofessionals providing competing services could lure potential clients and revenues away, pushing private practice owners to react with unethical professional and amoral organizational behavior.

One could infer, in Case Study 17.2, that Rhonda's motivation for treating clients after hours was fear of losing the client to a competitor, thus intrinsically impelling Rhonda to act unethically. Alternatively, the fear of subordination to the referring physician could have played a role. Rhonda may have wanted to keep good faith between all the stakeholders, thus sacrificing her own professional ethics. Regardless, Abigail was put in a position of having to act on the basis of her own sense of fidelity.

FRAMEWORK FOR ETHICAL DECISION MAKING IN PRIVATE PRACTICE

Historically, health care professionals have identified the deontological theory of ethics to represent the professional framework of ethical decision making in occupational therapy. This theory holds that one is acting ethically when one acts according to duties and rights (Purtilo & Doherty,

2011). In occupational therapy, duties and rights are defined by the principles of the profession.

Several frameworks are available and suitable for ethical decision making in private practice. Purtilo and Doherty (2011) used a six-step approach to ethical decision making. The AOTA Ethics Commission (2007) provided a seven-step approach. The 14-step Savage Facilitation Model of Ethical Contemplation offers a more detailed step-by-step process for ethical reasoning (cited in Opacich, 2003). Others have suggested a combination of several approaches to assist in eliminating personal bias and to promote fair and just consideration of all the involved stakeholders; a combined approach is described in Chapter 10 of this volume.

Previous management experience and ethical training may influence the selection of one of these systematic approaches. Managers who are less experienced and unfamiliar with fundamental documents providing professional and organizational guidance will benefit from the Savage Facilitation Model, whereas more seasoned managers with more resources may find the AOTA Ethics Commission's (2007) seven-step framework to be more applicable and efficient. The ultimate goal is to resolve an ethical situation with an administrative tool that uses ethical principles and various legal regulations to guide managers and owners to an ethical solution that will uphold the values and morals of the profession and fulfill the private practitioner's duty as a fiduciary organization to the primary stakeholder: the client.

The AOTA Ethics Commission's (2007) seven-step process for ethical decision making can assist the private practice owner in identifying, exploring, examining, and determining a solution or possible solutions to an ethical dilemma. The process follows the logic of clinical reasoning and therefore is easier to understand and implement than other professional frameworks available; each of the seven steps is briefly described in the sections that follow.

Step 1: Identify the Ethical Distress or Dilemma

Ethical distress is emotional or mental discomfort indicating awareness of a situation that is wrong but you are unsure what is wrong or are

prevented from performing the ethical actions to correct it (Purtilo & Doherty, 2011). An *ethical dilemma* is a problem that involves two morally correct choices that cannot both be followed (Purtilo & Doherty, 2011). In the first step, identify the source of the distress or dilemma, remembering that more than one type of distress or dilemma may be simultaneously occurring.

Step 2: Evaluate the Key Factors and Players in the Dilemma

Unraveling the facts and parts of the situation is necessary to delineate the moral issues and the duties of the stakeholders involved. Ask investigative questions about the situation until you have gathered all relevant information. In private practice, as exemplified by the case studies, consideration must be given to the additional factors inherent in health care business and small business operation. Examining both business and health care ethics is essential to unraveling dilemmas in private practice.

Step 3: Consider Alternatives and Consequences

Determine all the possible options for actions that can be taken. Confer with peers or colleagues whom you trust and who will not breach the client's confidentiality (Purtilo & Doherty, 2011) to thoroughly examine the available choices. On reflection, Jill would have found that many options were possible, all ethical and legal; examples include suggesting to the physician that she be added to his contracted policy with the third-party payers or pursuing an opt-out contract with the third-party payers directly.

Step 4: Examine the Code and Ethics Standards and Other Resources

Gather the Code and Ethics Standards and other legal and official documents necessary to direct further investigation, and use the process of objectivity to eliminate ethical solutions that fail to meet legal requirements in both common law and state licensure law. Then, apply professional standards and guidelines. A state licensure code of ethics is legally binding, so be sure to look at your state regulations and scope of practice first.

Step 5: Assess Resources and Ask Experts for Assistance as Needed

Interpretation of laws and guidelines is best handled by experts. Several sources of assistance are available, including state and national professional associations, professional liability insurance company advisors, the Service Corps of Retired Executives (SCORE), the Small Business Administration, and small business accountants and health care lawyers. In Case Study 17.2, Abigail would benefit from contacting a lawyer to assist her in renegotiating the employee contracts with special provisions as appropriate to achieve a win–win outcome.

Step 6: Make a Decision You Can Defend and Implement

Defense of a decision depends on a careful assessment of the legal and ethical considerations for all stakeholders involved in the dilemma and the development of a solution that is defensible both in legal court and to the stakeholders. Communicate the solution in a clear, understandable, accurate, and supported statement. Private practitioners take on additional risks by being business owners. They are not protected by the umbrella of a large enterprise, such as hospital institutions. More is at stake if dilemmas turn into lawsuits, so due diligence in the decision-making process with supportive documentation is important.

Step 7: Reflect on and Reevaluate the Effectiveness of the Solution

Not all solutions are going to be absolute, and outcomes may not turn out to be beneficial for all stakeholders. As stated in the introduction to this chapter, sometimes choosing the least detrimental of all solutions is the best available option, so you may find it helpful to look back and examine the approach and outcome for future use.

RISK MANAGEMENT FOR PREVENTION OF ETHICAL DILEMMAS

A plan to prevent or manage ethical tensions should be a part of an organization's risk management program. Basic prevention strategies include developing collaborative intervention plans driven by therapist and client, providing necessary skilled services, and employing competent therapists. Organizational strategies involve maintaining current knowledge of health care and business laws and regulations, promoting a positive and ethical organizational culture, adhering to reimbursement agencies' policies and guidelines, integrating core values, abiding by standards of ethics and ethical principles, and being familiar with the appropriate state practice acts, including ethical guidelines. Other elements of a risk management policy for ethical dilemmas include the following:

- Knowledge of Code and Ethics Standards and other official professional documents
- Employee ethics training
- Mission, vision, and value statements
- Policy and procedure manual
- Informed consent form
- HIPAA privacy statement
- Unusual occurrence form
- Employee handbook
- Code of conduct
- Tools for effective communication.

As Meadows (n.d.) noted, "Good management, open door policies, written conduct policies, training for leaders and staff, and confidential employee assistance programs help to manage situations before they start" (p. 24).

CONCLUSION

Unique moral challenges exist in private practice because of the myriad obligations and duties faced by a practitioner who is both a professional and a business owner. Ethical behavior in private practice is predicated on understanding the behavior guidance models of personal, professional, and organizational morality, regulated jointly by health care and business laws and regulations and guided by the values and principles of the Code and Ethics

Standards. Occupational therapy practitioners can resolve common private practice ethical dilemmas by using the AOTA seven-step ethical decision-making model. Prevention of ethical dilemmas in private practice is grounded in developing risk management policies and providing ethics training.

REFERENCES

American Occupational Therapy Association. (2010). Occupational therapy code of ethics and ethics standards (2010). *American Journal of Occupational Therapy, 64*(6 Suppl.), S17–S26. doi: 10.5014/ajot.2010.64S17

American Occupational Therapy Association Ethics Commission. (2007). *Everyday ethics: Core knowledge for occupational therapy practitioners and educators* (CEonCD). Bethesda, MD: AOTA Press.

American Occupational Therapy Association Ethics Commission. (2009). *AOTA advisory opinion for the ethics commission: Ethical considerations in private practice.* Retrieved from www.aota.org/Practitioners/Ethics/Advisory/Private-Practice.aspx

Gibbons, M. (1998, May 1). *A question of ethics.* Retrieved from http://physical-therapy.advanceweb.com/Article/a-question-of-ethics-6.aspx

Health Insurance Portability and Accountability Act of 1996, Pub. L. 104–191 110 Stat. 1936.

Individuals With Disabilities Education Act of 1990, Pub. L. 101–476, 20 U.S.C., Ch 33.

Kimberg, I. (2006, August 21). *Your moral compass.* Retrieved from http://occupational-therapy.advanceweb.com/Article/Your-Moral-Compass.aspx

Kornblau, B., & Burkhardt, A. (2012). *Ethics in rehabilitation: A clinical perspective* (2nd ed.). Thorofare, NJ: Slack.

Meadows, B. (n.d.). *Healthy patient–provider boundaries.* Retrieved from http://occupationaltherapy.advanceweb.com/Article/Healthy-Patient-Provider-Boundaries.aspx

Nosse, L. J., & Friberg, D. G. (2009). *Managerial and supervisory principles for physical therapists* (3rd ed.). Philadelphia: Lippincott Williams & Wilkins.

Nosse, L. J., Friberg, D. G., & Kovacek, P. R. (1999). *Managerial and supervisory principles for physical therapists.* Philadelphia: Lippincott Williams & Wilkins.

Opacich, K. (2003). Ethical dimensions of occupational therapy management. In G. L. McCormack, L. Jaffe, & M. Goodman-Lavey (Eds.), *The occupational therapy manager* (4th ed., pp. 491–510). Bethesda, MD: AOTA Press.

Purtilo, R., & Doherty, R. (2011). *Ethical dimensions in the health professions* (5th ed.). Philadelphia: Elsevier Saunders.

Scott, R. (1997). *Covering all bases obtaining informed consent.* Retrieved from http://physical-therapy.advanceweb.com/Article/covering-all-bases---obtaining-informed-consent.aspx

Slater, D., & Brandt, L. (2009, February 2). Combating moral distress. *OT Practice, 2,* 13–16.

Application of Ethics in Higher Education

18

Linda S. Gabriel, PhD, OTR/L

No one wants an unethical practitioner, least of all the client or client's family. No one wants a member of his or her profession to behave in a way that reduces the public's trust in that profession. The acquisition of ethical and virtuous habits does not begin when graduates sign their first contracts to work as occupational therapy practitioners. Habits need to be established and maintained through repetition within a supportive environment.

The habits necessary for ethical behavior specific to occupational therapy begin in the educational setting. Therefore, it is of utmost importance that ethical reasoning, ethical behavior, and moral courage be modeled and learned in educational settings. The literature pertinent to academic honesty and ethical behavior among students and faculty is reviewed in this chapter. The *Occupational Therapy Code of Ethics and Ethics Standards (2010)* (referred to as the "Code and Ethics Standards"; American Occupational Therapy Association [AOTA], 2010) are applied through case studies featuring a classroom student, a fieldwork student, and a faculty member.

BACKGROUND

One of the most basic ethical decisions confronting college students is whether "to cheat or not to cheat on their academic work" (McCabe, Treviño, & Butterfield, 2001, p. 220). The numbers are not encouraging. Cheating in college is prevalent, and some forms of cheating, such as unpermitted collaboration, have increased dramatically in the past 30 years (McCabe et al., 2001).

Personal as well as contextual factors contribute to academic dishonesty or cheating (McCabe et al., 2001). Examples of personal factors include pressure from family, society, and self; inadequate preparation; lack of understanding of what constitutes academic dishonesty; and values and beliefs. Contextual factors include the climate in the institution, program, and classroom and shared attitudes in peer relationships (McCabe et al., 2001).

To provide background and context for the case studies that follow, this section reviews the prevalence of cheating in higher education, requirements in accreditation standards, generational differences in ethical norms, and the role of faculty in preventing academic dishonesty.

Prevalence of Cheating in Higher Education

It would be comforting to think that the incidence of cheating among upper-level students in the health professions is lower than that of the total college population. Unfortunately, Fontana (2009) wrote, "this does not appear to be the case.

Not only are violations increasing, but methods of cheating are also becoming increasingly sophisticated" (p. 181). McCabe (2009) reached the same conclusion after analyzing surveys from 2,100 nursing students from 12 nursing schools and approximately 21,000 students majoring in other disciplines. He reported, "Approximately half of the graduate nursing students, in both the longitudinal survey and the nursing survey, self-reported one or more classroom cheating behaviors" (McCabe, 2009, p. 622).

How do occupational therapy students compare when it comes to academic honesty? Little has been published on cheating or plagiarism in the occupational therapy education literature. When I combined the search terms *occupational therapy* and *education* with *cheating* and *plagiarism* in a Cumulative Index to Nursing and Allied Health Literature search, I found only two articles. When I combined *occupational therapy* and *education* with *academic dishonesty,* I found no articles. In contrast, a search for *nursing* and *education* with *cheating* located 25 articles. Clearly, academic honesty in occupational therapy education warrants further investigation.

Another important area of investigation is the nature of the connection, if any, between honesty in the classroom and honesty in practice. Lovett-Hooper, Komarraju, Weston, and Dollinger (2007) administered the Academic Dishonesty Student Survey to a sample of psychology students to measure the frequency of 19 specific student behaviors that fell into the categories of plagiarism, being dishonest as an individual (e.g., copying from another student's test), and being dishonest as part of a group. The students in the study also completed the Imagined Futures Inventory, which involves rating the likelihood of a wide range of future life outcomes (i.e., the next 5 years). Lovett-Hooper et al. reported a pattern of significant positive correlations between scores on the Academic Dishonesty Student Survey and the Norm/Rule Violations portion of the Imagined Futures Inventory, "suggesting that those who show a lack of academic integrity in college may be more likely to violate norms and rules of society or the workplace in the future" (p. 330).

Papadakis et al. (2005) conducted a study to determine whether a relationship existed between poor professional behavior in medical school and

later problematic behavior as a licensed physician. They found that "disciplinary action by a medical board was strongly associated with prior unprofessional behavior in medical school" (p. 2673).

Requirements in Accreditation Standards

Educating students to be ethical practitioners is not only desirable but also a requirement for accreditation of occupational therapy education programs by the Accreditation Council for Occupational Therapy Education (ACOTE). Wording in the accreditation standards for educational programs for occupational therapists and occupational therapy assistants, specifically in Section B.9.0, makes it clear that occupational therapy programs are responsible for teaching "professional ethics, values, and responsibilities," including "an understanding and appreciation of ethics and values of the profession of occupational therapy" (ACOTE, 2012, p. S57). Standard B.9.10 states that students must have some level of knowledge of "strategies for analyzing issues and making decisions to resolve personal and organizational ethical conflicts" (ACOTE, 2012, p. S58). The expectation as to the depth of this ethics knowledge, however, varies by degree level (see Table 18.1). The need for ethical behavior also is included in the preamble to the ACOTE documents for all degree-level programs, which reads, "A graduate from an ACOTE-accredited . . . program must . . . uphold the ethical standards, values, and attitudes of the occupational therapy profession" (ACOTE, 2012, p. S7).

It is vital that occupational therapy faculty understand the nature and prevalence of academic misconduct and create environments that promote honesty and integrity during the training of future occupational therapy practitioners. Given

- The impact of workplace pressures and constraints that discourage occupational therapy practitioners from taking actions perceived to be ethical (Slater & Brandt, 2009),
- The high levels of cheating in high schools and colleges in the United States (Arhin,

TABLE 18.1
ACOTE Standards Addressing Ethical Conflicts, by Degree Program

Source of Standard	Wording
B.9.10, *Accreditation Standards for an Educational Program for the Occupational Therapy Assistant* (ACOTE, 2012)	"**Identify** strategies for analyzing issues and making decisions to resolve personal and organizational ethical conflicts." (p. S58)
B.9.10, *Accreditation Standards for a Master's-Degree-Level Educational Program for the Occupational Therapist* (ACOTE, 2012)	"**Demonstrate** strategies for analyzing issues and making decisions to resolve personal and organizational ethical conflicts." (p. S58)
B.9.10, *Accreditation Standards for a Doctoral-Degree-Level Educational Program for the Occupational Therapist* (ACOTE, 2012)	"**Demonstrate** strategies for analyzing issues and making decisions to resolve personal and organizational ethical conflicts." (p. S58)

Note. **Bold** font highlights the differences in the ACOTE standards by degree level. ACOTE = Accreditation Council for Occupational Therapy Education.

2009; Danielsen, Simon, & Pavlick, 2006; Fontana, 2009; Josephson Institute Center for Youth Ethics, 2010),

- The association between dishonest behaviors in college and dishonest behaviors in practice (Danielson et al., 2006; Lovett-Hooper et al., 2007; Papadakis et al., 2005), and
- The fact that ethics training is a requirement for accreditation (ACOTE, 2012),

helping students grow and develop ethical and moral behaviors while in academic programs must be a priority in occupational therapy curricula.

Generational Differences in Ethical Norms

One way to better understand academic misconduct is to consider the characteristics of the majority of current college students, who are sometimes known as the Millennial Generation or Generation Y. This cohort of students was born around 1980 (depending on the source), and many are the children of Baby Boomers. Millennials, as a group, grew up with a lot of structure in a busy world (Twenge, 2009). Twenge (2009) discussed the impact of what she called "Generation Me" on medical education. She noted that the generational changes that are likely to have the greatest impact on medical education include "higher expectations, higher levels of narcissism and entitlement, increases in anxiety and mental

problems, and a decline in the desire to read long texts" (p. 400).

Arhin (2009) examined the Generation Y perspective on academic dishonesty among nursing students. As they grew up, Generation Y students were taught to be resourceful, and they value social networks (Arhin, 2009). From their perspective, collaboration may be considered ordinary or morally acceptable in any situation, including one in which individual work is required. The classroom culture must actively identify and encourage academic integrity. According to Hutton (2006), faculty should recognize the importance of social networks and become a part of these networks by building relationships with students: "Creating and strengthening vertical connections between students and instructor is critical for maintaining the instructor's power base" (p. 175).

Occupational therapy students are commonly divided into small groups to work together on assignments. At other times, however, individual work is assigned to allow faculty to evaluate each student's competence in the subject matter. Sometimes the lines between collaboration, collusion, cheating, and plagiarism can be blurry (Savin-Baden, 2005). According to Savin-Baden (2005), "*collaboration* is seen as working together in some form of intellectual activity," whereas "*collusion* is more usually associated with copying work from a fellow student or the passing off of work done jointly as your own," and "*cheating* is trying to gain an unfair advantage or breaking a regulation" (p. 12, italics added). A more subtle form of collusion occurs when one student does not do his or her share of the work on a group project.

Faculty need to make sure that expectations are clear on assignments and that students understand the differences among collaboration, collusion, and plagiarism. Savin-Baden suggested asking groups of students to look at assignments, exams, and other assessments of their performance at the beginning of a course and to find all the ways they could plagiarize or collude. Then students could "be encouraged to contract with each other to collaborate rather than collude so that they all become stakeholders in both the agreement and the assessment" (p. 15).

Role of Faculty in Preventing Academic Dishonesty

One problem with plagiarism is that not all students understand the breadth of what is involved (Kiehl, 2006; Kolanko et al., 2006; Savin-Baden, 2005). Students must understand that plagiarism constitutes theft of ideas and goes beyond forgetting to put quotation marks on a passage. According to the AOTA Ethics Commission's Advisory Opinion, *plagiarism* involves "the taking of another's ideas, thoughts, and concepts from any source" (Kornblau, 2011, p. 205). Sources can include workshops, videos, and the Internet, as well as traditional printed material. Plagiarism also includes omitting quotation marks (even if the source is cited), citing the source inaccurately, or citing the incorrect source altogether.

Almost every university has a writing center, and most occupational therapy programs are in divisions or schools that offer advice to students (and faculty) on how to prevent plagiarism. Additionally, a plethora of Internet sites provide excellent guidance in this area. Many educational programs also provide students with assistance for poor time management, which can contribute to a temptation to plagiarize or otherwise cheat. In the midst of all these readily accessible resources, no one studying occupational therapy should engage in theft of another's ideas,

intentionally or unintentionally. However, faculty need to ensure that students know of the resources that are available and include these resources in course syllabi and on course sites supported by instructional technology.

A discussion of ethical issues in academia would be incomplete without also discussing the ethics and academic integrity of faculty. The Society for Teaching and Learning in Higher Education published *Ethical Principles for College and University Teaching* in Canada in 1996 (Murray, Gillese, Lennon, Mercer, & Robinson, 1996), which was reprinted in the *American Association for Higher Education and Accreditation Bulletin*. This document, intended to serve as a catalyst for discussion, listed nine principles for ethical teaching: (1) content competence, (2) pedagogical competence, (3) ways to deal with sensitive topics, (4) student development, (5) dual relationships with students, (6) confidentiality, (7) respect for colleagues, (8) valid assessment of students, and (9) respect for the institution. The document also includes examples of failure to fulfill each principle. Among the examples are faculty ignoring the power differential between students and faculty, intentionally or unintentionally exploiting students, engaging in favoritism, breaching student confidentiality, making "unwarranted derogatory comments in the classroom about the competence of another teacher" (Murray et al., 1996, para. 30) and "engaging in excessive work activity outside the university that conflicts with the university teaching responsibilities" (para. 36).

Malaski and Tarvydas (2002) explored the nine ethical principles as they relate to rehabilitation counseling educators. They made an important observation about the extra burden of teaching future professionals who will someday be working with patients and clients: Regarding Principle 4, student development, they wrote, "The educational process should not cause harm to students. However, this imperative must be balanced against the educator's responsibility to . . . ensure that the student may serve clients competently in the future as well as the profession overall" (p. 10).

Faculty are powerful role models for students; therefore, their behavior can have a significant impact on students' formation of academic integrity (Couch & Dodd, 2005; DiBartolo & Walsh, 2010; Malaski & Tarvydas, 2002; Tippitt et al., 2009). As Tippitt et al. (2009) observed, "Environments characterized by academic dishonesty are not the fault of students alone. Faculty, administrators, and the entire institutional culture share in the responsibility" (p. 241). In addition to role-modeling ethical behavior, faculty must act when they witness academic misconduct by students. McCabe et al. (2001) reported that faculty often overlook student transgressions because they "do not want to become involved in what they perceive as the bureaucratic procedures designed to adjudicate allegations of academic dishonesty on their campus" (p. 220).

Incivility among faculty, as well as among students, is also an ethical concern in higher education (Clark & Springer, 2007; Kolanko et al., 2006). Clark and Springer (2007) wrote, "Although addressing uncivil student behavior is imperative, it is important that attention is also given to contributions that faculty members may be making to incivility in the academic environment" (p. 7). Clark and Springer reported on incivility in nursing education in a descriptive study of the findings of the Incivility in Nursing Education survey. The respondents, 32 (of 36) faculty and 324 (of 467) nursing students, provided the following examples of faculty behaviors considered uncivil: belittling students through sarcasm, being distant or cold toward students, and ignoring disruptive students. Another category, "beyond uncivil," described behaviors considered more serious, the most frequent of which (cited by 43.5% of respondents) was faculty members' challenges to other faculty members' knowledge or credibility. This finding of incivility among faculty echoes the example used in *Ethical Principles for College and University Teaching* (Murray et al., 1996) under the category of respect for colleagues.

Aggression occurs in educational settings as well as in the workplace. Nursing, like occupational therapy, is a predominantly female profession, and women are more likely than men to express aggression relationally (Kolanko et al., 2006). Relational aggression is frequently played out as bullying or "mean girl games" (Kolanko et al., 2006). This type of aggression is harmful in any workplace, including institutions of higher education (Luparell, 2008). It harms the faculty who are the victims of bullying, compromises the functioning of the department, and can harm students who witness this behavior.

CASE STUDIES

The preceding discussion provides a foundation for the analysis of the three case studies that follow (see Case Studies 18.1–18.13). The first two case studies focus on student behavior, and the third addresses faculty behavior. After each case study, an analysis of the case using the principles of the Code and Ethics Standards is presented.

CASE STUDY 18.1. ADDRESSING ACADEMIC DISHONESTY AMONG OCCUPATIONAL THERAPY STUDENTS

Brittany and **Maddie**, best friends and roommates, were students in the last semester of an entry-level occupational therapy master's-degree program. They had gone to high school together and were very close. Brittany did well academically and was in the Pi Theta Honor Society. Maddie had great people skills but struggled on occasion with study skills and grades. Maddie's sister had a drug abuse problem, and Maddie had spent many hours with her sister in the weeks leading up to finals. She was reasonably prepared for final exams in all her courses except management. Brittany was helping Maddie study, but Maddie was still having difficulty concentrating.

Brittany was a student member on an occupational therapy department committee that met in the department office. Faculty members sent documents to a common printer in the office area. A few days before the management final, Brittany arrived early for a meeting, and the office area was vacant. While she was there, she noticed a copy of the occupational therapy management final exam on the printer. She pulled out her cell phone and took photographs of the exam with the intention of helping Maddie study. She knew it would be wrong to give Maddie the questions, but she decided she would use the questions to help Maddie focus her studying. Brittany didn't feel a need to have the questions because she already had a strong A in the management course and was well prepared for the final exam.

Brittany explained to Maddie that she wouldn't give Maddie the test questions but would use them to help her study. That night, after Brittany was asleep, Maddie got up and e-mailed herself the pictures of the exam questions from Brittany's phone. When Brittany found out, she was horrified and felt terrible. She wasn't sure what to do. If she turned Maddie in, it could end their friendship and her best friend could be kicked out of school, and Brittany would be putting herself in jeopardy as well. Maddie assured Brittany that there was no harm, and therefore no foul, and that this sort of thing happened all the time. Despite her best efforts, Brittany was unable to talk Maddie out of reading the test questions. She felt terribly guilty about having taken the photos in the first place, which was so out of character for her; what *was* she thinking? The exam was in 3 days. How, Brittany asked herself, should she proceed?

Brittany started by thinking about all the awful things that would happen to her and to Maddie and was almost immobilized with anxiety and guilt. Then she started picturing herself and Maddie in practice, working with patients who might be vulnerable and who put their trust in their occupational therapy practitioners. Although cutting a corner to gain an advantage in school might seem minor or inconsequential, what would happen if she or Maddie were under similar pressure in a job situation? Would they cut corners there, too? Brittany could not stand the thought of her coworkers or patients not being able to trust her. She recalled being taught that the Code and Ethics Standards applies to occupational therapy students as well as practitioners. She had practiced applying the Code and Ethics Standards to intervention situations, so she decided to try the same process with her current situation. She knew she had to do the right thing, but what exactly *was* the right thing?

Five of the seven principles of the Code and Ethics Standards have the greatest relevance to this case: Beneficence, Nonmaleficence, Procedural Justice, Veracity, and Fidelity. Principle 1, Beneficence, "requires taking action . . . by promoting good, by preventing harm, and by removing harm" (AOTA, 2010, p. S18). Specifically, Principle 1M states that occupational therapy personnel shall "report to appropriate authorities any acts in practice, education, and research that appear unethical or illegal" (p. S19). Even though Brittany felt fully prepared for the exam (and probably would have scored well), looking at the questions would give her, as well as Maddie, an unfair advantage and was clearly against the rules. In addition, she now had an obligation to prevent further harm (i.e., Nonmaleficence) from occurring through Maddie's use of the questions, which would violate the school's honor code and the Code and Ethics Standards.

Principle 5, Procedural Justice, requires that policies, regulations, and laws are followed to ensure fair treatment—in this case, fair treatment of all students. It would create an unfair advantage for Maddie and Brittany to use their knowledge of the test questions, despite Maddie's personal circumstances. Principle 6, Veracity, addresses the respect that is owed to others and is necessary to develop trust and maintain relationships. Veracity requires refraining from intentional deceit, whether that be lying, misleading someone, or omitting the truth. Brittany also was responsible for following Principle 7, Fidelity, and was therefore required to "discourage, prevent, expose, and correct any breaches of the Code and Ethics Standards, and report any breaches of the former to the appropriate authorities" (Principle 7C; AOTA, 2010, p. S25). This principle would require that, as painful as it may be, she report what had occurred to a faculty member. She decided to confide in **Sharon**, her academic advisor, with whom she had a relationship.

Now that Sharon knew the situation, how could the Code and Ethics Standards guide her decision making? Sharon would have the same obligation to ensure that the appropriate authorities were informed. In addition, Sharon needed to consider Beneficence for her student, particularly Principle 1K, which states that occupational therapy personnel shall "provide students . . . with . . . opportunities to discuss ethical conflicts and procedures for reporting unresolved ethical conflicts" (AOTA, 2010, p. S19). In addition to following enforcement procedures, which would result in disciplinary actions, it was important for Sharon to use the situation as a teaching opportunity. She also wanted to acknowledge and reinforce Brittany's decision to self-report her behavior before the exam.

Drawing on the core value of prudence, Sharon wanted Brittany to use her ethical reasoning skills and judgment to choose a course of action and then reflect on that course of action. Sharon decided to guide Brittany to review the school policies on academic misconduct and self-report to the instructor for the management course, the chair of the department, and the associate dean for academic affairs. Sharon also suggested that Brittany make an appointment at the Student Counseling Office. Sharon asked Brittany to come back to her office as needed for support. Brittany decided to give Maddie the same opportunity to self-report but also told her that if she did not self-report, Brittany would have to report Maddie's behavior. The instructor of the management course gave both students an F on the exam as a punishment for their behavior. The school's policies allowed the instructor to also fail one or both students in the course, but because the disclosure occurred before they took the exam, he opted to apply the consequences only to the theft of the exam questions.

CASE STUDY 18.2. CORRECTING UNWITTING PLAGIARISM BY A FIELDWORK STUDENT

Ben was nearing the end of his last Level II fieldwork at a large rehabilitation facility. He had already accepted a job offer after graduation and was looking forward to his transition from the student role to that of occupational therapist. One of the facility's last requirements for Level II fieldwork students was to provide an in-service to the department. Ben chose to present on the use of constraint-induced movement therapy to the 12 staff occupational therapists. He created a PowerPoint presentation and enjoyed being creative by including images from the Internet and YouTube clips. The presentation was packed with information and was very professional.

Afterward, Ben's fieldwork supervisor, **Andrea**, was interested in learning more about some of the information he presented. She looked up one journal article that he referenced in his presentation and found part of what he had attributed to this source, but he had attributed other information to this source that was not in the article. Andrea did a computer search on a sentence from this missing information. It took her to a Web site that contained an entire segment that Ben had included in his presentation word for word. She then did a similar search with several other passages and found that he had cut and pasted several chunks of information directly from two other Web sites. In neither case did he credit the Web sites or use quotation marks.

When Andrea brought this to Ben's attention, he immediately apologized. He said he had lost track of some of his sources in the process of editing for the final presentation. He also said he was surprised that information on Web sites needed to be referenced because many did not name a specific author.

When Andrea expressed her concern about his behavior as it related to scoring of the ethics portion of the AOTA Fieldwork Performance Evaluation for the Occupational Therapy Student (FWPEOTS; AOTA, 2002), Ben was shocked. He did not think that sharing good clinical information in a professional presentation was unethical, although he admitted it was sloppy on his part not to cite correctly. Andrea told him that even if someone who plagiarizes does not intend to break the law or violate ethical principles, plagiarism is still considered theft of another's ideas or intellectual property. As a result, Andrea explained to Ben that she had no option but to give him a score of unsatisfactory (i.e., 1) on the FWPEOTS Fundamentals of Practice item that reads, "Adheres to ethics: Adheres consistently to the American Occupational Therapy Association Code of Ethics and site's policies and procedures including, when relevant, those related to human subject research" (AOTA, 2002, p. 3). Furthermore, the following stipulation appears in bold font type on the FWPEOTS: "The ratings for the Ethics and Safety items must be scored at 3 or above on the final evaluation for the student to pass the fieldwork experience" (AOTA, 2002, p. 2).

Andrea called the academic fieldwork coordinator at Ben's university to discuss the options of extending Ben's fieldwork with the added requirement of a paper and presentation on plagiarism and asking the university to issue Ben a professional behavior citation that would be part of his academic record. The options would delay Ben's graduation and could affect his job offer, but the alternative would be that Ben receive a failing grade for this fieldwork experience and have to repeat it according to university policies.

The primary ethical principle that Ben violated was Veracity; "Veracity is based on respect owed to others" (AOTA, 2010, p. S23). Specifically, Ben violated Principle 6J, which states that "occupational therapy personnel shall not plagiarize the work of others," and Principle 6I, which directs one to "give credit and recognition when using the work of others in written, oral, or electronic media" (AOTA, 2010, p. S24). Veracity and respect are of utmost importance to maintain the integrity of individual practitioners and the profession.

Luebben (2010) recommended that educators emphasize copyright law violation, in addition to plagiarism, when teaching about intellectual property. Although not everything that is legal is also ethical, most things that are illegal are also unethical. Thus, Ben's action also violated the ethical principle of Procedural Justice. For additional information, see the AOTA Ethics Commission's Advisory Opinion on plagiarism (Kornblau, 2011).

CASE STUDY 18.3. AVOIDING THE DUTY TO REPORT CHEATING

Dr. Robinson had been teaching at a large state university for 10 years. During that time, her class sizes increased, and students seemed less prepared and less mature than when she started. She was knowledgeable in her area of occupational therapy and for the most part was a good teacher. However, Dr. Robinson had grown tired of dealing with what she considered rude behavior on the part of students. Confronting students about their behavior often led to counter-accusations, paperwork, and meetings that took time away from her other work.

Students took their examinations on laptop computers issued by the program using testing software. They were not allowed to have any other materials with them during exams. At a recent kinesiology exam, a student approached Dr. Robinson and said that another student, **Marybeth**, was looking at her cell phone in the pocket of her sweater and had entered insertions and attachments of muscles in her contacts. Dr. Robinson stood and walked around the room, occasionally looking in Marybeth's direction. She thought she might have seen Marybeth slip something into her pocket, but she wasn't sure and just didn't want to deal with the hassle that would ensue if Marybeth was caught cheating. After the exam, the students left the room, and Dr. Robinson headed back to her office. She knew she should have asked to see what was in Marybeth's pocket and to check her cell phone, but she really did not want to get involved.

As Lovett-Hooper et al. (2007) noted, "Teachers who are reluctant to take measures to address academic dishonesty in the classroom may be persuaded to do so when they realize that this behavior is likely to continue" (p. 332). If faculty do not model and take positive actions to promote academic integrity, it is more likely that students will exhibit incivility and misconduct (Clark & Springer, 2007; Hutton, 2006). Dr. Robinson's decision to look the other way could be seen as an act of implicit collusion. By not taking action, Dr. Robinson violated the principle of Beneficence, which states, "Beneficence requires taking action . . . by promoting good, by preventing harm, and by removing harm" (AOTA, 2010, p. S18). Beneficence also requires practitioners "to report to appropriate authorities any acts in practice, education, and research that appear unethical or illegal" (Principle 1M; p. S19).

Principle 5, Procedural Justice, also applies to this case. Specifically, Principle 5A states, "Occupational therapy personnel shall be familiar with and apply the Code and Ethics Standards to the work setting, and share them with employers, other employees, colleagues, students, and researchers" (AOTA, 2010, p. S22). In addition, Principle 5F directs occupational therapy personnel to "take responsibility for maintaining high standards and continuing competence in practice [and] education" (p. S23). Dr. Robinson's actions were a violation of the Code and Ethics Standards in her role as educator, just as not reporting unethical practice in a hospital would be a violation for a direct service provider. Frequently, ethical violations occur not because occupational therapy practitioners fail to recognize an ethical problem but because they choose not to take action. If students observe this type of behavior in the classroom, they may be less likely to demonstrate the moral courage necessary to address ethical issues in practice.

CONCLUSION

Occupational therapy educators have a special responsibility and opportunity to shape the ethical behavior of future occupational therapy practitioners. In addition to teaching about codes of conduct, honor, and ethics and other didactic content, faculty must find ways to promote academic integrity and ethical and civil behavior in the classroom. This content is especially important given the nature of the profession and the potential consequences of unethical practice for future clients.

Although dealing with student misconduct can be bothersome and time consuming, educators should keep in mind that both action and inaction can affect patient and client safety in the future (Danielson et al., 2006; Fontana, 2009; Malaski & Tarvydas, 2002) and that unethical conduct among students must be directly addressed at every opportunity. DiBartolo and Walsh (2010) noted,

> Much has been written about the prevalence of academic dishonesty in the past two decades. Despite the dialogue, incidents have not only increased in number, but also in complexity as students discover even more creative and technologically savvy ways to circumvent the system. (p. 543)

Faculty may need to know more about the ethical and moral maturity of students entering our professional programs. Couch and Dodd (2005) suggested that "instead of assuming that students come to higher education hard-wired with ethical principles, colleges should expand and refine new student orientation programs after first taking inventory of incoming students' understanding and application of ethical issues and behavior" (p. 25). They proposed adapting tools used by human resource managers in the business world to assess ethical or moral maturity.

Finally, faculty should consider any possible contributions they make to the problem of student misconduct by the manner in which they relate to other faculty and/or to students, and they should attempt to understand the issues associated with the current generation of college students. In conclusion, occupational therapy educators should heed the recommendations of Hutton (2006), who stated,

> Faculty attitudes, behavior, and actions can play a significant role in reducing the incidence of academic dishonesty by (1) reducing opportunities to cheat and increasing

the probability of being caught through greater vigilance, (2) overcoming our hesitancy to report cheaters, and (3) establishing and promoting academic integrity as the social norm among students through our relationships with students which, in turn, provides support for students who disapprove of cheating. (p. 175)

REFERENCES

Accreditation Council for Occupational Therapy Education. (2012). 2011 Accreditation Council for Occupational Therapy Education (ACOTE®) standards. *American Journal of Occupational Therapy, 66*(6 Suppl.), S6–S74. doi: 10.5014/ajot.2012.66S6

American Occupational Therapy Association. (2002). *Fieldwork performance evaluation for the occupational therapy student.* Bethesda, MD: Author.

American Occupational Therapy Association. (2010). Occupational therapy code of ethics and ethics standards (2010). *American Journal of Occupational Therapy, 64*(6 Suppl.), S17–S26. doi: 10.5014/ajot.2010.64S17

Arhin, A. O. (2009). A pilot study of nursing student's perceptions of academic dishonesty: A Generation Y perspective. *Association of Black Nursing Faculty in Higher Education Journal, 20,* 17–21.

Clark, C. M., & Springer, P. J. (2007). Incivility in nursing education: A descriptive study of definitions and prevalence. *Journal of Nursing Education, 46,* 7–14.

Couch, S., & Dodd, S. (2005). Doing the right thing: Ethical issues in higher education. *Journal of Family and Consumer Sciences, 97,* 20–27.

Danielson, R. D., Simon, A. F., & Pavlick, R. (2006). The culture of cheating: From the classroom to the exam room. *Journal of Physician Assistant Education, 17,* 23–29.

DiBartolo, M. C., & Walsh, C. M. (2010). Desperate times call for desperate measures: Where are we in addressing academic dishonesty? *Journal of Nursing Education, 49,* 543–544.

Fontana, J. S. (2009). Nursing faculty experiences of students' academic dishonesty. *Journal of Nursing Education, 48,* 181–185.

Hutton, P. A. (2006). Understanding student cheating and what educators can do about it. *College Teaching, 54,* 171–176.

Josephson Institute Center for Youth Ethics. (2010). *The ethics of American youth.* Retrieved from http://charactercounts.org/programs/reportcard/2010/index.html

Kiehl, E. M. (2006). Using an ethical decision-making model to determine consequences for student plagiarism. *Journal of Nursing Education, 45,* 199–203.

Kolanko, K. M., Clark, C., Heinrich, K. T., Olive, D., Serembus, J. F., & Sifford, K. S. (2006). Academic dishonesty, bullying, incivility, and violence: Difficult challenges facing nurse educators. *Nursing Education Perspectives, 27,* 34–42.

Kornblau, B. L. (2011). *Plagiarism.* In D. Y. Slater (Ed.), *Reference guide to the Occupational Therapy Code of Ethics and Ethics Standards* (2010 ed., pp. 205–208). Bethesda, MD: AOTA Press.

Lovett-Hooper, G., Komarraju, M., Weston, R., & Dollinger, S. J. (2007). Is plagiarism a forerunner of other deviance? Imagined futures of academically dishonest students. *Ethics and Behavior, 17,* 323–336.

Luebben, A. (2010, May). *Teaching and learning about intellectual property issues: Authorship, copyright, ownership, attribution, and plagiarism.* Poster session presented at the AOTA Annual Conference & Expo, Orlando, FL.

Luparell, S. (2008, April/May). Incivility in nursing education: Let's put an end to it. *National Student Nurses Association Imprint,* pp. 42–46.

Malaski, C., & Tarvydas, V. M. (2002). Teaching ethics and the ethics of teaching: Challenges for rehabilitation counselor educators. *Rehabilitation Education, 16,* 1–13.

McCabe, D. L. (2009). Academic dishonesty in nursing schools: An empirical investigation. *Journal of Nursing Education, 48,* 614–623.

McCabe, D. L., Treviño, L. K., & Butterfield, K. D. (2001). Cheating in academic institutions: A decade of research. *Ethics and Behavior, 11,* 219–232.

Murray, H., Gillese, E., Lennon, M., Mercer, P., & Robinson, M. (1996). *Ethical principles for college and university teaching.* Washington, DC: American Association for Higher Education and Accreditation. Retrieved from www.aahea.org/articles/Ethical+Principles.htm

Papadakis, M. A., Teherani, A., Banach, M. A., Knettler, T. R., Rattner, S. L., Stern, D. T., . . . Hodgson, C. S. (2005). Disciplinary action by medical boards and prior behavior in medical school. *New England Journal of Medicine, 353,* 2673–2682.

Savin-Baden, M. (2005). Why collaborate when you can cheat? Understanding plagiarism in OT education. *British Journal of Occupational Therapy, 68,* 11–16.

Slater, D., & Brandt, L. (2009). Combating moral distress. *OT Practice, 14*(2), 13–16, 18.

Tippitt, M. P., Nell, A., Kline, J. R., Tilghman, J., Chamberlain, B., & Meagher, P. G. (2009). Creating environments that foster academic integrity. *Nursing Education Perspectives, 30,* 239–244.

Twenge, J. M. (2009). Generational changes and their impact in the classroom: Teaching Generation Me. *Medical Education, 43,* 398–405.

Ethics in Occupational Therapy Research

19

Elizabeth Larson, PhD, OTR

Research is often viewed in U.S. culture as an objective way of discovering or validating knowledge. The popular belief is that immutable facts are revealed through carefully designed research that is executed and analyzed in precise and systematic ways. Although excellent research displays these hallmarks, designing and conducting high-quality research also requires a series of carefully considered ethical decisions. In addition, social scientists have pointed out that scientific inquiry is not a value-free activity but rather is shaped by cultural context and, at times, even political pursuit (Albert, Laberge, & Hodges, 2009). Consider the example of studies investigating genetically based differences in intelligence. Some applications of these studies' findings have been highly inflammatory and created widespread concern about their influence on social policies and on people's opportunities in society. As Gray and Thompson (2004) noted,

> Although the topic of race differences is only a minor area within the field of intelligence research, it has had a disproportionately large (and strongly negative) impact on the public perception of intelligence research. Science is generally perceived as a noble and honorable pursuit, yet "The field of intelligence itself is widely suspect" [Gottfredsen, 1994].

> Given the history of misuse of intelligence research, a statement about biology and intelligence that ignores the question of race can be mistaken as being complicit with a racist agenda. (p. 479)

Researchers' choices regarding framing questions and method selection are influenced by their current theoretical framework, their disciplinary and scholarly values, their methodological training, and the sociopolitical and historical contexts surrounding research. Scientific practices are formed by the disciplinary habitus (i.e., way of doing) and epistemic culture (i.e., valued way of knowing) of the discipline (Becher & Trowler, 2001; Bordieu, 2004). Schools of thought embracing specific theoretical orientations are often centered in different universities or research centers, each with its own cultural values. Through graduate training, new generations of researchers are enculturated into specific research values, roles, and approaches. This process may lead them to take for granted directives about what approach to take to research, what kinds of questions to ask, and how to conduct research (Albert et al., 2009).

The health care climate, the needs of occupational therapy consumers, and occupational therapy practitioners' professional values and beliefs shape how occupational therapy research is currently "produced" and used within our practice. All occupational therapists now enter the profession with graduate degrees. This move to advanced preparation for entry-level practice was predicated in part on the necessity for therapists to be competent in evaluating and using research evidence for best practice (Accreditation Council for Occupational Therapy Education [ACOTE], 2006). Three core ethical issues affecting research in occupational therapy are addressed in this chapter: (1) the centrality of research to professionalism and professional power, reflected in the identification and selection of specific research topics that produce knowledge of value to our profession and the general public (i.e., our epistemic culture); (2) the design and conduct of studies (i.e., our disciplinary habitus) in beneficent and principled ways, including in emerging areas of research in which fewer guidelines exist; and (3) publication of this knowledge to inform occupational therapy practice.

To better illustrate and understand the complexity of ethical decision making in the production of research, a vignette is provided. As these examples demonstrate, ethical practice in research requires more than simply following a prescribed set of behaviors or professional principles. Often situations arise that include competing interests among research stakeholders or conflicts in the application of ethical principles. In these circumstances, occupational therapy practitioners and researchers must carefully evaluate their own and others' interests and consider the balance among ethical principles to choose the most ethical response.

CENTRALITY OF RESEARCH TO PROFESSIONALISM AND PROFESSIONAL POWER

Science is the cornerstone of the forward-thinking *Centennial Vision* for occupational therapy: "We envision that occupational therapy is a powerful, widely recognized, science-driven, and evidence-based profession with a globally connected and diverse workforce meeting society's occupational needs" (American Occupational Therapy Association [AOTA], 2007, p. 613). The generation of a substantive knowledge base is viewed as

critical to supporting best practice, to increasing and broadening our reach to serve all those who can benefit from our services, and to allowing the profession to flourish within current and future health care climates. This vision emphasizes the need for science- and evidence-based practice that is supported by several principles found in the *Occupational Therapy Code of Ethics and Ethics Standards (2010)* (referred to as the "Code and Ethics Standards"; AOTA, 2010).

As the 100th anniversary of the founding of the occupational therapy profession approaches, the *Centennial Vision* is just one more indicator of the current spirit of both growth and renewal in occupational therapy. This vision accompanies what has been described as a renaissance or return to our occupational roots (Wood et al., 2000). In 1917, the founders articulated a need for a science of occupation to advance "occupation as a therapeutic measure for the study of the effect of occupation upon the human being; and for the scientific dispensation of this knowledge" (AOTA, 1967, p. 4). In the past several decades, scholars and occupational therapy practitioners have more keenly focused on articulating and demonstrating occupation as both a therapeutic means and end for promoting health and well-being (Gray, 1998). This focus on occupation is timely and in line with the current World Health Organization (2000) view of health as the ability of people to do what they wish to do. Respect for clients' autonomy is articulated in Principle 3 of the Code and Ethics Standards (AOTA, 2010).

Although occupational therapy has long claimed participation in occupation as the foundation of health and well-being, the study of participation has spread to other health professions across the world. For example, scientists in the fields of epidemiology, psychology, and other social sciences have developed participation measures (e.g., Brown et al., 2004; Van Brakel et al., 2006). How occupational therapy practitioners continue scholarship in occupation will influence how the profession is viewed and positioned within the larger realm of health and social professions. Whether occupational therapy practitioners are recognized as *the* or *key* experts in participation and health depends on how well we continue to generate relevant and high-quality evidence, promote public awareness of this research, and apply it for effective service delivery. It also depends on how research efforts are targeted. This targeting includes carefully considering what knowledge is needed and useful to professional practice and to society. The following epistemic questions must be addressed:

- What is worth knowing? Specifically, which theories or ideas should be investigated?
- How should this knowledge be generated?
- How should this knowledge be applied in practice?

These are all ethical questions. The first question addresses the unique niche we inhabit within health care. The decision as to what studies to pursue not only demonstrates what is valued but also shapes the way information is filtered in professional and nonprofessional settings. Occupational therapy practitioners think occupationally about their clients—in terms of doing. Hooper (2006), citing Palmer (1983), pointed out that values become a lens for viewing the world that influences what is seen, what rises to awareness, and what motivates actions. In turn, this "way of knowing" the world then shapes interactions such that "our epistemology is quietly transformed into our ethic" (Palmer, 1983, p. 21).

Occupational therapy practitioners hold a common belief in the power of occupation to foster health. In pursuing a core phenomenon, a profession may have competing paradigms that promote different theoretical approaches and research methods (Christiansen, 1981; Kuhn, 1962). In addition, tensions between influences inside and outside the profession, as well as pragmatic considerations, may act on the research agenda. For example, outside the profession, the agendas set by funders of research and their review panels control the available resources for research and historically have often promoted certain methodologies and research foci. In addition, funders of occupational therapy services and legislators are making demands for evidence of the efficacy of occupational therapy practice (Bernstein, Collette, & Pederson, 2010). This, too, is an outside influence that strongly influences the direction of our collective research efforts.

Leaders of the profession have waged a strong response to calls for data on the efficacy of

services. This response in turn has been encoded into our professional ethics in Principle 1N, "Occupational therapy personnel shall take responsibility for promoting and practicing occupational therapy on the basis of current knowledge and research and for further developing the profession's body of knowledge" (AOTA, 2010, p. S19). Indeed, demonstrating that our services promote improved functioning and well-being is an ethical imperative (Christiansen & Lou, 2001). Likewise, it is important that our services do no harm. Christiansen and Lou (2001) pointed out that although occupational therapy practitioners are less likely to cause harm by ineffective intervention than some other health care professionals, ineffective intervention still has psychological, financial, and other costs to clients. These costs may present in the form of diminished opportunities and abilities to succeed and wasted health care resources. Using the framework of evidence-based medicine (EBM) and assessment of levels of evidence, AOTA leaders forged a plan to promote the development and publication of specific kinds of research. The publication priorities developed by the *American Journal of Occupational Therapy (AJOT)* editorial board that are in alignment with the *Centennial Vision* (Gutman, 2008, 2010) are presented in Table 19.1.

The emphasis for these priorities is on producing the highest levels of evidence as outlined by Sackett and his colleagues' work in EBM (Sackett, Richardson, Rosenberg, & Haynes, 1997; Sackett, Straus, Richardson, Rosenberg, & Haynes, 2000). A pyramid of evidence showing what is considered increasing quality is displayed in Figure 19.1 (Dartmouth Biomedical Laboratories, 2008). The highest levels are critical analyses of compilations of studies. Systematic reviews, evidence syntheses, and critical appraisals of studies are judged the most powerful evidence. The best "unfiltered" evidence (in order of decreasing quality) is the randomized controlled trial (RCT), the cohort study, and the case control study. At the bottom of the pyramid is expert opinion. Proponents of evidence-based practice suggest that in some instances the best possible evidence for a particular question may not be an RCT; rather, the question should always direct the selection of study design (Sackett, Rosenberg, Gray, Haynes,

TABLE 19.1
Publication Priorities of the **American Journal of Occupational Therapy**

PRIORITY	SUGGESTED DESIGNS TO ADDRESS PRIORITIES
Evidence of efficacy and efficiency of clinical practices	Analysis of multiple studies (e.g., systematic reviews, meta-analyses, metasyntheses) Efficacy or outcome studies (e.g., randomized controlled trials, nonrandomized pretest–posttest designs, crossover or randomized block or follow-up designs, multiple baseline or participant single-subject designs, feasibility studies, case studies reporting novel interventions) Mixed-method studies of safety of, satisfaction with, adherence to, or tolerance of interventions Secondary analysis of large data sets to examine cost and time efficiency, patient satisfaction, safety, and adherence to interventions
Measures useful for occupational therapy practice and research	Instrument development and testing of psychometrics of tools
Evidence of the relationship of occupational engagement to development, health, and well-being throughout the life span	Studies that correlate specific health indicators with occupational engagement
Research on participation for people with disabilities that can be used to develop clinical practice guidelines testable for efficacy	Qualitative needs assessments of consumers in emerging practice areas
Scholarship guiding the profession's future growth and evolution	Analysis articles debating professional issues for "The Issue Is" section or other appropriate publications within the profession

Source. Gutman (2008).

& Richardson, 1996). In addition, they believe that the evidence must be considered in relation to client preferences and integrated with clinical expertise.

Heralded as a significant step forward for the health professions, the EBM model is not without critics. Critiques focus on questions of epistemology and application of EBM in practice professions. For example, Cohen, Stavri, and Hersch (2004) suggested a problematic imbalance in a focus on the empirical "purity" of studies (specifically, RCT methodologies) to the detriment of development of a core understanding of mechanisms and processes underlying health. They outlined three major points of concern: (1) the lack of evidence that RCTs and meta-analyses are more reliable than other research methods for answering clinical questions (which would entail research demonstrating better outcomes for clients of practitioners who apply evidence in practice); (2) the limited questions EBM is suited to answer; and (3) the lack of integration of EBM with "other, non-statistical, forms of medical information, such as professional experience and patient specific factors" (p. 39). Cohen and colleagues believed that defining evidence this way limits the questions that may be answered and leaves unanswered many questions essential to a practice profession:

Questions specific to small patient populations, or those that require subjective evaluation (such as improvement in the quality of life) . . . cannot be studied by the methods that EBM deems "best." Furthermore, since the methods

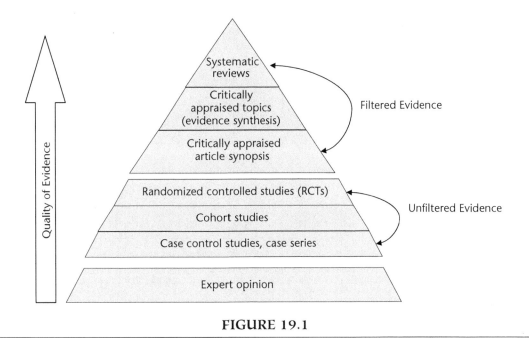

FIGURE 19.1

Quality of evidence in evidence-based medicine.
From EBM Pyramid and EBM Page Generator, Copyright © 2006–2011, Trustees of Dartmouth College and Yale University. All rights reserved. Produced by Jan Glover, David Izzo, Karen Odato and Lei Wang. Adapted with permission.

of EBM are epidemiological and statistical, clinically important details may be hidden, overlooked, or simply "averaged out" by the methods of the study. . . . Upshur describes a taxonomy that includes four types of evidence: qualitative–personal, qualitative–general, quantitative–personal, and quantitative–general. . . . Upshur's categorization conceptualizes the essential qualities of evidence as being the context of its use and its means of production, and does not rank one combination as inherently better than another. Of these four categories, EBM only specifically deals with the quantitative–general form of evidence. . . . Perhaps EBM should be renamed "methods of incorporating epidemiologic evidence into clinical practice." (p. 39)

These authors' insights suggest that, when generating evidence for practice, the means of best answering that question, and the context in which the resulting evidence will be used all need to be considered in the study's design. In prioritizing RCTs and meta-analyses as research designs for our profession, an emphasis is being placed on de-

veloping key evidence to demonstrate the efficacy of our services in populations of clients. This first step in generating population-based evidence of the efficacy of intervention needs to be followed by other research that focuses on client-centered implementation of these efficacious occupational therapy services.

Cochrane (2004), the grandfather of the EBM movement, recognized that some questions essential to health care practice do not lend themselves to "statistical manipulations." His book took a critical view of the efficiency and effectiveness of the British national health care system, noting that some common practices continued despite inefficiency or even possible patient harm. He noted that practitioners both *care* for and make efforts to *cure* their clients and that both the process and the methods for intervention were important to health care services. The diagram in Figure 19.2 illustrates the scope of information important to the client (Circle C) that is not believed to be "evidence based" (Cochrane, p. xxv, cited in Hope, 1997).

In her Eleanor Clarke Slagle Lecture, Rogers (1983), like Cochrane (2004), recognized this integrative interplay in practice as necessary for effective service delivery, which must

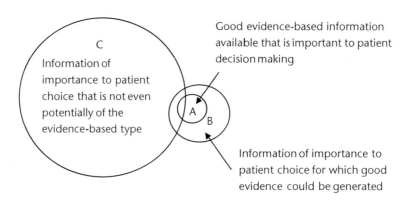

FIGURE 19.2

Availability of evidence-based information important to patient choice.
Adapted from "Random Reflections on Health Services" by T. Hope, in *Effectiveness and efficiency: Random reflections on health services*, (p. xxv), by A. J. Cochrane, 1972, London: Nuffield Provincial Hospitals Trust. (Reprinted in 2004 for Nuffield Trust by the Royal Society of Medicine Press, London)

include consideration of the dynamics of human relationships, an understanding of clients' preferences and capacities, and a process through which therapeutic change may occur. She noted that reflective, individualized practice results in ethical decisions about the approach and course of intervention. In her words, "Without science, clinical inquiry is not systematic; without ethics, it is not responsible; without art, it is not convincing" (Rogers, 1983, p. 616).

Occupational therapy scholars have debated what knowledge is useful and essential to our profession (Abreu, Peloquin, & Ottenbacher, 1998; Carlson & Clark, 1991; Spencer, 1993; Yerxa, 1992). In a seminal article on ethics and epistemology, Yerxa (1992) advocated that to be ethical, our science must be commensurate with our view of occupation. She outlined the following guidelines for knowledge generation in occupational therapy:

- Elucidate client capacities rather than limitations.
- Study people in context.
- Focus at the person level.
- Consider developmental and life span processes of occupation.
- Focus on the person's experience of occupation.
- Examine organization and balance of occupation in daily life.
- Synthesize knowledge across disciplines to address occupational complexity.

Research following these guidelines would require a contextualized approach to examine the person's experience while he or she is engaged in the world of everyday life activities. In this way, research produced would be both beneficent and socially just, providing knowledge about clients' occupational needs that is rooted in their unique personal, social, and cultural influences. In Yerxa's view, only qualitative methods have the breadth and depth to study occupation without losing its core essence. Similarly, Spencer (1993) advocated for the need to study meaning, context, and change processes within intervention. She advocated for efforts to enhance a practical understanding of how physical and cultural contexts influence recovery and daily functioning for people with disabilities. Research that fosters an understanding of consumers' perspectives is crucial to promoting effective life change.

Qualitative methods have an important role to play in our epistemic culture. As the *AJOT* Editorial Board pointed out in its priorities (Gutman, 2008, 2009), qualitative research can be both generative (producing new insights) and grounded (in the participant's perspective rather than the researcher's perspective or previous theory). As Yerxa (1992) and Spencer (1993) enjoined, these methods can increase our understanding of clients and their occupational choices and of what matters to them, how their experience evolves over time during the course of intervention, and what bolsters their healthy participation within their particular contexts. Qualitative methods also can help us understand why clients refuse or fail to use strategies or adaptive equipment, even after these interventions are demonstrated to be effective through various research methods. The rich descriptions generated through qualitative approaches provide sufficiently detailed information to allow occupational therapy practitioners to make decisions case by case about which clients may benefit from specific interventions and under what circumstances. These methods can be used in tandem with experimental designs or alone to better identify the critical person and process features that are vital to optimal outcomes.

The different views presented in this chapter about the kinds of research needed to foster the profession's growth and best serve clients diverge in significant ways. Factors both inside and outside the profession will influence how occupational science and occupational therapy research unfold in the next several decades. Schools of thought situated in specific universities, research societies, and public policies will all continue to shape the direction and use of research in the profession. Both clear vision and innovation are needed to direct research efforts in ways that are commensurate with the values of the profession.

Many research designs and methodologies can generate data for practice on occupational participation both in context and in relation to individual client factors. Several exemplars of occupational therapy research have used designs aligned with our professional values and focused on occupation and also have produced high-level evidence. The Tailored Activity Program (Gitlin et al., 2009) and the Well Elderly Study (Clark et al., 1997) are two examples of personalized, contextualized, occupation-based intervention programs that have been shown to be effective with elders. These studies used RCT designs with large populations and developed a standardized intervention protocol that was then personalized to each client's interests and desires. These exemplars are in line with our epistemology, professional values, and need for evidence.

Ethically, we owe it to the forces outside the profession demanding evidence of efficacy to pro-vide evidence that occupational therapy services are effective and socially useful. Current and accepted methods for demonstrating efficacy need to be used in ways that align with our epistemic culture. Unlike drug or other single treatments, occupational therapy is a complex, person-centered practice. When choosing the direction and methods of the profession's research agenda, it's important to consider the usefulness, limitations, and applicability of any approach used to generate evidence. Designs need to consider the person factors and the therapeutic relationship. In addition, we should not ignore critiques leveled in medicine that research intended to generate evidence for practice cannot be atheoretical in conceptualization or design. For occupational therapy, these considerations mean that practice evidence should contribute to an understanding of the processes underlying achieving health and well-being through occupational participation. One could argue that theoretical development and generation of evidence go hand in hand.

ETHICAL DESIGN AND CONDUCT OF RESEARCH

Over time, at key turning points in history, research has become increasingly regulated by international, national, and local agencies to ensure that researchers follow the principles of Beneficence, Nonmaleficence, Social Justice, Procedural Justice, and Veracity. Each of these principles is part of the Code and Ethics Standards of the occupational therapy profession (AOTA, 2010). Researchers must carefully consider the balance between potentially beneficial research outcomes and the costs to research participants when making decisions about the design, conduct, and publication of their research. In addition, to redress past limitations, current guidelines encourage more socially just approaches, such as the study of previously understudied or vulnerable groups. Throughout the process, following the established guidelines—Procedural Justice—is essential for ensuring the protection of human participants' rights. Finally, Veracity also permeates the entire research process, being essential to producing knowledge that in the end is useful, accurate, and ethical.

Historical Foundations of Research Ethics

Historically, public outcry surrounding unethical studies led to the development of guidelines for recruitment and treatment of research participants (National Institutes of Health [NIH], 2004). In several infamous studies in the early 20th century, researchers embraced a utilitarian ethical principle; they believed that despite the high costs to the few participants, the studies' findings would benefit the many. This end often outweighed their consideration of the participants' health and well-being.

For example, some medical researchers intentionally induced diseases or failed to treat disease in the people participating in their studies (Corbie-Smith, 1999; Hornblum, 1997). They sought to recruit readily available or easily influenced populations such as prisoners, institutionalized people with mental retardation, debilitated elders in institutions, or illiterate or poor members of minority populations (Hornblum, 1997). Prisoners and residents of treatment centers were considered both convenient and desirable participants for research because they lived in "controlled settings."

Following the Nuremberg trials of Nazi physicians, the first worldwide code for research was generated (see Appendix 19.A). The Nuremburg Code (1949) laid the foundation for core ethical principles in use today and included key provisions to protect participants and to ensure that studies were reasonable, necessary, and likely to produce humanitarian benefits. Specifically, this code required studies to be rooted in prior knowledge or research, to be conducted by qualified researchers, to have a potential humanitarian benefit that exceeded the potential risks to participants, to be conducted only if a priori evidence suggested that participation would not result in potential death or disability, and to be terminated at any time continuation was believed to be harmful to participants.

Unfortunately, after World War II, some U.S. physicians did not believe that the Nuremberg Code applied to their research. In some of these studies, researchers encouraged prisoners' participation by offering early release or other privileges in exchange for participation in studies that involved intentional exposure to deadly diseases,

cancer, or radiation or unnecessary surgeries (Hornblum, 1997). The reasoning of the time suggested that prisoners' research participation was moral, allowing them to right a wrong (their crime) or to contribute (during World War II) to the war effort by being "human guinea pigs" for various studies, including radiation studies. Historical evidence suggests that many prison participants were not informed of the potential risks and that their participation was not voluntary by the Nuremberg Code standards.

Likewise, psychological studies have evoked concern, especially when deception was used as part of the design. Milgram's (1968) study on authority, aimed at examining Nazis' justifications for their war conduct, is one example. His experiments studied the conditions under which and likelihood with which people would follow an authority figure's demands. In multiple studies, he found that when an authority figure wearing a white coat stood nearby, 65% of participants provided increasing and even deadly levels of electrical current to an actor they believed was a coparticipant who made learning mistakes. Following the study, participants were not debriefed on the deception. They were left to deal with altered self-perceptions of their capacity to do or not do harm to another person when influenced by a person in power.

Later, again in response to highly publicized abuses in the 1960s and 1970s, global and U.S. scientific councils outlined additional ethical standards for the conduct of research studies. The Declaration of Helsinki (World Medical Association, 2008), the Belmont Report (NIH, 2004), and the Office for Human Research Protections of the U.S. Department of Health and Human Services (DHHS; 2005) rules for the protection of human participants provided additional guidelines and requirements for researchers. The first Declaration of Helsinki was the first effort of the worldwide medical community to regulate medical and clinical research. The Belmont Report emphasized three core ethics: respect for persons, beneficence, and justice (NIH, 2004). Carefully balancing the needs of a vulnerable population with the importance of studying their health, the DHHS rules specifically addressed the manner and method for inclusion of vulnerable and underresearched populations in research (see

Appendix 19.B; Office for Human Research Protections, DHHS, 2005). These guidelines address the ethical treatment of participants through all steps of the research, beginning with the study's conceptualization and continuing through the steps of design, consent, conduct, conclusion, analysis, and publication. These codes are meant to assist researchers in designing studies that ensure that "serious efforts have been made to protect the rights and welfare of research subjects" (NIH, 2004, p. 4).

Ethics in Design

Study design begins with the identification of a significant and socially valuable question. The question must be of sufficient importance to justify the participants' time and exposure to risks (Gilliam, Guillemin, Bolitho, & Rosenthal, 2009). The study design and methods selected to address the question must also be scientifically rigorous. Poorly designed or shoddy research violates basic ethical guidelines (Gilliam et al., 2009).

Questions for research are often rooted in current social concerns. Presently, investigating and explaining the underlying roots of health disparities among ethnic groups that cannot be accounted for by variations in resources, such as education or income, is a key priority in U.S. health research (DHHS, 2000). This priority has spurred funding of studies inclusive across age, gender, ethnicity, sexual orientation, socioeconomic status, and educational attainment. Equitable inclusion of diverse people requires study designs that address a more complex heterogeneous participant selection. In the past, researchers often excluded female participants in medical research in an effort to control for variability attributable to hormone cycles. This practice led to the current problem of limited and insufficient understanding of women's responses to different treatments, including those for leading causes of mortality and disability. Efforts to control variability must be balanced against the need to produce research that benefits people of all groups, especially those most likely to have the specific conditions under study.

Researchers must weigh choices to study vulnerable groups against the benefits likely to accrue to members of those groups and others from their participation and from the potential outcomes of the proposed studies. Concerns about past exploitation have led to strict guidelines for the participation of vulnerable people in research. Institutional review board (IRB) applications require investigators to document whether a vulnerable population will be included and require evidence that the study safeguards and procedures will address the specific needs of the vulnerable population. Measures may include specially designed recruitment material, simplified language in the informed consent form, alternative procedures for nonliterate participants, or justification of the use of incentives to recruit or reward participants after study completion.

Planning and designing procedures for informed consent are a critical part of the research process. Many online Web resources are available to assist in developing informed consent forms with all of the essential components and in assessing the grade level of language used, such as the SMOG Formula and the Fry Readability Graph (Centers for Disease Control and Prevention, 2009). A common guideline is that the informed consent should be at a 6th- to 8th-grade reading level. In cases in which participants' literacy is known to be more limited, the consent should be at a reading level appropriate to the group's comprehension of language. For example, when working with a group of Native American caregivers, I knew that the literacy of some was at the 4th-grade level, and I therefore created consents with simpler vocabulary and paragraph structure and more active language. Consents for non-English-speaking participants also may need to be translated and back translated (i.e., translated to the participants' first language and translated again to English to check the accuracy of the translation) to ensure that they understand the expectations and procedures of the study.

In the case of research with children, minors generally are not able to consent to research participation, so their parents must consent on their behalf. Still, assent procedures are highly recommended, especially for children ages 10 years or older. To obtain assent, researchers describe the study to a child in language he or she can understand and then give the child the option to sign or otherwise note his or her agreement or refusal to participate.

In all studies, the written consent is only one part of the consent process. The research team also is obligated to discuss and explain study procedures to the participant. Both the oral presentation, either in person or by phone, and the signing of the consent are important steps in ensuring that the participant understands and agrees to participate in the study. In addition, a review of recruitment materials and processes is part of the IRB steps for approval of the study. The advertising scripts used to recruit participants must explain the study in clear and accurate ways, and wording of the risks and benefits must carefully parallel the wording used in the informed consent.

Progressive researchers are now also assessing participants' understanding of the informed consent process. This additional step of surveying participants' understanding of the study's aims, the activities expected of them, and their rights helps ensure and verify that vulnerable study participants truly understand the import of their consent (Buccini, 2009; Dunn, 2006). Following such a survey, researchers can then provide further education in areas the participant did not understand well. This step is particularly useful in adult populations in which people's medical or health conditions are believed to potentially impair their capacity for autonomous decision making.

The design of study procedures is an important step in conducting an ethical research project. Throughout the design of a study, multiple decisions must be made to ensure that the best and most ethical options are chosen. This process often entails weighing ideal scientific design against the participants' interests and pragmatic considerations that constrain or limit the research design and conduct of the study.

Impact of Research on Participants

Even with well-designed consents, surveys of consent comprehension, and considerable forethought in addressing expected consequences of participation, research may have unintended effects on participants. For this reason, researchers must continue to monitor participants throughout the study for any ill effects, which must be reported to the IRB in yearly reviews. Intervention studies must provide participants with information about viable alternatives to those offered in the study, and researchers may need to provide treatment if undesired outcomes occur. In treatment studies in which positive outcomes result from the intervention, ethical researchers typically offer the intervention to people who participated in control groups. This offer requires advance planning to ensure that the research budget includes control group treatment.

Little research has been done to examine the effects of study participation, even effects whose risks are typically considered minimal. In a follow-up of research on occupational therapy practitioners' ethical dilemmas in practice, Barnitt and Partridge (1999) interviewed therapists about their experience participating in the ethics study. Two therapists provided very different accounts of the experience of participating:

[The researcher] asked me to describe an ethical problem I had encountered at work. I had had notice of this and had decided which one to report on. She just left me to talk, and I found that I was getting out of my depth, revealing things I didn't want exposed. (p. 256)

My colleagues are nervous of discussing the dilemma [discharge of a confused elderly patient] because we can never agree. It was nice to talk about it without being judged. (p. 257)

Although the first therapist felt vulnerable and overexposed, the second felt the study provided an open and affirming forum. In both cases, participating in research was neither objective nor neutral from the participating therapists' perspectives. Some may argue that the participants had disparate reactions because it was qualitative research and addressed a sensitive topic; nevertheless, evidence on the impact of research on the people who participate in it remains insufficient. Researchers need to recognize that participation can have life-altering effects on participants, and more study is warranted in this area.

VIGNETTE 19.1. CONFRONTING THE RISKS OF RESEARCH FOR PARTICIPANTS: A PERSONAL STORY

While in graduate school in California, I received a call from my sister-in-law in Wisconsin telling me that **my mother** had been hospitalized. I flew home to find her in a hospital bed, her left side black and blue from head to toe and a baseball-sized hematoma over her left eye. She looked as if she'd survived a bad car wreck. Because of a "shower" of pulmonary embolisms, she'd passed out in her home and fallen from midstair onto a concrete basement floor. Doctors said she'd beaten the odds; they'd given her only a 30% chance of survival when she arrived in the emergency room. Using a textbook to guide them, they administered a new "clot-busting" drug that saved her life.

My mom was one of the many volunteers participating in the longitudinal **Women's Health Initiative (WHI) Study** examining the effects of hormone replacement therapy (HRT) and other supplements on the incidence of heart disease and stroke. We suspected this life-threatening event was related to medication she received from the study. We called the WHI study coordinator, who refused to provide any information about what medications she was receiving via the study. Only after her physician contacted the research team did they break the double-blind group assignments to reveal that she was indeed receiving HRT.

My mother's experience and the experiences of others led to the early termination of the hormone replacement part of the study in 2002, although she continued in the study until its completion. Despite practitioners' intuition that HRT was beneficial to women's health, this randomized controlled trial demonstrated that HRT was not beneficial for many and caused harm for some (National Heart, Lung, and Blood Institute, 2002).

Do you agree with the research team's response to my family? Was the team's behavior consistent with the principles of the Code and Ethics Standards? How and when should a "negative event" such as the one my mother experienced lead to an alteration of study procedures? How should my mother's and other participants' consent to this study be reevaluated following an aversive reaction?

Issues in the Use of Innovative Methodology and Confidentiality of Data

Several advances in research methods have highlighted the need for additional safeguards and study to determine how to ethically manage research participants' confidential information. For example, genetics researchers are currently concerned about third-party consent. People who consent to genetics studies, by nature of the information analyzed, provide information about their family members. Incidental identification of conditions may be a risk the participant chooses to assume, but what of the family members who do not choose to participate in the study? The immediate or extended family may experience both the information sharing and the evaluation results as both unwelcome and life changing.

Another arena provoking discussion is the online environment for research. Online surveys are increasingly being used to gather data. Such surveys have the benefits of being easily administered across wide geographic areas and of enabling simultaneous data compilation. Researchers typically promise anonymity to participants in Web surveys. Yet with increasingly sophisticated software, some people are able to "mine" Web interactions. These issues must be resolved to ensure participants' confidentiality and protection of their medical and other personal information. New technologies, such as the Internet, bring both opportunities and challenges in research methods.

ETHICS IN PUBLISHING RESEARCH

Publishing, the last step in the process of research, is nonetheless an essential one. When an article is published, the researcher's choices throughout the process, as well as the findings, are documented and distributed for public consumption. Publication is vitally important because the dissemination of research efforts to a wider audience can create major shifts in practice or policy and provide evidence for practice.

Research findings are often presented in neat and tidy ways in publications, yet behind-the-scenes accounts of research processes are informative about the many dilemmas that exist in describing the design, implementation, and findings published in research. Choices on how to describe the methods, which analyses to perform, what visual displays to use, and which findings to publish are all shaped by ethical decisions. Typically, multiple articles may be published from a given study, with each focused on a specific aspect. Thus, researchers may limit descriptions of methods or refer readers to earlier published descriptions of methods to save space. This balance between providing depth of description of methods versus dedicating more space to findings is one that researchers consider in publications. The analyses that are selected need to be guided by scientific traditions and ethics. It's problematic for researchers to run multiple analyses in a "fishing expedition" for statistically significant findings. Analyses should be based on the theoretical assumptions about the relationships between variables guiding the study. In addition, null findings often are not published, despite the contribution they make to the knowledge base. In many instances, null findings are important to patient care—for example, in studies of the efficacy of specific treatments or medications. Knowing that a specific approach is not effective is important knowledge for practice.

Many times the focus at the publication stage is solely on considerations of the originality and veracity of the publication. Although in rare cases researchers have intentionally published false or misleading research (Farthing, 1998), these instances can have a widespread impact. One recent infamous case includes the retraction of a *Lancet* article that suggested an association between the emergence of regressive autism and administration of a childhood vaccination (Deer, 2010). This discredited study has been responsible for worldwide decreases in the numbers of children being immunized and for increases in preventable diseases (e.g., measles, mumps, rubella) that previously were rarely seen.

Similarly, plagiarism or duplicate data publications, also considered to be research misconduct, are rare but problematic. Errami et al. (2008) used a text analysis to identify an incidence of 0.04% potential plagiarism and 1.35%, or 117,550, duplicate publications in articles in the Medline database. Martinson, Anderson, and de Vries (2005) surveyed 3,247 NIH-funded scientists who reported engaging in plagiarism and duplicate data publications, as well as keeping inadequate records, dropping observations or data outliers on the basis of gut instincts, changing study design because of external pressures (e.g., funding sources), or ignoring human participant provisions. These problematic actions reflect inadequate attention to procedures and veracity, violating Principles 5, Procedural Justice, and 6, Veracity, of the Code and Ethics Standards.

It is the function of peer review to carefully consider the quality of manuscripts submitted to journals, judge originality, and identify unintended errors in analyses or misleading narrative. Still, peer reviewers may miss self-plagiarism, use of large sections of a prior publication in a new one, or inaccurate citation of others' work or failure to cite foundational work. Using a complex analysis program, Simkin and Roychowdhury (2003) tracked inaccurate duplicate citations through generations of publications. They argued that these persistent errors represented researchers' repeated use of others' analyses of the literature without returning to the original sources and that only a paltry 20% of citers read the original source. This, too, is problematic because persistent errors can be transmitted through the literature.

Several other ethical considerations exist at publication, including timely dissemination of findings, selection of publication venue and audience for the information, and choices in reporting the data (e.g., how to visually display data in figures, whether to report null results, how to fairly represent the importance of the findings). For example, in occupational therapy, the researcher's choice of journal to submit to may be driven by a variety of inside and outside pressures. The journal that represents the ideal audience for an article may not have a sufficiently high impact rating to support the researcher's progress in an academic career at a high-productivity university. This consideration has been a challenge in occupational therapy and occupational science; many of our professional journals have not been rated for impact or have relatively low impact factor ratings.

The researcher is thus torn between reaching occupational therapy practitioners, the ideal consumers of the research, and succeeding in academia.

CONCLUSION

Leaders and policymakers advocate that translation of research into practice is a high priority for occupational therapy practitioners. Because of this priority, entire courses in occupational therapy curricula are dedicated to the evaluation of the quality and use of research in practice. The implementation of knowledge in service of our clients is being viewed both within and outside the profession as a moral imperative. Occupational therapy practitioners must make a lifelong professional commitment to keep abreast of and use new knowledge in practice. Recognizing the appropriate uses and limits of knowledge translation, not merely its addition to practice, and addressing the gaps and needs in the knowledge base are essential to moving the profession forward.

REFERENCES

Abreu, B. C., Peloquin, S. M., & Ottenbacher, K. (1998). Competence in scientific inquiry and research. *American Journal of Occupational Therapy, 52,* 751–759. doi: 10.5014/ajot.52.9.751

Accreditation Council for Occupational Therapy Education. (2012). 2011 Accreditation Council for Occupational Therapy Education (ACOTE®) standards. *American Journal of Occupational Therapy, 66*(6 Suppl.), S6–S74. doi: 10.5014/ajot.2012.66S6

Albert, M., Laberge, S., & Hodges, B. D. (2009). Boundary-work in the health research field: Biomedical and clinician scientists' perceptions of social science research. *Minerva, 47,* 171–194.

American Occupational Therapy Association. (1967). *American Occupational Therapy Association: Then and now! 1917–1967.* Rockville, MD: Author.

American Occupational Therapy Association. (2007). AOTA's *Centennial Vision* and executive summary. *American Journal of Occupational Therapy, 61,* 613–614. http://dx.doi.org 10.5014/ajot.61.6.613

American Occupational Therapy Association. (2010). Occupational therapy code of ethics and ethics standards (2010). *American Journal of Occupational Therapy, 64*(6, Suppl.), S17–S26. http://dx.doi.org 10.5014/ajot.2010.64S17

Barnitt, R., & Partridge, C. (1999). The legacy of being a research subject: Follow-up studies of participants in therapy research. *Physiotherapy Research International, 4,* 250–261.

Becher, T., & Trowler, P. R. (2001). *Academic tribes and territories: Intellectual enquiry and the culture of disciplines* (2nd ed.). Philadelphia: Society for Research into Higher Education and Open University Press.

Bernstein, J., Collette, D., & Pederson, S. (2010). Basing healthcare on empirical evidence. *Mathematica, 3,* 1–4.

Bordieu, P. (2004). *Science of science and reflexivity.* Cambridge, England: Polity Press.

Brown, M., Dijkers, M. P., Gordon, W. A., Ashman, T., Charatz, H., & Chen, Z. (2004). Participation objective, participation subjective: A measure of participation combining outsider and insider perspectives. *Journal of Head Trauma Rehabilitation, 19,* 459–481.

Buccini, L. D. (2009). *Developing an instrument to measure informed consent in non-cognitively impaired adults.* Doctorate of Public Health thesis, University of Wollongong, New South Wales, Australia.

Carlson, M. E., & Clark, F. A. (1991). The search for useful methodologies in occupational science. *American Journal of Occupational Therapy, 45,* 235–241. doi: 10.5014/ajot.45.3.235

Centers for Disease Control and Prevention. (2009). *Simply put: A guide for creating easy-to-understand materials* (3rd ed.). Atlanta: Author. Retrieved from www.cdc.gov/healthliteracy/pdf/Simply_Put.pdf

Christiansen, C. (1981). Toward the resolution of crisis: Research requisites in occupational therapy. *Occupational Therapy Journal of Research, 1,* 115–124.

Christiansen, C., & Lou, J. Q. (2001). Ethical considerations related to evidence-based practice. *American Journal of Occupational Therapy, 55,* 345–349. doi: 10.5014/ajot.55.3.345

Clark, F., Azen, S. P., Zemke, R., Jackson J., Carlson, M., Mandel D., . . . Lipson, L. (1997). Occupational therapy for independent-living older adults: A randomized controlled trial. *JAMA, 278,* 1321–1326.

Cochrane, A. J. (2004). *Effectiveness and efficiency: Random reflections on health services.* London: Royal Society of Medicine Press. (Original work published 1972)

Cohen, A. M., Stavri, P. Z., & Hersch, W. R. (2004). A categorization and analysis of the criticisms of evidence-based medicine. *International Journal of Medical Informatics, 73,* 35–43.

Corbie-Smith, G. (1999). The continuing legacy of the Tuskegee syphilis study: Considerations for clinical investigation. *American Journal of Medical Science, 317,* 5–8.

Dartmouth Biomedical Libraries. (2008). *Evidence-based medicine (EBM) resources.* Available from www.dartmouth.edu/~biomed/resources.htmld/guides/ebm_resources.shtml

Deer, B. (2010). Secrets of the MMR scare: How the case against the MMR vaccine was fixed. *British Medical Journal, 342,* c5347. Retrieved from www.bmj.com/content/342/bmj.c5347.full

Dunn, L. (2006). Capacity to consent to research in schizophrenia: The expanding evidence base. *Behavioral Sciences and the Law, 24,* 431–445.

Errami, M., Hicks, J. M., Fisher, W., Trusty, D., Wren, J. D., Long, T. C., & Garner, H. R. (2008). Déjà vu: A study of duplicate citations in Medline. *Bioinformatics, 24,* 243–249.

Farthing, M. (1998). The COPE report: Coping with fraud. *Lancet, 352,* 10–11.

Gilliam, L., Guillemin, M., Bolitho, A., & Rosenthal, D. (2009). Human research ethics in practice: Deliberative strategies, process and perceptions. *Monash Bioethics Review, 28,* 7.1–7.17.

Gitlin, L. N., Winter, L., Earland, T. V., Herge, E. A., Chernett, N. L., Piersol, C. V., & Burke, J. P. (2009). The Tailored Activity Program to reduce behavioral symptoms in individuals with dementia: Feasibility, acceptability, and replication potential. *Gerontologist, 49,* 428–439.

Gray, J. M. (1998). Putting occupation into practice: Occupation as ends, occupation as means. *American Journal of Occupational Therapy, 52,* 354–364. doi: 10.5014/ajot.52.5.354

Gray, J. R., & Thompson, P. M. (2004). Neurobiology of intelligence: Science and ethics. *Nature Reviews Neuroscience, 5,* 471–482.

Gutman, S. (2008). From the Desk of the Editor—Research priorities of the profession. *American Journal of Occupational Therapy, 62,* 619–622. doi: 10.5014/ajot.62.5.499

Gutman, S. (2009). From the Desk of the Editor—State of the journal, 2009. *American Journal of Occupational Therapy, 63,* 667–673. doi: 10.5014/ajot.63.6.667

Gutman, S. (2010). From the Desk of the Editor—State of the journal, 2010. *American Journal of Occupational Therapy, 64,* 832–840. doi: 10.5014/ajot.2010.064601

Hooper, B. (2006). Epistemological transformation in occupational therapy: Educational implications and challenges. *OTJR: Occupation, Participation and Health, 26,* 15–24.

Hope, T. (1997). Evidence-based patient choice and the doctor–patient relationship. In *But will it work, doctor?* (pp. 20–24). London: Kings Fund.

Hornblum, A. M. (1997). They were cheap and available: Prisoners as research subjects in twentieth century America. *British Medical Journal, 315,* 1437–1341.

Kuhn, T. S. (1962). *The structure of scientific revolutions* (3rd ed.). Chicago: University of Chicago Press.

Martinson, B. C., Anderson, M. S., & de Vries, R. (2005). Scientists behaving badly. *Nature, 435,* 737–738.

Milgram, S. (1968). Some conditions of obedience and disobedience to authority. *International Journal of Psychiatry, 6,* 259–76.

National Heart, Lung, and Blood Institute. (2002, July 9). *NHLBI stops trial of estrogen plus progestin due to increased breast cancer risk, lack of overall benefit.* Retrieved from www.nhlbi.nih.gov/news/press-releases/2002/nhlbi-stops-trial-of-estrogen-plus-progestin-due-to-increased-breast-cancer-risk-lack-of-overall-benefit.html

National Institutes of Health. (2004). *Guidelines for the conduct of research using human subjects at the National Institutes of Health* (Publication No. ADM 00-4783). Washington, DC: U.S. Government Printing Office. Retrieved from http://sourcebook.od.nih.gov/ethic-conduct/Conduct%20Research%206-11-07.pdf

Nuremburg Code. (1949). Retrieved from http://history.nih.gov/research/downloads/nuremberg.pdf

Office for Human Research Protections, U.S. Department of Health and Human Services. (2005). *Protection of human subjects.* 45 C.F.R. §46.111. Retrieved from www.hhs.gov/ohrp/humansubjects/guidance/45cfr46.html/

Rogers, J. C. (1983). Clinical reasoning: The ethics, science, and art (Eleanor Clarke Slagle Lecture). *American Journal of Occupational Therapy, 37,* 601–616. doi: 10.5014/ajot.37.9.601

Sackett, D. L., Richardson, W. S., Rosenberg, W., & Haynes, R. B. (1997). *Evidence-based medicine: How to practice and teach EBM.* London: Churchill Livingstone.

Sackett, D. L., Rosenberg, W. M. C., Gray, J. A., Haynes, R. B., & Richardson, W. S. (1996). Evidence based medicine: What it is and what it isn't. *British Medical Journal, 312,* 71.

Sackett, D. L., Straus, S. E., Richardson, W. S., Rosenberg, W., & Haynes, B. (2000). *Evidence-based medicine: How to practice and teach EBM* (2nd ed.). Edinburgh, Scotland: Churchill Livingstone.

Simkin, M. V., & Roychowdhury, V. P. (2003). Read before you cite! *Complex Systems, 14,* 269.

Spencer, J. C. (1993). The usefulness of qualitative methods in rehabilitation: Issues of meaning, of context, and of change. *Archives of Physical Medicine and Rehabilitation, 74,* 119–126.

U.S. Department of Health and Human Services. (2000). *Healthy people 2010: Understanding and improving health* (2nd ed.). Washington, DC: U.S. Government Printing Office.

Van Brakel, W. H., Anderson, A. M., Mutatakar, R. K., Bakirtzief, Z., Nicholls, P. J., Raju, M. S., & Das-Pattanayak, R. K. (2006). The Participation Scale: A key concept in public health. *Disability and Society, 28,* 193–203.

Wood, W., Nielson, C., Humphry, R., Coppola, S., Baranek, G., & Rourk, J. (2000). A curricular renaissance: Graduate occupation centered on occupation. *American Journal of Occupational Therapy, 54,* 586–597. http://dx.doi.org/10.5014/ajot.54.6.586

World Health Organization. (2000). *International classification of functioning, disability and health.* Geneva: Author.

World Medical Association. (2008). *WMA Declaration of Helsinki—Ethical principles for medical research involving human subjects.* Retrieved from www.wma.net/en/30publications/10policies/b3/17c.pdf

Yerxa, E. J. (1992). Some implications of occupational therapy's history for its epistemology, values, and relation to medicine. *American Journal of Occupational Therapy, 46,* 79–83. http://dx.doi.org/10.5014/ajot.46.1.79

APPENDIX 19.A. THE NUREMBERG CODE (1947)

1. The voluntary consent of the human subject is absolutely essential.

   This means that the person involved should have legal capacity to give consent; should be so situated as to be able to exercise free power of choice, without the intervention of any element of force, fraud, deceit, duress, overreaching, or other ulterior form of constraint or coercion; and should have sufficient knowledge and comprehension of the elements of the subject matter involved as to enable him to make an understanding and enlightened decision. This latter element requires that before the acceptance of an affirmative decision by the experimental subject there should be made known to him the nature, duration, and purpose of the experiment; the method and means by which it is to be conducted; all inconveniences and hazards reasonably to be expected; and the effects upon his health or person which may possibly come from his participation in the experiment.

   The duty and responsibility for ascertaining the quality of the consent rests upon each individual who initiates, directs, or engages in the experiment. It is a personal duty and responsibility which may not be delegated to another with impunity.

2. The experiment should be such as to yield fruitful results for the good of society, unprocurable by other methods or means of study, and not random and unnecessary in nature.

3. The experiment should be so designed and based on the results of animal experimentation and knowledge of the natural history of the disease or other problem under study that the anticipated results justify the performance of the experiment.

4. The experiment should be so conducted as to avoid all unnecessary physical and mental suffering and injury.

5. No experiment should be conducted where there is an a priori reason to believe that death or disabling injury will occur; except, perhaps, in those experiments where the experimental physicians also serve as subjects.

6. The degree of risk to be taken should never exceed that determined by the humanitarian importance of the problem to be solved by the experiment.

7. Proper preparations should be made and adequate facilities provided to protect the experimental subject against even remote possibilities of injury, disability or death.

8. The experiment should be conducted only by scientifically qualified persons. The highest degree of skill and care should be required through all stages of the experiment of those who conduct or engage in the experiment.

9. During the course of the experiment the human subject should be at liberty to bring the experiment to an end if he has reached the physical or mental state where continuation of the experiment seems to him to be impossible.

10. During the course of the experiment, the scientist in charge must be prepared to terminate the experiment at any stage, if he has probable cause to believe, in the exercise of good faith, superior skill and careful judgment required of him that a continuation of the experiment is likely to result in injury, disability or death to the experimental subject.

Note. Reprinted from *Nuremberg Code* (1949).

APPENDIX 19.B. CRITERIA FOR INSTITUTIONAL REVIEW BOARD (IRB) APPROVAL OF RESEARCH FROM THE CODE OF FEDERAL REGULATIONS

§46.111 Criteria for IRB approval of research.

(a) In order to approve research covered by this policy the IRB shall determine that all of the following requirements are satisfied:
1. Risks to subjects are minimized: (i) By using procedures which are consistent with sound research design and which do not unnecessarily expose subjects to risk, and

(ii) whenever appropriate, by using procedures already being performed on the subjects for diagnostic or treatment purposes.

2. Risks to subjects are reasonable in relation to anticipated benefits, if any, to subjects, and the importance of the knowledge that may reasonably be expected to result. In evaluating risks and benefits, the IRB should consider only those risks and benefits that may result from the research (as distinguished from risks and benefits of therapies subjects would receive even if not participating in the research). The IRB should not consider possible long-range effects of applying knowledge gained in the research (for example, the possible effects of the research on public policy) as among those research risks that fall within the purview of its responsibility.

3. Selection of subjects is equitable. In making this assessment the IRB should take into account the purposes of the research and the setting in which the research will be conducted and should be particularly cognizant of the special problems of research involving vulnerable populations, such as children, prisoners, pregnant women, mentally disabled persons, or economically or educationally disadvantaged persons.

4. Informed consent will be sought from each prospective subject or the subject's legally authorized representative, in accordance with, and to the extent required by §46.116.

5. Informed consent will be appropriately documented, in accordance with, and to the extent required by §46.117.

6. When appropriate, the research plan makes adequate provision for monitoring the data collected to ensure the safety of subjects.

7. When appropriate, there are adequate provisions to protect the privacy of subjects and to maintain the confidentiality of data.

(b) When some or all of the subjects are likely to be vulnerable to coercion or undue influence, such as children, prisoners, pregnant women, mentally disabled persons, or economically or educationally disadvantaged persons, additional safeguards have been included in the study to protect the rights and welfare of these subjects.

Source. Reprinted from Office for Human Research Protections, U.S. Department of Health and Human Services (2005).

Internal Relationships: Ethical Issues Within Institutions

20

S. Maggie Reitz, PhD, OTR/L, FAOTA

Potential ethical issues can arise both within and between institutions. In this chapter, the term *institution* refers to any workplace (e.g., clinic, hospital, school system, skilled nursing facility, university) or association (e.g., local, state, national, international professional association). Ethical issues, resolutions, and consequences that occur inside institutions are the topic of this chapter. Ethical situations that extend beyond an individual institution to involve multiple external business and professional partners are addressed in Chapter 21.

It is commonly accepted that there is greater strength in numbers, as when people come together to successfully solve a complex problem or situation. However, even a group of competent, usually ethical people can make poor choices (American Occupational Therapy Association [AOTA], 2011). *Groupthink* occurs when group members feel pressure to conform at the expense of logical thinking, thereby negatively influencing the group's effectiveness. This diminished level of function can damage individuals and groups inside the institution and even the institution itself (Engleberg & Wynn, 2007); most important, groupthink can bring harm to the clients or students the institution is designed to serve.

Ethical issues can arise in any institution, so all institutions should take steps to minimize their occurrence. Administrators of an organization or leaders of an association should lead by example in this regard; the *Occupational Therapy Code of Ethics and Ethics Standards (2010)* (referred to as the "Code and Ethics Standards"; AOTA, 2010b), together with other resources (AOTA, 2009, 2011; Glennon & Van Oss, 2010; Slater, 2011), can help guide ethical behavior within institutions.

ETHICAL TENSIONS WITHIN INSTITUTIONS

Ethical tensions within institutions can result from behaviors that include the following:

- Conflict of commitment (see Vignette 20.1);
- Disrespect for colleagues (see Vignette 20.2), students (American Medical Association, [AMA] 2011), coworkers, covolunteers, or clients;
- Disrespect for institutional rules (see Vignette 20.3);
- Discriminatory behavior (see Case Study 20.1);
- Bullying (see Case Study 20.2); and
- Sabotaging and mobbing (see Case Study 20.3).

Preventive strategies include transparency in decision making, disclosure of potential conflicts of interest, self-monitoring of motivations and possible conflicts of commitment, respect for colleagues and others, and use of a framework for analysis of ethical dilemmas when an issue arises (AOTA Ethics Commission, 2011).

Conflict of Commitment

VIGNETTE 20.1. RECTIFYING A CONFLICT OF COMMITMENT

Myra, the senior occupational therapist in an occupational therapy department of a county hospital, was concerned about the deteriorating performance of **Kiki**, who had been one of the most efficient and effective occupational therapists in the department. Besides patient care, Kiki also was responsible for coordinating the department's mentoring program. Kiki's departmental mentoring and continuing education verification logs were becoming sloppy, and she was arriving increasingly late for staff meetings. Myra knew that Kiki was serving on the hospital's Ethics Board and was becoming concerned that this responsibility, although important for the department's visibility and patient autonomy, was affecting her job performance and might soon compromise patient care.

Myra approached Kiki with her concerns. Kiki disclosed that one of the vice presidents who served on the Ethics Board had asked her also to serve on the Patient Satisfaction Committee, to which she had agreed. Kiki realized that she should have shared this information with Myra because she now was unable to perform all of her responsibilities to the expected level of performance. They agreed to delegate the mentoring program responsibilities to another therapist who was eager and able to take on additional responsibilities. In addition, they agreed to monitor Kiki's performance together to determine if she should relinquish one of the two hospital committee responsibilities. These actions are supported by Principle 2, Non-maleficence, of the Code and Ethics Standards, particularly Principle 2G, which obligates practitioners to avoid situations in which they are "unable to maintain clear professional boundaries . . . to ensure the safety and well-being of recipients of service" (AOTA, 2010b, p. S20).

Disrespect for Colleagues

VIGNETTE 20.2. SHOWING RESPECT FOR COLLEAGUES

Jack, a new occupational therapist and new employee in a rehabilitation medicine department in a university hospital, was perplexed about the manner in which staff addressed each other in front of patients and their families. The occupational, physical, and speech therapists addressed each other as Dr., Ms., or Mr., but they referred to the occupational therapy assistants, physical therapy assistants, and aides by their first name. Jack thought this was disrespectful and in violation of Principle 7, Fidelity, of the Code and Ethics Standards, which states, "Occupational therapy personnel shall treat colleagues and other professionals with respect, fairness, discretion, and integrity" (AOTA, 2010b, p. S24). He decided to address all staff in the same formal manner when with patients and their families. Within a short time, he noticed a shift in the norm of the department to the more respectful treatment of support staff.

Disrespect for Institutions

VIGNETTE 20.3. ENSURING RESPECT FOR INSTITUTIONAL RULES

Virginia, an occupational therapy student, was enrolled in an evening kinesiology lab section. She chose that particular section because she wanted to have a class with an instructor who was "in the trenches" as a currently employed full-time practitioner. Virginia was excited to meet **Leneida**, the course instructor, who came to class in scrubs and looked like the vision that Virginia imagined for herself in the future. Virginia did not mind that Leneida let the first class out early because Virginia wanted to get to a friend's birthday celebration. When Leneida let the next two classes out early, however, Virginia became concerned that she was not having the same educational experience as the students in the daytime lab section, which had been meeting for the entire designated time period.

Before Virginia could decide what to do, **Bart**, a full-time professor, came to observe the class as part of the department's regular peer evaluation process.

Bart saw that Leneida was behind on the course content timetable, so during a break, he inquired as to why Leneida was behind. She responded that the students just needed more time to absorb the material. A half-hour after the break, Bart saw that many of the students were packing up their materials and looking at the clock. Leneida, seeing Bart's concern, decided to announce that the students should be prepared to stay the entire class time that night and in the future and that they might need to take shorter breaks in the future to catch up on the required material. Virginia was glad that she did not need to take action that time but made a commitment to herself that in the future she would take action if a teacher was not following departmental procedures and policies.

Discrimination and Lack of Inclusion

One hallmark of the profession is its commitment to nondiscrimination and inclusion. This commitment is supported by the Code and Ethics Standards and detailed in the AOTA (2009) position paper "Occupational Therapy's Commitment to Nondiscrimination and Inclusion." This commitment not only extends to clients but also guides relationships among and opportunities within the occupational therapy professional community: "Inclusion requires that we ensure not only that everyone is treated fairly and equitably but also that all individuals have the same opportunities to participate in the naturally occurring activities of society, such as . . . participating in professional organizations" (AOTA, 2009, p. 819).

CASE STUDY 20.1. COMBATING DISCRIMINATORY AND NONINCLUSIVE BEHAVIOR IN A VOLUNTEER ROLE

Nancy and **Philip**, who worked together at a skilled nursing facility, decided they would like to be more active in their state occupational therapy association. Nancy shared an e-mail notice soliciting volunteers to join the conference committee to support the planning of an upcoming state association conference. With Philip, she reviewed the commitments and timing of the conference, and they concluded the work was manageable. Nancy and Philip were

excited about the opportunity to contribute to the profession. Together they approached their supervisor, **Reina**, to see if they could modify their work schedule so that they could travel to the planning committee meetings.

As they drove to the first scheduled meeting of the committee, Nancy and Philip talked about how excited they were to meet other occupational therapy practitioners around the state and become involved. They arrived and were scanning the room for familiar faces when someone yelled out, "Oh look, great! We have a guy. Now we have someone to fetch the coffee and carry the boxes." The comment was received with giggles and whispered comments. Both Nancy and Philip were taken aback, but they started introducing themselves to the other people present.

After the meeting, Nancy and Philip discussed the comment and hoped it was simply an isolated event and someone's poor attempt at humor after a long workday. At the next meeting, however, additional male-bashing comments were made. Both Nancy and Philip believed that their technology and social media skills could benefit the group's planning and ultimately the success of the state conference. However, they were uncomfortable with the group's repeated disparaging and discriminatory remarks about men. They decided to consult with their work supervisor, Reina, regarding possible responses to this unprofessional behavior.

Together with Reina, they identified the potential actions outlined in Table 20.1. They decided that the best approach was to suggest that the conference committee offer an educative program, such as the Speak Up! program developed by the Southern Poverty Law Center (2005), both at a conference committee meeting and at the conference itself. Nancy and Philip had received Speak Up! training when they were student leaders at the university where they received their occupational therapy education, so they were able to lead the training. At the presentation to the conference committee, group members initially were defensive and then became embarrassed about the impact of their behavior; however, they accepted that their behavior needed to change. A well-attended Speak Up! session was conducted at conference, and its success was evident from conference evaluation data. To their delight, Nancy and Philip were asked to co-chair the following year's conference committee.

TABLE 20.1
Decision Table for Case Study 20.1

POSSIBLE ACTION	POSITIVE OUTCOMES	NEGATIVE CONSEQUENCES
No action; quit the conference planning committee	Nancy and Philip avoid an uncomfortable situation and the potential conflict resulting from addressing their concerns with the group.	This action does not confront the discriminatory behaviors and thus fails to uphold Principles 4D, 7, 7C, and 7G. The committee loses the benefit of Nancy's and Philip's technology skills without knowing the true reason behind their decision to quit. Committee members are likely to continue their unethical behaviors.
No action; continue to participate on the committee	Nancy and Philip avoid an uncomfortable situation and the potential conflict resulting from addressing their concerns with the group. Nancy and Philip continue to contribute their technology expertise to planning the state conference.	Philip may continue to be subjected to an uncomfortable group environment. This action does not confront the discriminatory behaviors and thus fails to uphold Principles 4D, 7, 7C, and 7G.
Contact the chair of the committee to discuss their concerns and ask for support in addressing behaviors	Nancy and Philip attempt to uphold Principles 2H, 4D, 7, 7C, and 7G. This action is transparent with the committee chair and minimizes meeting disruption.	The conference chair might dismiss their concerns. Committee members may feel defensive.
Offer to provide an educative program, such as the Speak Up! program developed by the Southern Poverty Law Center (2005), for the committee and at the conference to help people develop skills to address discrimination in a nonconfrontational manner	This action upholds Principles 2H, 4D, 7, 7C, and 7G.	Committee members may feel defensive.

Note. A variety of possible actions to address this situation and analyses of each are provided in this table; however, other actions or analyses are possible depending on the decision-making model and specific ethics theory or approach used (see Chapter 10).

Bullying

Bullying at school and in the workplace is getting increased attention (AMA, 2011; Briles, 1994; Seeley, Tombari, Bennett, & Dunkle, 2011; U.S. Department of Health and Human Services, n.d.; Workplace Bullying Institute [WBI], 2010). Briles (1994), in her studies of workplace abuse among female health care workers, reported unprofessional gossiping, sabotaging, and other abusive behaviors among women in health care workplaces. Consistently in this research and in previous research across other professions, Briles found that women reported being mistreated at work more by other women than by men. This finding is consistent with the research of the WBI, which reported that women tend to bully women more than they do men. In addition, people with college educations reported being bullied more often than those with less education (WBI, 2010).

Given that the majority of occupational therapy practitioners are college-educated women (AOTA, 2010c), institutions need to take measures to prevent and confront bullying. Occupational therapy practitioners are not immune from experiencing moments of lack of judgment and unprofessional behavior with students, each other, colleagues from other disciplines, or clients. This type of behavior becomes increasingly troublesome when the behaviors turn into a pattern or the behavior escalates.

CASE STUDY 20.2. CONFRONTING BULLYING IN THE WORKPLACE

Darlene was hired as the new occupational therapy manager at a large outpatient clinic 1 month before the conclusion of the annual performance review period. Darlene was told that the previous manager had left the position to provide care to an aging family member. Because Darlene was new to the facility, **Becky**, the rehabilitation medicine director, completed the performance review process, and she summarized each review using a written evaluation form that she shared with employees. One of the seven occupational therapists, **Lolita**, thought she had been unfairly rated. She demanded, in a hostile tone and within earshot of the other staff, to meet with Darlene, the new manager.

Darlene agreed to a meeting with Lolita and was prepared to support her, even though Lolita had treated her disrespectfully. Before the meeting, Darlene reviewed the evaluation policy and procedures and found that there was a mechanism for appeal. At the beginning of the meeting, Darlene informed Lolita that she did not appreciate Lolita's tone and attitude when she demanded the meeting. Although Darlene understood that Lolita was upset, she stressed, Lolita needed to consider the impact of her behavior on others. Next, Darlene explained the appeal process that was in place and suggested that Lolita schedule a meeting with

Becky to begin the appeal process. Lolita chuckled at this and said, "You're preciously naïve. Soon you will see—I am the one really in charge here. You wait and see."

The appeal meeting took place a week later. After the meeting, Lolita burst into Darlene's office, yelling, "I cannot believe that witch Becky. She lied to me, and I have it on tape!" Darlene attempted to calm Lolita down and get a sense of what had happened at the meeting. Lolita screamed, "That witch promised me a good evaluation if I was acting manager until we could hire someone! I did a stellar job. No disrespect meant, but we really do not need you. I can do this job, and better than you. I have control of these folks!"

Darlene sat calmly, not taking the remarks personally, and asked Lolita about the outcome of the meeting. Lolita chuckled, "Becky would not change my evaluation, but I have her! I taped our summer meeting, so this is not the end of this!" At first Darlene sat speechless, knowing that it was against state law to audiotape anyone without their permission. She reminded Lolita of this fact; Lolita stormed out of the office sneering, "You will be the next to leave to 'take care of an aging family member'!"

Darlene consulted a variety of resources, including the Code and Ethics Standards and the *Reference Guide to the Occupational Therapy Code of Ethics and Ethics Standards* (Slater, 2011). After thoughtful reflection, Darlene took action. She decided to first call and describe the situation to the hospital attorney. The attorney's first response was, "Oh, so she is up to her usual tricks. If she was not such a great therapist, she would have been fired years ago!" Afterward, Darlene asked Lolita to come to her office, where she presented her with a copy of the Code and Ethics Standards and reviewed the principles she believed Lolita had violated: Principle 2, Nonmaleficence; Principle 5, Procedural Justice; Principle 6, Veracity; and Principle 7, Fidelity. She informed Lolita that she had 48 hours in which to meet with Becky, confess that she had taped the meeting, apologize, and destroy the tape and any transcripts. If she did not comply, Darlene would report Lolita's behavior to both Becky and the state regulatory board (SRB).

Darlene then told Lolita that she would be contacting human resources to establish the next steps in the disciplinary action process. In addition,

Darlene informed Lolita that if she further threatened or bullied her or anyone else in the department or engaged in other unethical behavior, she would report the behavior to Becky, the hospital vice president for human resources, the SRB, the National Board for Certification in Occupational Therapy (NBCOT) if she held certification, and AOTA if she was a member.

Darlene's behavior throughout the incident was supported by the Code and Ethics Standards. First, she remained professional when confronted in a hostile manner. This behavior is consistent with Principle 7, Fidelity. Second, she took time to ensure that she was following institutional rules by contacting the hospital attorney; this action is supported by Principle 5, Procedural Justice. Third, she made sure to inform Lolita how her behavior was in violation of the Code and Ethics Standards, which is dictated by Principle 5L. In addition, she attempted to resolve the situation internally before escalating to the SRB or other entities. From the discussion with the attorney, it became obvious that this employee had a pattern of bullying behavior that the institution had overlooked because of the top-quality care she provided to patients. Darlene's action was supported by Principle 7D: "Occupational therapy personnel shall attempt to resolve perceived institutional violations of the Code and Ethics Standards by utilizing internal resources first" (AOTA, 2010b, pp. S24–S25).

Darlene's next action required her to balance two conflicting principles: Principles 7B and 7C. According to Principle 7B, "occupational therapy personnel shall preserve, respect, and safeguard private information about employees, colleagues, and students unless otherwise mandated by national, state, or local laws or permission to disclose is given by the individual" (AOTA, 2010b, p. S24). Principle 7C states that "occupational therapy personnel shall take adequate measures to discourage, prevent, expose, and correct any breaches of the Code and Ethics Standards, and report any breaches of the former to the appropriate authorities" (AOTA, 2010b, pp. S24–S25). Darlene decided, on reflection, that the most ethical outcome she would pursue was to maintain the viability of an employee who was an exceptional provider of client care while ensuring that the bullying behavior ceased. If the bullying behavior did not cease, Darlene was committed to report Lolita to all appropriate bodies.

Sabotaging and Mobbing

Florence Clark, while AOTA Vice President, observed that the use of lateral attacks is one of the obstacles to women-dominated health professions securing power and using their expertise to enhance quality of life and save health care dollars (Clark, 2009). A *lateral attack*, also known as *lateral* or *horizontal violence* or *abuse*, "is the disruptive, disrespectful or antagonistic behavior of others on the same hierarchical level within an organization" (Fuimano-Donley, 2011, p. 5). Bullying, launching lateral attacks, and mobbing are examples of *workplace sabotage*, in which an employee or group distracts energy and attention from tasks that could move a department, unit, team, task force, commission, professional organization, or profession ahead. According to Briles (1994), "In healthcare, women's sabotaging behavior will definitely be directed toward other women" (p. 57). Examples from Briles's research included "lying, spreading rumors about personal matters and professional abilities," ganging up on someone before a meeting, or making them a target of gossiping or backstabbing, among other behaviors (pp. 57–58).

Mobbing, or bullying or sabotaging by a group, has been described as "emotional abuse in the workplace" through "malicious, nonsexual, nonracial, general harassment" (Mobbing-USA, 2010, para. 1). Like other forms of bullying, mobbing disrupts productivity and harms the target's health and well-being (Lovell & Lee, 2011; Niedhammer et al., 2011) and professional reputation. Mobbing perpetrators can include supervisors and subordinates, as well as coworkers at the same level in the organization, and is usually done to force the target to leave the place of employment (Mobbing-USA, 2010). Occupational therapy practitioners are susceptible to engaging in this behavior.

CASE STUDY 20.3. CONFRONTING MOBBING IN THE WORKPLACE

An occupational therapy department with 24 employees within a large county hospital had undergone a series of staff changes over the previous 3 years. Two new recent graduates, **Keira** and **Teri**, who had been classmates, were hired to replace the latest two employees who had abruptly resigned. Keira and Teri were invited to have lunch with three of the current staff, **Rosalyn**, **Ursula**, and **Desdemona**. They were excited to be asked to join what seemed to be the popular group. During lunch, Keira and Teri were told to steer clear of **Inga** because she "never carried her weight" and was the physical therapy director's "pet." This information was followed by smirks and other innuendos. After the first week, Keira was assigned to the stroke care team and Teri to the orthopedic team; these two teams had different lunchtimes, so they did not get to see as much of each other as they thought they would when they accepted the positions.

Keira was assigned to the same unit as Inga. At first, Keira was deeply suspicious of Inga and avoided her; however, one day she was having a difficult time with a complex patient, and Inga came over and offered her assistance. Later that day, after Inga had left for the day, Rosalyn, Ursula, and Desdemona started imitating her accent and insinuating that Inga had left to "hook up" with the physical therapy director. Keira became upset because she had believed Inga when she told Keira that she had to leave to pick up her sick child from school. Keira thought she had been duped by Inga, as the others had warned her. As she prepared to leave, Keira turned and said to the others, "I wish I had listened to your advice. I can't believe I fell for her ruse!"

As Keira was leaving the hospital, she walked by the pharmacy, where she saw Inga with a young child at the prescription pickup counter. Inga was trying to manage her wallet and purse while holding the child, who obviously was not feeling well. Keira went in and asked if she could help and walked with Inga to her car, carrying the prescriptions and a humidifier, while Inga carried the child. After Keira got home, she reflected on how she had so quickly jumped to the wrong conclusion and had readily joined a mob that was spreading malicious rumors without merit. The following week, Keira started to have lunch with Inga and found her to be an excellent mentor and, as a single mother of three children, too busy to be having an affair with anyone.

Teri routinely went to lunch with Rosalyn, Ursula, and Desdemona and was shocked to hear them being critical of Keira for becoming friends with Inga and saying how they were going to give a negative report of Keira's first-month performance to the occupational therapy director. They further shared that they were angry with Keira because before Keira came, they had almost "broken" Inga and gotten her to leave. Teri sat stunned, but not as stunned as she was by the next information they shared: Ursula said, "We know that Keira and Inga are having a joint affair with the physical therapy director." Teri tried not to laugh out loud. Teri had roomed with Keira, a self-proclaimed prude, for over 4 years before Keira married, and she was confident that Keira was still madly in love with her spouse, who was currently deployed for combat duty.

Ursula saw a slight grin on Teri's face and misread the reason. She stated, "That's right, Teri, we have your back. We will get rid of Inga and Keira. We are experts at weeding out those who don't listen or work too hard. With Inga and Keira gone, you will gain more seniority when we hire the next crop in a couple of months. Stick with us; you will be safe, and we can get coworkers who speak English and work to the rule!" Teri realized that Rosalyn, Ursula, and Desdemona were targeting Inga and Keira out of fear and prejudice, but she was terrified and did not know what to do.

After work, Teri texted Keira and asked if they could get together and discuss their new jobs. After they shared their experiences interacting with Rosalyn, Ursula, and Desdemona, they sat back and pondered what to do. They decided that they should first let Inga know of the plot. Inga was mortified when she heard. As a single mother, Inga did not want to risk being unemployed or receiving a bad reference. After the three of them talked for a while, they determined that the best form of employment security and the most ethical step to take was to request a meeting with the occupational therapy and physical therapy directors.

The meeting was scheduled for the following week. The next day, as Keira was changing into her scrubs, Ursula slammed Keira's locker closed, yelling, "I heard about your meeting. Who do you think you are? You'd better get in line, or the next time, I will slam that locker door on your fingers. Then see how much longer you will be working!" Two of the other occupational therapists who had been working at the hospital for a while were getting changed on the other side of the lockers. They heard the exchange and approached Keira, who was now shaking and sobbing. One of them, **Priscilla**, said "OK; this has gone too far. We, and I mean *we*, cannot wait for a week to have this meeting. We are going to human resources now!" An immediate meeting was called, and Rosalyn, Ursula, and Desdemona were placed on paid leave pending an investigation. Priscilla lamented that she wished she had spoken up sooner. Keira responded, "At least you had the guts to do so when I really needed you. I was ready to walk out and quit the minute she slammed my locker door, and I would have if you had not supported me."

As part of the investigation, the occupational therapy staff was interviewed. A culture of fear was uncovered. All of the occupational therapy staff, including Rosalyn and Desdemona, shared that they were fearful of Ursula and either participated in the mobbing or ignored it because of this fear. Although Ursula resigned before the investigation was completed, the occupational therapy director reported Ursula's behavior to the SRB, AOTA, and NBCOT. Keira, Teri, and Inga secured restraining orders against Ursula. Rosalyn and Desdemona received a reprimand and were placed on probation for a year for sharing privileged information inappropriately (i.e., gossiping), and the rehabilitation executive secretary who had informed Ursula of the meeting also was placed on probation. The executive secretary and the rest of the occupational therapy staff were encouraged to seek counseling if they found that they had difficulty coping with the outcomes of their actions or inactions. The hospital hired a consultant in workplace violence who recommended that all current and newly hired staff receive in-service training on bullying and mobbing prevention and that policies on workplace bullying be implemented and monitored.

The actions taken by Keira, Teri, Inga, Priscilla, and the occupational therapy director were supported by the Code and Ethics Standards, specifically Principles 2 (Nonmaleficence), 4D (advocate for fair treatment for all), 5 (Procedural Justice), 6B (refrain from participating in false communication), 7 (Fidelity), and 7D (attempt to resolve violations internally). The failure to report Ursula's behavior earlier by Rosalyn, Desdemona, and the other occupational therapy staff put them all in violation of Principles 2, Nonmaleficence; 6, Veracity; and 7, Fidelity. However, whether they were either coconspirators or unwitting bystanders in fear of intimidation should be weighed against their failure to report Ursula's actions.

In addition, the occupational therapy director's actions were supported by Principles 2A (avoid inflicting harm) and 2C and 2J (avoid exploitative relationships). The director chose not to report the failure to report of Rosalyn, Desdemona, and the other occupational therapy staff because of their dual roles as victims. Although Principle 7G directs occupational therapy practitioners to "use conflict resolution and/or alternative dispute resolution resources to resolve organizational and interpersonal conflicts" (AOTA, 2010b, p. S25), the director reported Ursula to the SRB, AOTA, and NBCOT because of the egregiousness of her actions.

CONCLUSION

Occupational therapy practitioners have a role to play in fostering healthy, meaningful relationships in the workplace (Glennon & Van Oss, 2010) and in professional organizations. This proactive preventive behavior is supported by the Code and Ethics Standards, specifically Principles 1, Beneficence; 2, Nonmaleficence; and 7, Fidelity.

As a profession, we communicate strategies to the public to prevent bullying of school-age students (AOTA, 2008, 2011, 2012, n.d.); we also need to consider what we can do as a profession to stop bullying, sabotaging, and mobbing at the workplace and among ourselves. We must always be vigilant and reflective to avoid engaging in behaviors that take time and attention from our responsibilities to students and clients. If we become aware of any such behaviors, we must be prepared to confront the perpetrators and take appropriate action consistent with the Code and Ethics Standards and the *Enforcement Procedures for the Occupational Therapy Code of Ethics and Ethics Standards* (AOTA, 2010a). Our profession and those we serve deserve nothing less.

REFERENCES

American Medical Association. (2011, August). One in five medical school grads report mistreatment; AMA taking action. *AMA MedEd Update.* Retrieved from www.ama-assn.org/ama/pub/meded/2011-august/2011-august.shtml

American Occupational Therapy Association. (2008). AOTA's societal statement on youth violence. *American Journal of Occupational Therapy, 62,* 709–710. doi: 10.5014/ajot.62.6.709

American Occupational Therapy Association. (2009). Occupational therapy's commitment to nondiscrimination and inclusion. *American Journal of Occupational Therapy, 63,* 819–820. doi: 10.5014/ajot.63.6.819

American Occupational Therapy Association. (2010a). Enforcement procedures for the *Occupational Therapy Code of Ethics and Ethics Standards. American Journal of Occupational Therapy, 64*(6 Suppl.), S4–S16. doi: 10.5014/ajot.2010.64S4

American Occupational Therapy Association. (2010b). Occupational therapy code of ethics and ethics standards (2010). *American Journal of Occupational Therapy, 64*(Suppl.), S17–S26. doi: 10:5014/ajot2010.62S17

American Occupational Therapy Association. (2010c). *2010 occupational therapy compensation and workforce study.* Bethesda, MD: Author.

American Occupational Therapy Association. (2011). *Mental health in children and youth: The benefit and role of occupational therapy* [Fact sheet]. Retrieved from www.aota.org/Practitioners-Section/Children-and-Youth/Role-of-OT/Fact-Sheets-on-the-Role-of-OT/44479.aspx?FT=.pdf

American Occupational Therapy Association. (2012). *Children and youth: Bullying.* Retrieved from www.aota.org/Practitioners/PracticeAreas/EmergingAreas/CY/Bullying.aspx

American Occupational Therapy Association. (n.d.). *Pediatric virtual chats: Prevention of and intervention for bullying* [Audio presentation]. Retrieved from www.talkshoe.com/talkshoe/web/audioPop.jsp?episodeId=380320&cmd=apop

American Occupational Therapy Association Ethics Commission. (2011). *Everyday ethics: Core knowledge for occupational therapy practitioners and educators* (CEonCD; 2nd ed.). Bethesda, MD: Author.

Briles, J. (1994). *The Briles report on women in healthcare: Changing conflict to collaboration in a toxic workplace.* San Francisco: Jossey-Bass.

Clark, F. (2009). *The Centennial Vision: Power, branding, and OT state associations* (PowerPoint presentation at the Spring Program Directors Meeting). Bethesda, MD: American Occupational Therapy Association.

Engleberg, A. N., & Wynn, D. R. (2007). *Working in groups* (4th ed.). Boston: Houghton Mifflin.

Fuimano-Donley, J. (2011). What is "lateral violence"? *Advance for Occupational Therapy Practitioners, 27*(16), 5–6.

Glennon, T. J., & Van Oss, T. V. (2010). Identifying and promoting professional behavior. *OT Practice, 15*(17), 13–16.

Lovell, B. L., & Lee, R. T. (2011). Impact of workplace bullying on emotional and physical well-being: A longitudinal collective case study. *Journal of Aggression, Maltreatment and Trauma, 20,* 344–357.

Mobbing-USA. (2010). *Mobbing is . . .* Retrieved from www.mobbing-usa.com

Niedhammer, I., David, S., Degioanni, S., Drummond, A., Philip, P., Acquarone, D., . . . Vital, N. (2011). Workplace bullying and psychotropic drug use: The mediating role of physical and mental health status. *American Occupational Hygiene, 55,* 152–163.

Seeley, K., Tombari, M. L., Bennett, L. J., & Dunkle, J. B. (2011). Bullying in schools: An overview. *Juvenile Justice Bulletin.* Retrieved from www.ojjdp.gov/pubs/234205.pdf

Slater, D. L. (Ed.). (2011). *Reference guide to the Occupational Therapy Code of Ethics and Ethics Standards* (2010 ed.). Bethesda, MD: AOTA Press.

Southern Poverty Law Center. (2005). *Responding to everyday bigotry: Speak up!* Montgomery, AL: Author.

U.S. Department of Health and Human Services. (n.d.). *stopbullying.gov.* Retrieved from www.stopbullying.gov/index.html

Workplace Bullying Institute. (2010). *The WBI U.S. workplace bullying survey.* Retrieved from http://workplacebullying.org/multi/pdf/WBI_2010_Natl_Survey.pdf

External Relationships: Ethical Issues in Interactions Among Institutions

21

Marian K. Scheinholtz, MS, OT/L, and
Janie B. Scott, MA, OT/L, FAOTA

Most occupational therapy practitioners in the United States work within either the health care or education industries (American Occupational Therapy Association [AOTA], 2010c). The U.S. health care industry has evolved into a complex system of for-profit and not-for-profit agencies and organizations that attempt to meet the health care needs of the public. Other occupational therapy practitioners are employed in the education system, another complex series of institutions. This system provides education to children and youth from kindergarten through the 12th grade as well as to students in higher education. Occupational therapy practitioners employed in higher education work as faculty in occupational therapy academic programs as educators or researchers or in a combination of these two roles and in administrative positions such as department chair and dean.

Occupational therapy practitioners working in such systems interact *internally,* within their immediate work setting, with institutional professionals, paraprofessionals, staff, and consumers; internal relationships are discussed in Chapter 20 of this volume. They also interact with a variety of *external* organizations and bodies, defined as those that are outside the specific settings where occupational therapy practice and education directly occur. Ethical issues related to interactions with external organizations and bodies are the focus of this chapter.

Occupational therapy practitioners in the health care industry interact with such external entities as independent providers or provider groups who work at other settings, health care provider organizations, external health care settings and facilities, health products and equipment suppliers, pharmaceutical companies, long-term care providers (e.g., nursing homes, assisted living facilities, adult day care, hospice), government agencies, and regulatory and standard-setting organizations. In the education system, external organizations include ancillary professionals in the community such as mental health or other health care professionals, educational provider associations, accreditation bodies, government agencies, parent groups (e.g., parent–teacher associations), educational and therapeutic material suppliers, and advocacy or specialty organizations (e.g., Easter Seals).

Academic faculty and administrators also collaborate with external entities such as accreditation bodies, professional associations, fieldwork placement sites, and other academic and scientific institutions. Researchers interact with funding agencies at the local, state, or federal levels; foundations; other public and private research institutions; and proprietary research companies.

In addition, nontraditional organizations provide equipment, supplies, and services to health care and education systems. These organizations include grocery stores, spas, government-sponsored educational institutions (e.g., county health departments, consumer protection and information providers), and specialized service providers (e.g., massage therapists). Regulatory bodies are an important component of the health care industry and education systems; they include private, state, and federal regulatory and accreditation bodies.

All occupational therapy practitioners are governed by federal, state, city, and/or county legislative bodies that establish laws and regulations directing the day-to-day functions of professionals and citizens. Directly or indirectly, occupational therapy practitioners interact with these external organizations or individuals in the practice of their profession. In their everyday interactions and functions, occupational therapy practitioners encounter ethical issues, distress, and dilemmas, some of which involve people or organizations external to their specific practice setting. Guidance is provided in this chapter regarding ethical decision making with respect to external bodies and organizations. Six case studies and one vignette are provided to challenge readers to reflect on ethical issues and problems that occupational therapy practitioners encounter in service delivery and funding involving external groups.

HEALTH CARE SYSTEM ISSUES

Spending in the health care industry is considerable, and factors related to profit making and accumulation of funds by not-for-profit organizations are significant drivers of ethical dilemmas and problems for occupational therapy practitioners (Brandt, 2010). Health care is one of the largest and fastest growing industries in the United States. In 2009, $2.5 trillion was spent on health care, accounting for 17.6% of the country's gross domestic product, and it is estimated that spending will reach $4.3 trillion by 2018 (Austin & Wetle, 2012). With such significant expenditures, it is no wonder that ethical issues abound in the development and provision of health care and related services.

In the 20th century, health care expanded from professions focused on caretaking of medical needs and problems to a business in which health care services are a commodity (Austin & Wetle, 2012). Another step in the evolution of health care was legislation establishing the entitlement benefits of Medicare (for those ages 65 or older or severely disabled) and Medicaid (for those with low incomes). Just as in corporate businesses, fraud, waste, abuse, and greed impinge on the appropriate, ethical, and legal conduct of both the not-for-profit and profit-making arms of the health care industry.

In addition to the cost of health care, access is another issue that influences health care provision and decision making. Equality and justice are ethical theories considered by policy makers in deciding how to address access, specifically the allocation of health care. Within occupational therapy, these core values are articulated in Principle 4, Social Justice; Principle 5, Procedural Justice; and Principle 7, Fidelity, of the *Occupational Therapy Code of Ethics and Ethics Standards* (referred to as the "Code and Ethics Standards"; AOTA, 2010b). Equalities in health care are not easy to achieve (Austin & Wetle, 2012). Many people living in the United States have no health insurance, and federally qualified health care clinics and other low-cost government or private clinics are unable to fully address their needs (Austin & Wetle, 2012). Overcrowding in emergency rooms and soaring health care costs are inevitable outcomes of this situation. Passed in 2010, the landmark Patient Protection and Affordable Care Act will hopefully alleviate this situation. It mandates insurance coverage and is an attempt to increase equality in the health care system by reducing the number of people in the United States who are uninsured and receiving no health care benefits or services.

Quality of care and services is the third issue that affects the provision of health care. Quality encompasses several ethical attributes, including ensuring the safety of the patient, addressed in Principle 2, Nonmaleficence, and providing the best possible care, covered in Principle 1, Beneficence.

The organizational culture of a specific health care business, agency, organization, or system may be influenced by one or all of these issues discussed. For example, a clinic located in a low-income neighborhood may be driven by its mission to serve all people who present for health care services. In another instance, a hospital associated with a research institution may have an admission policy based in part on the research studies it is conducting. The quality of services of these two health care organizations may vary because of differences in the amount of funding, access to a qualified workforce, and ability to understand and respond to the immediate needs of patients.

Organizational cultures also have differences in ethical standards and practices. An example of such a difference is the ethical approach to patients with terminal illnesses provided by a hospice organization versus a community-based hospital. Both institutions intend to provide high-quality care. For the hospital, this means providing as much care as possible to alleviate the patients' disease or disorder, despite the pain or suffering this care may cause as a side effect. For the hospice, however, care is palliative, serving to support the patient in dying with dignity and as painlessly as possible.

In addition to the impact of the values of equality and justice on health care, the principles of Veracity (Principle 6) and Autonomy and Confidentiality (Principle 3) in the Code and Ethics Standards form the basis of professional standards of practice and duty to patients. Austin and Wetle (2012) articulated the virtues of professional behavior—namely, compassion, integrity, trustworthiness, and wisdom.

EDUCATION SYSTEM ISSUES

The U.S. education system can be divided into two parts; one serves infants and children from birth to age 21 years, and the other serves people with high school diplomas who attend institutions of higher education. Twenty-six percent of occupational therapy practitioners work in early intervention and schools and 5% in higher education (AOTA, 2010c). Similar issues and problems to those found in health care systems exist in education systems, including the cost of education, access to quality education, and the impact of poor academic preparation on the health and

well-being of people and families in the United States.

External relationships exist between occupational therapy practitioners who serve children and youth and the local education agency, the state department of education, and the U.S. Department of Education. Funding to pay for "related services" typically comes from government sources, and providers are subject to state and federal regulations that influence practice. In institutions of higher education, faculty are employed primarily to teach, perform service, and conduct research. The cost of this education is paid for by the student, the student's family, public funding (e.g., taxes, grants), and in some cases private endowment. Educational services are designed to enable students to learn, succeed academically or professionally, and attain a degree or certificate. Although educational institutions are not businesses per se, they can be considered, like health care institutions, as a specialized type of business. Thus, business ethics codes, directives, and dilemmas, as well as general ethical issues, dilemmas, theories, and frameworks, apply to educational institutions.

ETHICAL GUIDELINES AND EXTERNAL ORGANIZATIONS

Most institutions have principles and standards that govern and determine ethical parameters for the institution. These may be expressed in a code of conduct for employees, contractors, consultants, volunteers, and boards of directors (Joint Commission, 2009). Organizations also have policies and procedures that direct the structure, format, and content of activities conducted in the health care or educational institution. The principles, standards, policies, and procedures may originate in ethical principles governing professional behavior in a certain culture (e.g., health care, school system, or higher education).

Accrediting bodies also may impose standards and requirements with which an organization must comply to attain the accreditation or certification. Often accreditation is required to receive funds (e.g., a hospital must be accredited by Medicare to receive Medicare funding for patient services delivered in that hospital). Through an arrangement with the Centers for Medicare and Medicaid Services (CMS), the Joint Commission has "deemed status" to conduct the accreditation process for certain health care organizations. Standards for such accreditation include compliance with federal and state laws and regulations and other standards set by CMS. The Joint Commission may go above and beyond these standards—for example, in promoting higher quality of services—but organizations must be compliant at least with the required and relevant laws, regulations, and standards.

In addition, professionals working within the institution may have their own professional code of ethics or conduct that governs their practice in the setting. Institutions and organizations that represent professionals and nonprofessionals often have specific procedures for enforcing their code of conduct. For example, AOTA has the *Enforcement Procedures for the Occupational Therapy Code of Ethics and Ethics Standards* (AOTA, 2010a) to inform members and the public about steps that can be taken to address breaches of the Code and Ethics Standards. In the sections that follow, we discuss institutional and professional standards and ethical principles within the context of case examples of interactions with external bodies and organizations. Before each case study, a short introduction to provide context and a foundation for decision making appear. Readers are encouraged to use one of the ethical decision-making models presented in Chapter 10 to analyze each case.

LEGAL COMPLIANCE

Organizational activities and employee conduct are to be in compliance with all applicable laws and regulations. Principle 5, Procedural Justice, of the Code and Ethics Standards states, "Occupational therapy personnel shall comply with institutional rules, local, state, federal, and international laws and AOTA documents applicable to the profession of occupational therapy" (AOTA, 2010b, p. S22). Under regulations governing grants given by the U.S. Department of Health and Human Services (DHHS), DHHS is required to ensure that recipients of service be citizens or have legal status in the United States

(U.S. Code of Federal Regulations, 1999). To provide services to people who do not have legal status is in violation of these regulations and may be considered fraudulent and an abuse of the system. In Case Study 21.1, an occupational therapist weighs consideration of the legal status of a client against the principle of Social Justice.

CASE STUDY 21.1. ENSURING LEGAL COMPLIANCE WITH A FUNDER'S REQUIREMENTS

Jane, an occupational therapist, provided services part-time to an early intervention program for developmentally challenged infants and toddlers. The program billed Medicaid for screening of the infants and toddlers and private insurance for screenings and intervention when possible. The program also received federal government funds to pay for other program services and for clients who did not have Medicaid or other insurance, including consultation by the occupational therapist. Jane received a referral to see **Kiku**, a 2-year-old girl whom a neighbor referred to the clinic's doctor because she was not crawling and failed to make eye contact with the parents or the neighbor. Kiku's parents did not have insurance; her father worked as a day laborer. Kiku had two school-age siblings who attended a local elementary school. Her mother was a full-time homemaker and used a cane because she had lost a limb following an attack by a terrorist guerrilla.

As part of her assessment, Jane learned that Kiku's parents, **Mr. and Mrs. San**, were Somalian and had been in the United States for 6 years. They fled Somalia when militant gangs threatened their city. Her father and mother had been interviewed at intake, and they both spoke limited English. **Sondra** was the team member who provided social work services, and she approached Jane to ask about the parents. She had been unable to get Mr. San to bring in his pay stub or give her sufficient information about his or his wife's background to enable her to assist the family in applying for government benefits (i.e., food stamps, special supplemental nutrition program for Women, Infants, and Children) and explore whether they might be eligible for Medicaid because of Mrs. San's disability. Sondra suspected that Mr. and Mrs. San did not have legal status and knew Jane had an upcoming home visit. She wanted

Jane to see what more she could find out to determine if Mr. and Mrs. San were illegal immigrants.

The administrator of the program had indicated that funding was "tight" these days because many people in the community were losing their jobs and seeking care at the clinic. Jane even feared that her job as a contractor might be in jeopardy if funding was lost. She was unsure whether her program was legally permitted to provide services to illegal immigrants under their funding contract. Jane reviewed the Code and Ethics Standards in an effort to understand her ethical responsibilities to the child, the family, and her employer. In particular, she wondered if she had any ethical responsibility as an occupational therapist under the ethical principle of Social Justice.

The questions about the family's legal status had Jane and the agency feeling cautious. In Principle 3, Autonomy, Confidentiality—"Occupational therapy personnel shall respect the right of the individual to self-determination" (AOTA, 2010b, p. S20; specifically, Principles 3G, 3I, and 3J)—Jane recognized her obligation to respect the family's right to privacy and try to avoid placing them or the agency she worked for in legal jeopardy. Jane also needed to make sure that she understood the family and they her, as well as the process. In addition, Principle 4, Social Justice, states that "Occupational therapy personnel shall provide services in a fair and equitable manner" (p. S21; see also Principles 4D and 4G). Jane had a duty to advocate for the services that might be legally available to Kiku.

According to Principle 5, Procedural Justice, "Occupational therapy personnel shall comply with institutional rules, local, state, federal, and international laws and AOTA documents applicable to the profession of occupational therapy" (AOTA, 2010b, p. S22; see also Principles 5B, 5C, 5L, and 5P). Jane thus had a legal and ethical obligation to comply with current laws, regulations, AOTA association policies, and her employer's organizational guidelines. Jane, and possibly the agency, therefore was obligated to learn or seek consultation with experts regarding Kiku's legal entitlement to services. Jane also had a responsibility to inform the agency of her obligations under the Code and Ethics Standards, particularly if her compliance with her employer's policies placed her activities in conflict with the Code and Ethics Standards. The Code and Ethics Standards, which emphasize values, would support Jane's efforts to

seek alternative avenues to providing Kiku's care if traditional means were unavailable.

BUSINESS ETHICS PRINCIPLES

Business ethics principles include honest and accurate communication, appropriate use of proprietary information, and prohibition of activities that are fraudulent, including dishonest or deceptive acts. Fraud may occur when inappropriate or deceptive activities are conducted to increase the profit of a business, obtain services or property, or violate the requirements of a funding agency or organization. Medicare suggests that *fraud* be defined as intentional deception or misrepresentation that a person makes in the belief that there will be some benefit to himself or herself or to another person, business, or cause (DHHS, 1998, para. 1).

One of the occupational therapy profession's seven core values is truth: "In all situations, occupational therapists, occupational therapy assistants, and students must provide accurate information, both in oral and written form" (AOTA, 2010b, p. S18). In essence, then, fraud is the opposite of truth. Furthermore, occupational therapy practitioners are bound by Principle 6, Veracity, of the Code and Ethics Standards, which states, "Occupational therapy personnel shall provide comprehensive, accurate, and objective information when representing the profession" (p. S23). Case Study 21.2 describes an occupational therapist's efforts to avoid fraud in representing her ability to administer assessments.

CASE STUDY 21.2. ENGAGING IN DUE DILIGENCE TO AVOID FRAUD

Jessica had completed her occupational therapy degree 1 year previously, passed the National Board for Certification in Occupational Therapy (NBCOT) exam, and became licensed in her home state; she had obtained a degree in psychology before entering her occupational therapy program. Before beginning her present position, she completed a fieldwork experience in pediatrics working under the supervision of **Lena**, an occupational therapist in a school system. In addition, on the weekends, Jessica assisted

Lena as an occupational therapy aide in her private pediatric practice. Lena was certified to perform a psychological battery that provides an assessment of intelligence in children. During Jessica's fieldwork, she observed and had a chance to practice some of these assessments. This activity complemented her occupational therapy academic and Level I fieldwork training, which also addressed psychosocial assessment of young children.

Jessica's husband was in the armed services and was transferred to Nevada, so Jessica was looking for a new job where she would be living. She applied for a position as an occupational therapist at a specialized pediatric program that provided contract therapists to school systems and operated a private practice for young children with autism and other developmental disabilities. When the program interviewer learned of Jessica's background and exposure to conducting psychological testing, she felt this might help the private practice with their certification as a psychosocial rehabilitation provider for the State of Nevada. The program planned to notify their accrediting body that they had certified personnel who could conduct psychological and intelligence testing on the basis of Jessica's experience and training to date. Jessica was unsure whether this claim would be ethical, but the interviewer assured her that this practice was consistent with Nevada state licensure for occupational therapists and offered her a sign-on bonus to cover moving expenses and a good salary for a 12-month position.

Jessica recognized that she had a great deal of training and some experience in psychosocial intervention, but she questioned whether she could ethically present herself as certified to conduct intelligence testing services. In this job, Jessica realized, she could be a great help to the program in maintaining their accreditation while gaining experience in an area of great interest to her. What were her ethical responsibilities to the accrediting organization and to the state occupational therapy licensure board? Was what the organization proposed fraud?

Jessica identified her first step as contacting the State of Nevada board of occupational therapy and reading the statutes and regulations to understand the profession's scope of practice in that state. Second, Jessica realized, she needed to contact the developer of the assessments to learn whether there were any certification requirements. Undertaking these activities and reviewing the Code and Ethics Standards helped Jessica determine a legal and ethical way to address the agency's hiring requests. Whether or not the organization was proposing fraud was uncertain and a matter for legal interpretation. Jessica planned to take advantage of the organization's interest in her to educate them about what she'd learned and what alternatives might be available.

RELATIONS WITH GOVERNMENT AGENCIES

In addition to compliance with federal, state, and local laws, employees are required to be compliant with rules and requirements of government agencies, even when the relationship is not contractual. This obligation is relevant to federal grants and cooperative agreements (U.S. Code of Federal Regulations, 1999). State laws vary, and all practicing occupational therapy practitioners should be aware of the laws and regulations that govern practice in their state. The state licensure board and membership in the state occupational therapy association are recommended as sources of information on state laws, regulations, and information concerning requirements of state funding sources. Occupational therapy practitioners may engage with government agencies in many ways.

Local, state, and federal agencies, including hospitals and universities, have rules regarding the use of human research participants. For example, in 1991, the *Federal Policy for the Protection of Human Subjects*, or "Common Rule," was adopted as regulations that are applicable across many federal agencies (Office for Human Research Protections, DHHS, 2005). Ethical principles are identified in the Belmont Report, which formed the basis for the federal policy (see U.S. Department of Education, 2011).

The U.S. Department of Education's Rehabilitation Services Administration, in conjunction with states, provides grant funding to support the work of centers for independent living (CILs). Occupational therapy students and practitioners are sometimes involved with CILs as volunteers, staff, or board members. People with disabilities must form 51% of the members of the board of directors of a CIL. This percentage requirement also is applied to community boards, advisory councils, and commissions. The government also may pose requirements for racial and geographic diversity on boards.

The federal government, through the Individuals With Disabilities Education Act of 1990, helps families and individualized education program team members (which include occupational therapy practitioners) resolve ethical and legal disputes with the help of a mediator. The impartial mediator is considered external to the occupational therapist and his or her role. For example, if parents request an increase in the frequency and intensity of occupational therapy services for their child that is not supported by the school, a mediator may help the parties resolve the dispute (Scott, 2007).

In Case Study 21.3, an occupational therapy researcher must decide how to handle communication with the funders of his research regarding the difficulties he encounters in his study.

CASE STUDY 21.3. DEALING ETHICALLY WITH FUNDING AGENCIES AND ORGANIZATIONS

Paul was an occupational therapist with a doctoral degree in disability studies. He was a faculty member and researcher in the occupational therapy department of a large university, where he was seeking tenure. Following a pilot study, Paul received a federal research grant to examine occupational therapy's role in health promotion in a program integrating primary care and behavioral health (i.e., mental health and substance abuse) to serve the needs of people diagnosed with serious and persistent behavioral health disorders. The research study protocol required patient consent and had defined selection criteria for diagnosis and level of functioning of each research participant. In his proposal, Paul indicated that in his 3-year study, he would enroll 75 participants in a subgroup of the program that had an occupational therapist working as the health promotion specialist and 75 control participants in another subgroup in which social workers provided the health promotion services. Previously, social workers had run other health promotion activities in a nonintegrated behavioral health system, but the program saw limited change in participants' overall health status.

Because of hiring and licensing difficulties, Paul's research program had a slow start. In addi-

tion, the program experienced difficulties integrating services because of differences in organizational culture between the primary care and behavioral health care practices.

In the 8th month of the program, the occupational therapist was hired and began providing services to clients who entered the integrated practice and elected to join the health promotion group program on a rolling basis. By the end of the 2nd year, trends indicating an improvement in health status were noted in the research group; the lack of a statistically significant difference was attributed to the small size of the group run by the occupational therapist because of low enrollment in the overall integrated program. Paul's government project officer (GPO) and his department director were concerned about the low enrollment of participants in the research study. Paul tried numerous tactics to increase enrollment in the health promotion group program, but to no avail, and he was counting on success in this study to further his aspirations for tenure and demonstrate that he could responsibly administer and use federal funds.

A colleague suggested that "there are ways" for Paul to seem to improve his results, in spite of low enrollment. This colleague had tenure and several significant grants completed in his portfolio and might potentially be on the committee that reviewed Paul's dossier for tenure in the future. Paul wondered whether he could improve his results through alternate means but stay within the confines of his study parameters. He realized that most of the questions he faced could be answered through a review of the Code and Ethics Standards and a discussion with the GPO or grants manager.

Paul considered the options of falsifying his outcomes, lowering the study's entry criteria, or changing the methods used in his groups. Principle 2G of the Code and Ethics Standards reminded Paul to remain objective because altering the admission criteria might have a negative impact on the type and benefit of participation; Principle 2G states, "Avoid situations in which a practitioner, educator, researcher, or employer is unable to maintain clear professional boundaries or objectivity to ensure the safety and well-being of recipients of service, students, research participants, and employees" (AOTA, 2010b, p. S20). If Paul altered the selection criteria or the group interventions, the study outcomes also would be altered. If he decided to "fudge" the outcomes, future study participants might not be helped. If the admission criteria or group interventions were weakened to produce better outcomes, current or future participants might be harmed. If future researchers attempted to replicate Paul's work and wasted time and money, this might ultimately harm the public's perception of occupational therapy. Principle 1L states, "Ensure that occupational therapy research is conducted in accordance with currently accepted ethical guidelines and standards for the protection of research participants and the dissemination of results" (p. S19).

He also reflected on Principles 6A and 6B, which address misrepresentation of the facts. The expectation articulated in these principles is to "represent the credentials, qualifications, education, experience, training, roles, duties, competence, views, contributions, and findings accurately in all forms of communication about recipients of service, students, employees, research participants, and colleagues" and "refrain from using or participating in the use of any form of communication that contains false, fraudulent, deceptive, misleading, or unfair statements or claims" (AOTA, 2010b, p. S24).

Even though Paul was motivated to establish a positive working relationship with participants, faculty, his project officer, and potential funding agencies, it was imperative that Paul familiarize himself with all relevant policies, institutional and ethical, that might affect his work. His understanding was clarified after reading Principle 5B: "Be familiar with and seek to understand and abide by institutional rules, and when those rules conflict with ethical practice, take steps to resolve the conflict" (AOTA, 2010b, p. S22).

If Paul's colleague also was an occupational therapy practitioner, Paul should share the Code and Ethics Standards with him (Principle 5A). If Paul believed that his colleague was engaged in wrongdoing, his first step would be to follow Principle 7D (attempt to resolve violations using internal resources first). He also should consider the implications of Principles 1L (ensure that research is conducted in line with ethical guidelines) and 1M (report acts that appear unethical or illegal) before revealing his personal and ethical conflicts with this situation. This information might highlight to Paul's colleague vulnerabilities in his thinking and behavior while keeping Paul compliant with the principles. If Paul's colleague were to threaten him with a negative tenure review recommendation in the future,

Paul would need to follow up with his supervisor and attempt to handle the situation locally without escalating to the state regulatory board, AOTA's Ethics Commission, or NBCOT, unless necessary.

However, what should Paul tell his project officer? What were his ethical responsibilities to the federal government for accepting their grant funds? Are there any differences in responsibilities to government funders versus private foundations? Principle 6, Veracity, of the Code and Ethics Standards states, "Occupational therapy personnel shall provide comprehensive, accurate, and objective information when representing the profession" (AOTA, 2010b, p. S23). Occupational therapy practitioners represent themselves and the profession in a wide variety of situations in which they are communicating information. They have an obligation to deliver reports, testimony, research outcomes, recommendations, and verbal and written materials in an honest and factual manner. Falsifying one's credentials or experiences is unethical and likely a breach of one's licensure law.

On further discussion, Paul believed that what his colleague was suggesting was unethical, and he considered how he might proceed. For both his government and private funders, Paul decided to contact the GPO and grants manager and accurately communicate the problems and difficulties he was experiencing as early as possible so they were aware of the situation and could suggest ways for Paul to proceed within the confines of his funding. Waiting for an extended period for things to improve might result in negative results and a lack of further support. Communication might be through a phone call, report, or other type of communication. This communication could result in positive assistance. For example, Paul's GPO might suggest he meet with the staff working on implementing the overall integrated project to determine why their enrollment was so low and ways to improve engagement of clients in the health promotion program that were ethical and allowed by the funding agency or organization.

CONFLICT OR DUALITY OF INTEREST

The ethical principle of avoiding conflict or duality of interest requires that an occupational therapy practitioner be loyal to his or her institution and employer. It prohibits practitioners from using their position to profit personally or to help others profit via their connection with the institution: "Having a financial interest in a business venture such as product sales related to occupational therapy while providing occupational therapy services to the client may be perceived as a conflict of interest" (Austin, 2010, p. 135). Conflict of interest is mentioned in Principles 2 and 7. According to Principle 2, "Occupational therapy personnel shall intentionally refrain from actions that cause harm" (AOTA, 2010b, p. S19); Principles 2C, 2J, and 2K provide more detail. Additionally, Principle 7, "Occupational therapy personnel shall treat colleagues and other professionals with respect, fairness, discretion, and integrity" (p. S24), and specifically Principle 7E, are relevant to discussions of conflict of interest. In Case Study 21.4, an occupational therapy assistant weighs an opportunity for advancement against his obligations to his employer.

CASE STUDY 21.4. EXAMINING A DUALITY OF INTEREST

Gaines Rehabilitation Services was a freestanding rehabilitation company that provided physical and occupational therapy services in a suburban community. A husband–wife team who were physical therapists owned the company. **Ed** managed the business, and his wife, **Leora**, supervised the day-to-day operations and provided physical therapy evaluation and intervention to patients. Staff included **Calvin**, an occupational therapist; two other physical therapists; **Lloyd**, an occupational therapy assistant; and two physical therapy aides. The clients of the company included patients recovering from neurological conditions, including brain trauma; orthopedic injuries, surgeries, and disorders; and acute and chronic pain syndromes.

Lloyd, the occupational therapy assistant, had worked for the practice for 6 months. He liked Calvin and enjoyed the clients served by the program. In addition to direct intervention, Calvin and Lloyd ran a work tolerance program designed to help injured workers return to work after injury or surgery. Many of these clients were being seen in the practice under workers' compensation insurance, and others were referred by a managed health care company with which the practice had

a contract to provide return-to-work services for injured workers. Ed sometimes encouraged the therapy staff to "keep the patients on program" for extended periods when the therapists believed the clients were ready for discharge from the work therapy or tolerance program.

Lloyd was uncomfortable with this situation and planned to discuss it with Calvin. In the meantime, **Harold**, a client case manager from the managed care company and old school friend of Lloyd's, stopped by to check on his patients' progress and afterward to have dinner with Lloyd. At dinner, Harold mentioned that the company's patients seemed to be having trouble when they returned to work and that it would be good if a service could be provided to assist the workers on the job. Lloyd said he would talk to his employer about this, but Harold said he thought that the managed care company was not very satisfied with Gaines Rehabilitation Services but might be interested in contracting independently with Lloyd to assist workers when they returned to their jobs.

This seemed like an opportunity for Lloyd to advance himself, although he was concerned about whether he could take Harold up on his offer without the supervision of an occupational therapist. He also was concerned about being disloyal to Gaines Rehabilitation Services and wondered if he had any legal obligation to the company. Lloyd knew he should review his contract with the company and, if he had any questions, seek the services of an attorney. (FindLaw.com could help him identify attorneys in his area and with the skill set he needed.)

Was Lloyd obligated to tell his employer about his conversation with Harold (e.g., negative feedback about Gaines Rehabilitation Services and his potential job offer with the managed care company), even though he did not specifically sign anything that bound him to the company? Unless the contract or work agreement includes restrictive covenants or noncompete clauses, employees may resign at will. However, they should abide by previously agreed on resignation notification time frames. Although no specific ethical principle required Lloyd to inform Calvin of the other company's dissatisfaction with their services, reporting this information would be supported by the Code and Ethics Standards, specifically Principle 7: "Occupational therapy personnel shall treat colleagues and other professionals with respect, fairness, discretion, and integrity" (AOTA,

2010b, p. S24). Specifically, Principle 7E ("avoid conflicts of interest . . . in employment"; p. S25) and Principle 7F ("avoid using one's position . . . or knowledge gained from that position in such a manner that gives rise to real or perceived conflict of interest among the person [and] the employer"; p. S25) provide guidance regarding a conflict of interest in this situation. Researching standards set by state boards of occupational therapy practice and AOTA might guide Lloyd's responses to this situation.

How should Lloyd resolve his discomfort with carrying out Ed's suggestions to keep clients on his caseload longer than Lloyd believed was appropriate and warranted? First, Lloyd needed to decide whether a client had reached maximum benefit in collaboration with the occupational therapist. Lloyd's professional and ethical responsibility in collaboration with the occupational therapist is discussed in Principles 1H (terminate services when goals have been met), 4D (advocate for just, fair, ethical treatment), 6B (refrain from false, fraudulent, or deceptive communication), and 6D (ensure that documentation is in accordance with regulations) of the Code and Ethics Standards. Keeping clients on one's caseload who have reached their goals and are no longer benefitting from occupational therapy intervention is a violation of these principles.

GIFTS

Organizations typically have principles or policies that govern when employees may accept or give gifts, both within the organization and from and to outside sources. This guidance is necessary because gifts must be distinguished from bribes. As defined by the Markkula Center for Applied Ethics, "a *gift* is something of value given without the expectation of return; a *bribe* is the same thing given in the hope of influence or benefit" (Nadler & Schulman, 2006, para. 3, italics added).

For example, federal government employees may accept gifts only if they are of nominal worth or value. At the state level, employees may have to complete a financial disclosure statement and comply with restrictions on the value of gifts received (State of Maryland, 2010). Similarly, accepting meals may be addressed within organizational and government rules; for example,

meals may be accepted only if they are part of a scheduled event or meeting or if they have nominal worth (U.S. Department of Justice, n.d.) The Code and Ethics Standards address this topic in Principle 5J: "Report all gifts and remuneration from individuals, agencies, or companies in accordance with employer policies as well as state and federal guidelines" (AOTA, 2010b, p. S23). In Case Study 21.5, an occupational therapist must assess an offer of gifts to her organization.

CASE STUDY 21.5. ASSESSING AN OFFER OF GIFTS

Joanette was the director of an occupational therapy department of a large, freestanding, not-for-profit rehabilitation hospital. Patients seen by the occupational therapy practitioners included those diagnosed with neurological disorders such as brain injury and stroke, traumatic disorders such as amputation and spinal cord injury, and orthopedic surgeries. The occupational therapy practitioners worked as part of a rehabilitation team with physiatrists, physical therapists, and speech–language pathologists. Many patients required wheelchairs, augmentative communication devices, or adaptive equipment to function independently in their home on discharge. Joanette worked closely with local universities to provide fieldwork training for both occupational therapy and occupational therapy assistant students.

While attending a rehabilitation conference, Joanette met the sales manager of a large rehabilitation equipment and supplies dealer. He offered to provide training on wheelchair prescription and the use of new adaptive devices for people who have had traumatic injuries. Joanette was very interested; she saw it as good training for her entry-level therapy staff, students, and more advanced practitioners. **Mr. Miller**, the sales manager, invited Joanette out for dinner that night. At dinner, Mr. Miller suggested that his company could provide further training at no cost to the occupational therapy department featuring noted speakers, videos, and hands-on training in basic neurology and anatomy review, neurological injuries, splinting, and other topics. In addition, he shared that his company was an approved provider of medical education and could thus provide continuing education credits for occupational therapy practitioners.

In return for this training, Mr. Miller expressed that his company would refer patients and "work closely" with these patients and their treatment team to provide electric and manual wheelchairs and other adaptive and augmentative equipment. He indicated that many other occupational therapy and physical therapy departments across the country had taken advantage of this opportunity and that he hoped Joanette could see the value of such an arrangement. Joanette told him she would consult with her colleagues and then let him know.

Joanette explored the different resources available to her to determine the appropriate and ethical course of action. Her first step was to discuss the situation with her supervisor and review hospital policies regarding the acceptance of gifts (e.g., staff training and education, dinner, the potential agreement with Mr. Miller's company for equipment and referrals). Joanette also reviewed the Code and Ethics Standards to make sure that she and her occupational therapy students and staff would remain compliant with the ethical standards established for the profession pertaining to conflict of interest, exploitation, and adherence to existing institutional policies.

Was Mr. Miller's offer to provide free training worth entering into the proposed arrangement? Was this an informal agreement, a formal agreement, or a bribe? Mr. Miller's offer to provide education and training for referrals might be considered a form of fee splitting. Fremgen (2012) discussed fee splitting and used the following example: "Fee splitting occurs when one physician offers to pay another physician for the referral of patients" (p. 86). Fremgen indicated that if Medicare or Medicaid is a direct or indirect payment source, the billers might be guilty of a felony. This example suggests that some issues an occupational therapy practitioner encounters may have both legal and ethical implications. It is important to review the ethical principles and seek legal opinions to ensure that agreements such as that presented to Joanette do not lead to breaches in ethical conduct and existing laws. The wheelchair referrals might lead to purchases paid by Medicare and a violation of their rules.

Which ethical principles should Joanette consider? Joanette's review of the Code and Ethics Standards helped her identify Principles 2C (avoid relationships that exploit others), 2K (avoid bartering for services), 5J (report all gifts), and 7F (avoid using one's position in a way that leads to a conflict of interest) as relevant. Joanette's personal research, discussions with her su-

pervisor, and review of hospital policies and Medicare guidelines helped her conclude that the opportunity Mr. Miller proposed would be outside the realm of ethical behavior and potentially illegal. Both Joanette and the hospital declined the offer.

NONMALEFICENCE AND BENEFICENCE

Nonmaleficence and Beneficence are two of the seven principles of the AOTA Code and Ethics Standards. They are core principles for occupational therapy practitioners that are included in the codes of ethics or behavior for many health care and other professionals (Austin & Wetle, 2012). *Beneficence* means doing good and considering the possibility of one's actions creating a harmful situation; a corollary to beneficence is *nonmaleficence,* which means not to cause harm or the possibility of harm to a client.

During external relationships, these principles extend beyond the individual patient to the organization or client served within the external relationship. In Case Study 21.6, the occupational therapist must consider the possible harm done to the patient, the relationship between the clinic and the referring physician, and the possible harmful impact on the arrangement with payers.

CASE STUDY 21.6. PROMOTING NONMALEFICENCE AND BENEFICENCE IN A BUSY CLINIC

Dr. Letinger was a primary care physician who worked in a large clinic where other medical specialists also practiced. He often referred patients to the local community hospital's outpatient rehabilitation clinic. The clinic staff included occupational therapy, physical therapy, and speech–language pathology practitioners, as well as rehabilitation counselors and licensed social workers. Frequently, Dr. Letinger sent referrals for occupational therapy that said "knee replacements—evaluate and treat for 6 weeks, 2×/ week." Sometimes his referrals were more specific and included "gait training, back strengthening, or shoulder taping to decrease pain."

Atep was the occupational therapist in the rehabilitation clinic. He noted that Dr. Letinger and other physicians sometimes made similarly inappropriate referrals to the physical therapists and speech–language pathologists that would be most appropriate for occupational therapy. For example, Atep knew from the speech–language pathologist that she had recently received a referral to screen a patient who had a stroke for ability to continue to drive.

Several of the staff of the rehabilitation clinic were very overworked because they also provided backup to the inpatient service of the hospital, and several vacancies had not been filled. For this reason, they did not meet as a team and rarely communicated other than through their documentation about patients. Overall, it seemed that many patients needed to be seen, but Atep sometimes found himself having a low monthly census. The director of the clinic indicated that Atep's low productivity might affect the continuation of his full-time position. Therefore, Atep accepted Dr. Leitinger's referrals rather than considering whether the patients' referrals should be directed to another therapy provider.

What ethical concerns should Atep have with regard to his state licensure board? Atep needed to make sure he was practicing as an occupational therapist within his scope of practice and according to licensure regulations. What ethical concerns should Atep have with regard to the patients he served? Patients deserve to receive the appropriate interventions from qualified practitioners. To this end, Atep could operate for the greater good of all patients by offering to conduct a staff in-service to discuss issues to improve the flow of referrals. What ethical concerns should Atep have with regard to the physicians who made referrals to him? Principles 1E, 1G, 6A, and 7A inform occupational therapy practitioners that failure to live up to the expectations of competence may cause harm to the patient, the public's perception of occupational therapy, and professionals external to occupational therapy practice.

Finally, Atep had a professional responsibility to his clients to practice within the bounds of his license and his skills. He needed to validate that his interventions were helping patients in the same way a colleague might, that he was practicing according to legal and ethical standards, and that no harm might result from his service delivery. Atep also needed to recognize that if his caseload wasn't adequate to provide him with the income he needed, he could consider working elsewhere part-time or resigning and finding full-time employment that would meet his financial needs without challenging his standards for ethical behavior.

AUTONOMY, CONFIDENTIALITY

As stated earlier, Principle 3 of the Code and Ethics Standards, Autonomy and Confidentiality, specifies the patient's right to self-determination and includes recognition of and respect for the person's right to privacy and maintenance of confidentiality. Patients have the right to decide to allow disclosure or not; health care professionals must not disclose personal information, medical information, or educational information without the permission of the person served. Employees of an organization are generally expected to maintain employee and financial information and any other proprietary information confidential. However, as in Vignette 21.1, sometimes the rules governing consent to disclose or disclosure of organizational information are challenged.

VIGNETTE 21.1. WEIGHING DISCLOSURE OF PERSONAL INFORMATION

Victoria was an occupational therapy assistant for a community behavioral health service in Florida, where she provided services to a broad range of patients under the direction of an occupational therapist. In September, a significant hurricane was predicted to affect the area where Victoria practiced, and preparations were being made to address the needs of the patients. Victoria had been through a similar situation in another state where she lived a year previously. To enable the evacuation of her patients who were in dire need, Victoria provided fire and rescue personnel with these patients' names and addresses and the nature of their disorder or disability. At the time, it seemed necessary, but she later wondered how she might have handled the situation differently given that the community behavioral health service had some advance notice of the impending storm. Victoria sat down with her supervising therapist to discuss her concerns.

Based on your reading of this chapter on external relationships and a review of the Code and Ethics Standards, consider the following questions:

- What should Victoria and her supervisor consider in their discussion?
- Are crisis situations a special case in which rules of confidentiality do not apply?

- Is there a way to prepare for the hurricane but also protect the privacy of the patients receiving care from the community behavioral health service?
- What other ethical issues do crisis situations raise?

CONCLUSION

Occupational therapy practitioners engage in numerous external relationships throughout their academic and professional lives. These relationships are established through organizations, agencies, governments, and institutions that have policies, procedures, and regulations that occupational therapy students and practitioners must follow. In addition to compliance with each set of standards, practitioners must adhere to ethical principles governing occupational therapy during service delivery. Occupational therapy practitioners are encouraged to continually update their knowledge of guidelines that have an impact on their relationships with external entities.

REFERENCES

American Occupational Therapy Association. (2010a). Enforcement procedures for the *Occupational Therapy Code of Ethics and Ethics Standards (2010)*. *American Journal of Occupational Therapy,* S4–S16. doi: 10.5014/ajot.2010.64S4

American Occupational Therapy Association. (2010b). Occupational therapy code of ethics and ethics standards (2010). *American Journal of Occupational Therapy* (6 Suppl.), S17–S26. doi: 10:5014/ajot2010.62S17

American Occupational Therapy Association. (2010c). *2010 occupational therapy compensation and workforce study,* Bethesda, MD: AOTA Press.

Austin, A., & Wetle, V. (2012). *The United States health care system: Combining business, health and delivery* (2nd ed.). Upper Saddle River, NJ: Pearson Education.

Austin, D. (2010). Ethical considerations when occupational therapists engage in business transactions with clients. In D. Y. Slater (Ed.), *Reference guide to the Occupational Therapy Code of Ethics and Ethics Standards* (2010 ed., pp. 135–139). Bethesda, MD: AOTA Press.

Brandt, L. C. (2010). *Organizational ethics: Occupational therapy practice in a complex health environment* [CEonCD]. Bethesda, MD: American Occupational Therapy Association.

Fremgen, B. F. (2012). *Medical law and ethics* (4th ed). Upper Saddle River, NJ: Pearson Education.

Individuals With Disabilities Education Act of 1990, Pub. L. 101–476, 20 U.S.C., Ch 33.

Joint Commission. (2009). *The Joint Commission code of conduct*. Oakdale, IL: Author. Retrieved from www.jointcommission.org/assets/1/18/TJC_Code_of_Conduct_09.pdf

Nadler, J., & Schulman, M. (2006). *Gifts and bribes*. Santa Clara, CA: Markkula Center for Applied Ethics, Santa Clara University. Retrieved from www.scu.edu/ethics/practicing/focusareas/government_ethics/introduction/gifts.html

Office for Human Research Protections, U.S. Department of Health and Human Services. (2005). *Protection of human subjects*. 45 C.F.R. §46.111. Retrieved from www.hhs.gov/ohrp/humasubjects/guidance/45cfr46.html/

Patient Protection and Affordable Care Act, H.R. 3590, Pub. L. 111–148, signed into law 3/23/10, as modified by the Health Care and Education Reconciliation Act, H.R. 4872, Pub. L. 111–152, signed into law 3/30/10 C.F.R. (2010).

Scott, J. B. (2007). Ethical issues in school based and early intervention practice. In L. L. Jackson (Ed.), *Occupational therapy services for children and youth under IDEA* (3rd ed., pp. 213–227). Bethesda, MD: AOTA Press.

State of Maryland. (2010). Title 15. Public ethics. *Maryland Public Ethics Law* Retrieved from http://ethics.gov.state.md.us/Ethics%20Law.pdf

U.S. Code of Federal Regulations, 45, Part 72 and Part 94. Revised as of October 1, 1999. Retrieved from www.archives.gov/federal-register/cfr/subject-title-45.html

U.S. Department of Education. (2011). *Information about the protection of human subjects in research supported by the Department of Education—Overview*. Retrieved from www2.ed.gov/policy/fund/guid/humansub/overview.html

U.S. Department of Health and Human Services. (1998). Medicare definition of fraud. *FindLaw for Legal Professionals*. Retrieved from http://library.findlaw.com/1998/Feb/19/131383.html

U.S. Department of Justice. (n.d.). *Do it right*. Retrieved from www.justice.gov/jmd/ethics/generalf.htm

Appendix A
Occupational Therapy Code of Ethics and Ethics Standards (2010)

PREAMBLE

The American Occupational Therapy Association (AOTA) *Occupational Therapy Code of Ethics and Ethics Standards (2010)* ("Code and Ethics Standards") is a public statement of principles used to promote and maintain high standards of conduct within the profession. Members of AOTA are committed to promoting inclusion, diversity, independence, and safety for all recipients in various stages of life, health, and illness and to empower all beneficiaries of occupational therapy. This commitment extends beyond service recipients to include professional colleagues, students, educators, businesses, and the community.

Fundamental to the mission of the occupational therapy profession is the therapeutic use of everyday life activities (occupations) with individuals or groups for the purpose of participation in roles and situations in home, school, workplace, community, and other settings. "Occupational therapy addresses the physical, cognitive, psychosocial, sensory, and other aspects of performance in a variety of contexts to support engagement in everyday life activities that affect health, well-being, and quality of life" (AOTA, 2004, p. 694). Occupational therapy personnel have an ethical responsibility primarily to recipients of service and secondarily to society.

The *Occupational Therapy Code of Ethics and Ethics Standards (2010)* was tailored to address the most prevalent ethical concerns of the profession in education, research, and practice. The concerns of stakeholders including the public, consumers, students, colleagues, employers, research participants, researchers, educators, and practitioners were addressed in the creation of this document. A review of issues raised in ethics cases, member questions related to ethics, and content of other professional codes of ethics were utilized to ensure that the revised document is applicable to occupational therapists, occupational therapy assistants, and students in all roles.

The historical foundation of this Code and Ethics Standards is based on ethical reasoning surrounding practice and professional issues, as well as on empathic reflection regarding these interactions with others (see e.g., AOTA, 2005, 2006). This reflection resulted in the establishment of principles that guide ethical action, which goes beyond rote following of rules or application of principles. Rather, *ethical action* is a manifestation of moral character and mindful reflection. It is a commitment to benefit others, to virtuous practice of artistry and science, to genuinely good behaviors, and to noble acts of courage.

While much has changed over the course of the profession's history, more has remained the same. The profession of occupational therapy remains grounded in seven core concepts, as identified in the *Core Values and Attitudes of Occupational Therapy Practice* (AOTA, 1993): *altruism, equality, freedom, justice, dignity, truth,* and *prudence. Altruism* is the individual's ability to place the needs of others before their own. *Equality* refers to the desire to promote fairness in interactions with others. The concept of *freedom* and personal choice is paramount in a profession in which the desires of the client must guide our interventions. Occupational therapy practitioners, educators, and researchers relate in a fair and impartial manner to individuals with whom they interact and respect and adhere to the applicable laws and standards regarding their area of practice, be it direct care, education, or research *(justice)*. Inherent in the practice of occupational therapy is the promotion and preservation of the individuality and *dignity* of the client, by assisting him or her to engage in occupations that are meaningful to him or her regardless of level of disability. In all situations, occupational therapists, occupational therapy assistants, and students must provide accurate information, both in oral and written form *(truth)*. Occupational therapy personnel use their clinical and ethical reasoning skills, sound judgment, and reflection to make decisions to direct them in their area(s) of practice *(prudence)*. These seven core values provide a foundation by which occupational therapy personnel guide their interactions with others, be they students, clients, colleagues, research participants, or communities. These values also define the ethical principles to which the profession is committed and which the public can expect.

The *Occupational Therapy Code of Ethics and Ethics Standards (2010)* is a guide to professional conduct when ethical issues arise. Ethical decision making is a process that includes awareness of how the outcome will impact occupational therapy clients in all spheres. Applications of Code and Ethics Standards Principles are considered situation-specific, and where a conflict exists, occupational therapy personnel will pursue responsible efforts for resolution. These Principles apply to occupational therapy personnel engaged in any professional role, including elected and volunteer leadership positions.

The specific purposes of the *Occupational Therapy Code of Ethics and Ethics Standards (2010)* are to

1. Identify and describe the principles supported by the occupational therapy profession.
2. Educate the general public and members regarding established principles to which occupational therapy personnel are accountable.
3. Socialize occupational therapy personnel to expected standards of conduct.
4. Assist occupational therapy personnel in recognition and resolution of ethical dilemmas.

The *Occupational Therapy Code of Ethics and Ethics Standards (2010)* define the set of principles that apply to occupational therapy personnel at all levels.

Definitions

- **Recipient of service:** Individuals or groups receiving occupational therapy.
- **Student:** A person who is enrolled in an accredited occupational therapy education program.
- **Research participant:** A prospective participant or one who has agreed to participate in an approved research project.
- **Employee:** A person who is hired by a business (facility or organization) to provide occupational therapy services.
- **Colleague:** A person who provides services in the same or different business (facility or organization) to which a professional relationship exists or may exist.
- **Public:** The community of people at large.

Beneficence

Principle 1. Occupational therapy personnel shall demonstrate a concern for the well-being and safety of the recipients of their services.

Beneficence includes all forms of action intended to benefit other persons. The term *beneficence* connotes acts of mercy, kindness, and charity

(Beauchamp & Childress, 2009). Forms of beneficence typically include altruism, love, and humanity. Beneficence requires taking action by helping others, in other words, by promoting good, by preventing harm, and by removing harm. Examples of beneficence include protecting and defending the rights of others, preventing harm from occurring to others, removing conditions that will cause harm to others, helping persons with disabilities, and rescuing persons in danger (Beauchamp & Childress, 2009).

Occupational therapy personnel shall

A. Respond to requests for occupational therapy services (e.g., a referral) in a timely manner as determined by law, regulation, or policy.

B. Provide appropriate evaluation and a plan of intervention for all recipients of occupational therapy services specific to their needs.

C. Reevaluate and reassess recipients of service in a timely manner to determine if goals are being achieved and whether intervention plans should be revised.

D. Avoid the inappropriate use of outdated or obsolete tests/assessments or data obtained from such tests in making intervention decisions or recommendations.

E. Provide occupational therapy services that are within each practitioner's level of competence and scope of practice (e.g., qualifications, experience, the law).

F. Use, to the extent possible, evaluation, planning, intervention techniques, and therapeutic equipment that are evidence-based and within the recognized scope of occupational therapy practice.

G. Take responsible steps (e.g., continuing education, research, supervision, training) and use careful judgment to ensure their own competence and weigh potential for client harm when generally recognized standards do not exist in emerging technology or areas of practice.

H. Terminate occupational therapy services in collaboration with the service recipient or responsible party when the needs and goals of the recipient have been met or when services no longer produce a measurable change or outcome.

I. Refer to other health care specialists solely on the basis of the needs of the client.

J. Provide occupational therapy education, continuing education, instruction, and training that are within the instructor's subject area of expertise and level of competence.

K. Provide students and employees with information about the Code and Ethics Standards, opportunities to discuss ethical conflicts, and procedures for reporting unresolved ethical conflicts.

L. Ensure that occupational therapy research is conducted in accordance with currently accepted ethical guidelines and standards for the protection of research participants and the dissemination of results.

M. Report to appropriate authorities any acts in practice, education, and research that appear unethical or illegal.

N. Take responsibility for promoting and practicing occupational therapy on the basis of current knowledge and research and for further developing the profession's body of knowledge.

Nonmaleficence

Principle 2. Occupational therapy personnel shall intentionally refrain from actions that cause harm.

Nonmaleficence imparts an obligation to refrain from harming others (Beauchamp & Childress, 2009). The principle of nonmaleficence is grounded in the practitioner's responsibility to refrain from causing harm, inflicting injury, or wronging others. While beneficence requires action to incur benefit, nonmaleficence requires non-action to avoid harm (Beauchamp & Childress, 2009). Nonmaleficence also includes an obligation to not impose risks of harm even if the potential risk is without malicious or harmful intent. This principle often is examined under the context of *due care*. If the standard of due care outweighs the benefit of treatment, then refraining from treatment provision would be ethically indicated (Beauchamp & Childress, 2009).

Occupational therapy personnel shall

A. Avoid inflicting harm or injury to recipients of occupational therapy services, students, research participants, or employees.

B. Make every effort to ensure continuity of services or options for transition to appropriate services to avoid abandoning the service recipient if the current provider is unavailable due to medical or other absence or loss of employment.

C. Avoid relationships that exploit the recipient of services, students, research participants, or employees physically, emotionally, psychologically, financially, socially, or in any other manner that conflicts or interferes with professional judgment and objectivity.

D. Avoid engaging in any sexual relationship or activity, whether consensual or nonconsensual, with any recipient of service, including family or significant other, student, research participant, or employee, while a relationship exists as an occupational therapy practitioner, educator, researcher, supervisor, or employer.

E. Recognize and take appropriate action to remedy personal problems and limitations that might cause harm to recipients of service, colleagues, students, research participants, or others.

F. Avoid any undue influences, such as alcohol or drugs, that may compromise the provision of occupational therapy services, education, or research.

G. Avoid situations in which a practitioner, educator, researcher, or employer is unable to maintain clear professional boundaries or objectivity to ensure the safety and well-being of recipients of service, students, research participants, and employees.

H. Maintain awareness of and adherence to the Code and Ethics Standards when participating in volunteer roles.

I. Avoid compromising client rights or well-being based on arbitrary administrative directives by exercising professional judgment and critical analysis.

J. Avoid exploiting any relationship established as an occupational therapist or occupational therapy assistant to further one's own physical, emotional, financial, political, or business interests at the expense of the best interests of recipients of services, students, research participants, employees, or colleagues.

K. Avoid participating in bartering for services because of the potential for exploitation and conflict of interest unless there are clearly no contraindications or bartering is a culturally appropriate custom.

L. Determine the proportion of risk to benefit for participants in research prior to implementing a study.

Autonomy, Confidentiality

Principle 3. Occupational therapy personnel shall respect the right of the individual to self-determination.

The principle of autonomy and confidentiality expresses the concept that practitioners have a duty to treat the client according to the client's desires, within the bounds of accepted standards of care and to protect the client's confidential information. Often *autonomy* is referred to as the *self-determination* principle. However, respect for autonomy goes beyond acknowledging an individual as a mere agent and also acknowledges a "person's right to hold views, to make choices, and to take actions based on personal values and beliefs" (Beauchamp & Childress, 2009, p. 103). Autonomy has become a prominent principle in health care ethics; the right to make a determination regarding care decisions that directly impact the life of the service recipient should reside with that individual. The principle of autonomy and confidentiality also applies to students in an educational program, to participants in research studies, and to the public who seek information about occupational therapy services.

Occupational therapy personnel shall

A. Establish a collaborative relationship with recipients of service including families, significant others, and caregivers in setting goals and priorities throughout the intervention process. This includes full disclosure of the benefits, risks, and potential outcomes of any intervention; the personnel who will be providing the intervention(s); and/or any reasonable alternatives to the proposed intervention.

B. Obtain consent before administering any occupational therapy service, including evaluation, and ensure that recipients of service (or their legal representatives) are kept informed of the progress in meeting goals specified in the plan of intervention/care. If the service recipient cannot give consent, the practitioner must be sure that consent has been obtained from the person who is legally responsible for that recipient.

C. Respect the recipient of service's right to refuse occupational therapy services temporarily or permanently without negative consequences.

D. Provide students with access to accurate information regarding educational requirements and academic policies and procedures relative to the occupational therapy program/educational institution.

E. Obtain informed consent from participants involved in research activities, and ensure that they understand the benefits, risks, and potential outcomes as a result of their participation as research subjects.

F. Respect research participants' right to withdraw from a research study without consequences.

G. Ensure that confidentiality and the right to privacy are respected and maintained regarding all information obtained about recipients of service, students, research participants, colleagues, or employees. The only exceptions are when a practitioner or staff member believes that an individual is in serious foreseeable or imminent harm. Laws and regulations may require disclosure to appropriate authorities without consent.

H. Maintain the confidentiality of all verbal, written, electronic, augmentative, and non-verbal communications, including compliance with HIPAA regulations.

I. Take appropriate steps to facilitate meaningful communication and comprehension in cases in which the recipient of service, student, or research participant has limited ability to communicate (e.g., aphasia or differences in language, literacy, culture).

J. Make every effort to facilitate open and collaborative dialogue with clients and/or responsible parties to facilitate comprehension of services and their potential risks/benefits.

Social Justice

Principle 4. Occupational therapy personnel shall provide services in a fair and equitable manner.

Social justice, also called *distributive justice,* refers to the fair, equitable, and appropriate distribution of resources. The principle of social justice refers broadly to the distribution of all rights and responsibilities in society (Beauchamp & Childress, 2009). In general, the principle of social justice supports the concept of achieving justice in every aspect of society rather than merely the administration of law. The general idea is that individuals and groups should receive fair treatment and an impartial share of the benefits of society. Occupational therapy personnel have a vested interest in addressing unjust inequities that limit opportunities for participation in society (Braveman & Bass-Haugen, 2009). While opinions differ regarding the most ethical approach to addressing distribution of health care resources and reduction of health disparities, the issue of social justice continues to focus on limiting the impact of social inequality on health outcomes.

Occupational therapy personnel shall

A. Uphold the profession's altruistic responsibilities to help ensure the common good.

B. Take responsibility for educating the public and society about the value of occupational therapy services in promoting health and wellness and reducing the impact of disease and disability.

C. Make every effort to promote activities that benefit the health status of the community.

D. Advocate for just and fair treatment for all patients, clients, employees, and colleagues, and encourage employers and colleagues to abide by the highest standards of social justice and the ethical standards set forth by the occupational therapy profession.

E. Make efforts to advocate for recipients of occupational therapy services to obtain needed services through available means.

F. Provide services that reflect an understanding of how occupational therapy service delivery can be affected by factors such as economic status, age, ethnicity, race, geography, disability, marital status, sexual orientation, gender, gender identity, religion, culture, and political affiliation.

G. Consider offering *pro bono* ("for the good") or reduced-fee occupational therapy services for selected individuals when consistent with guidelines of the employer, third-party payer, and/or government agency.

Procedural Justice

Principle 5. Occupational therapy personnel shall comply with institutional rules, local, state, federal, and international laws and AOTA documents applicable to the profession of occupational therapy.

Procedural justice is concerned with making and implementing decisions according to fair processes that ensure "fair treatment" (Maiese, 2004). Rules must be impartially followed and consistently applied to generate an unbiased decision. The principle of procedural justice is based on the concept that procedures and processes are organized in a fair manner and that policies, regulations, and laws are followed. While *the law* and *ethics* are not synonymous terms, occupational therapy personnel have an ethical responsibility to uphold current reimbursement regulations and state/territorial laws governing the profession. In addition, occupational therapy personnel are ethically bound to be aware of organizational policies and practice guidelines set forth by regulatory agencies established to protect recipients of service, research participants, and the public.

Occupational therapy personnel shall

A. Be familiar with and apply the Code and Ethics Standards to the work setting, and share them with employers, other employees, colleagues, students, and researchers.

B. Be familiar with and seek to understand and abide by institutional rules, and when those rules conflict with ethical practice, take steps to resolve the conflict.

C. Be familiar with revisions in those laws and AOTA policies that apply to the profession of occupational therapy and inform employers, employees, colleagues, students, and researchers of those changes.

D. Be familiar with established policies and procedures for handling concerns about the Code and Ethics Standards, including familiarity with national, state, local, district, and territorial procedures for handling ethics complaints as well as policies and procedures created by AOTA and certification, licensing, and regulatory agencies.

E. Hold appropriate national, state, or other requisite credentials for the occupational therapy services they provide.

F. Take responsibility for maintaining high standards and continuing competence in practice, education, and research by participating in professional development and educational activities to improve and update knowledge and skills.

G. Ensure that all duties assumed by or assigned to other occupational therapy personnel match credentials, qualifications, experience, and scope of practice.

H. Provide appropriate supervision to individuals for whom they have supervisory responsibility in accordance with AOTA official documents and local, state, and federal or national laws, rules, regulations, policies, procedures, standards, and guidelines.

I. Obtain all necessary approvals prior to initiating research activities.

J. Report all gifts and remuneration from individuals, agencies, or companies in accordance with employer policies as well as state and federal guidelines.

K. Use funds for intended purposes, and avoid misappropriation of funds.

L. Take reasonable steps to ensure that employers are aware of occupational therapy's ethical obligations as set forth in this Code and Ethics Standards and of the implications of those obligations for occupational therapy practice, education, and research.

M. Actively work with employers to prevent discrimination and unfair labor practices, and advocate for employees with disabilities to ensure the provision of reasonable accommodations.

N. Actively participate with employers in the formulation of policies and procedures to ensure legal, regulatory, and ethical compliance.

O. Collect fees legally. Fees shall be fair, reasonable, and commensurate with services delivered. Fee schedules must be available and equitable regardless of actual payer reimbursements/contracts.

P. Maintain the ethical principles and standards of the profession when participating in a business arrangement as owner, stockholder, partner, or employee, and refrain from working for or doing business with organizations that engage in illegal or unethical business practices (e.g., fraudulent billing, providing occupational therapy services beyond the scope of occupational therapy practice).

Veracity

Principle 6. Occupational therapy personnel shall provide comprehensive, accurate, and objective information when representing the profession.

Veracity is based on the virtues of truthfulness, candor, and honesty. The principle of *veracity* in health care refers to comprehensive, accurate, and objective transmission of information and includes fostering the client's understanding of such information (Beauchamp & Childress, 2009). Veracity is based on respect owed to others. In communicating with others, occupational therapy personnel implicitly promise to speak truthfully and not deceive the listener. By entering into a relationship in care or research, the recipient of service or research participant enters into a contract that includes a right to truthful information (Beauchamp & Childress, 2009). In addition, transmission of information is incomplete without also ensuring that the recipient or participant

understands the information provided. Concepts of veracity must be carefully balanced with other potentially competing ethical principles, cultural beliefs, and organizational policies. Veracity ultimately is valued as a means to establish trust and strengthen professional relationships. Therefore, adherence to the Principle also requires thoughtful analysis of how full disclosure of information may impact outcomes.

Occupational therapy personnel shall

A. Represent the credentials, qualifications, education, experience, training, roles, duties, competence, views, contributions, and findings accurately in all forms of communication about recipients of service, students, employees, research participants, and colleagues.

B. Refrain from using or participating in the use of any form of communication that contains false, fraudulent, deceptive, misleading, or unfair statements or claims.

C. Record and report in an accurate and timely manner, and in accordance with applicable regulations, all information related to professional activities.

D. Ensure that documentation for reimbursement purposes is done in accordance with applicable laws, guidelines, and regulations.

E. Accept responsibility for any action that reduces the public's trust in occupational therapy.

F. Ensure that all marketing and advertising are truthful, accurate, and carefully presented to avoid misleading recipients of service, students, research participants, or the public.

G. Describe the type and duration of occupational therapy services accurately in professional contracts, including the duties and responsibilities of all involved parties.

H. Be honest, fair, accurate, respectful, and timely in gathering and reporting fact-based information regarding employee job performance and student performance.

I. Give credit and recognition when using the work of others in written, oral, or electronic media.

J. Not plagiarize the work of others.

Fidelity

Principle 7. Occupational therapy personnel shall treat colleagues and other professionals with respect, fairness, discretion, and integrity.

The principle of fidelity comes from the Latin root *fidelis* meaning loyal. *Fidelity* refers to being faithful, which includes obligations of loyalty and the keeping of promises and commitments (Veatch & Flack, 1997). In the health professions, fidelity refers to maintaining good-faith relationships between various service providers and recipients. While respecting fidelity requires occupational therapy personnel to meet the client's reasonable expectations (Purtilo, 2005), Principle 7 specifically addresses fidelity as it relates to maintaining collegial and organizational relationships. Professional relationships are greatly influenced by the complexity of the environment in which occupational therapy personnel work. Practitioners, educators, and researchers alike must consistently balance their duties to service recipients, students, research participants, and other professionals as well as to organizations that may influence decision making and professional practice.

Occupational therapy personnel shall

A. Respect the traditions, practices, competencies, and responsibilities of their own and other professions, as well as those of the institutions and agencies that constitute the working environment.

B. Preserve, respect, and safeguard private information about employees, colleagues, and students unless otherwise mandated by national, state, or local laws or permission to disclose is given by the individual.

C. Take adequate measures to discourage, prevent, expose, and correct any breaches of the Code and Ethics Standards, and report any breaches of the former to the appropriate authorities.

D. Attempt to resolve perceived institutional violations of the Code and Ethics Standards by utilizing internal resources first.

E. Avoid conflicts of interest or conflicts of commitment in employment, volunteer roles, or research.

F. Avoid using one's position (employee or volunteer) or knowledge gained from that position in such a manner that gives rise to real or perceived conflict of interest among the person, the employer, other Association members, and/or other organizations.

G. Use conflict resolution and/or alternative dispute resolution resources to resolve organizational and interpersonal conflicts.

H. Be diligent stewards of human, financial, and material resources of their employers, and refrain from exploiting these resources for personal gain.

REFERENCES

American Occupational Therapy Association. (1993). Core values and attitudes of occupational therapy practice. *American Journal of Occupational Therapy, 47,* 1085–1086.

American Occupational Therapy Association. (2004). Policy 5.3.1: Definition of occupational therapy practice for state regulation. *American Journal of Occupational Therapy, 58,* 694–695.

American Occupational Therapy Association. (2005). Occupational therapy code of ethics (2005). *American Journal of Occupational Therapy, 59,* 639–642.

American Occupational Therapy Association. (2006). Guidelines to the occupational therapy code of ethics. *American Journal of Occupational Therapy, 60,* 652–658.

Beauchamp, T. L., & Childress, J. F. (2009). *Principles of biomedical ethics* (6th ed.). New York: Oxford University Press.

Braveman, B., & Bass-Haugen, J. D. (2009). Social justice and health disparities: An evolving discourse in occupational therapy research and intervention. *American Journal of Occupational Therapy, 63,* 7–12.

Maiese, M. (2004). *Procedural justice.* Retrieved July 29, 2009, from http://www.beyondintractability. org/essay/procedural_justice/

Purtilo, R. (2005). *Ethical dimensions in the health professions* (4th ed.). Philadelphia: Elsevier/Saunders.

Veatch, R. M., & Flack, H. E. (1997). *Case studies in allied health ethics.* Upper Saddle River, NJ: Prentice Hall.

Authors

Ethics Commission (EC):

Kathlyn Reed, PhD, OTR, FAOTA, MLIS,
   Chairperson

Barbara Hemphill, DMin, OTR, FAOTA,
   FMOTA, *Chair-Elect*

Ann Moodey Ashe, MHS, OTR/L

Lea C. Brandt, OTD, MA, OTR/L

Joanne Estes, MS, OTR/L

Loretta Jean Foster, MS, COTA/L

Donna F. Homenko, RDH, PhD

Craig R. Jackson, JD, MSW

Deborah Yarett Slater, MS, OT/L, FAOTA,
   AOTA Staff Liaison

Adopted by the Representative Assembly 2010CApr17.

Note. This document replaces the following rescinded Ethics documents 2010CApril18: the *Occupational Therapy Code of Ethics (2005) (American Journal of Occupational Therapy, 59, 639–642)*; the *Guidelines to the Occupational Therapy Code of Ethics (American Journal of Occupational Therapy, 60, 652–658)*; and the *Core Values and Attitudes of Occupational Therapy Practice (American Journal of Occupational Therapy, 47, 1085–1086)*.

Copyright © 2010 by the American Occupational Therapy Association.

Citation. American Occupational Therapy Association. (2010). Occupational therapy code of ethics and ethics standards (2010). *American Journal of Occupational Therapy,* 64(Suppl.), S17–26. doi: 10.5014/ajot.2010.64S17

Appendix B
Enforcement Procedures for the *Occupational Therapy Code of Ethics and Ethics Standards* (2010)

1. INTRODUCTION

The principal purposes of the *Occupational Therapy Code of Ethics and Ethics Standards* (hereinafter referred to as the "Code and Ethics Standards") are to help protect the public and to reinforce its confidence in the occupational therapy profession rather than to resolve private business, legal, or other disputes for which there are other more appropriate forums for resolution. The Code and Ethics Standards also is an aspirational document to guide occupational therapists, occupational therapy assistants, and occupational therapy students toward appropriate professional conduct in all aspects of their diverse roles. It applies to any conduct that may affect the performance of occupational therapy as well as to behavior that an individual may do in another capacity that reflects negatively on the reputation of occupational therapy.

The *Enforcement Procedures for the Occupational Therapy Code of Ethics and Ethics Standards* (formerly the *Enforcement Procedures for the Occupational Therapy Code of Ethics*) have undergone a series of revisions by the American Occupational Therapy Association's (AOTA's) Ethics Commission (hereinafter referred to as the *EC*) since their initial adoption. The most recent update was in 2009. This public document articulates the procedures that are followed by the EC as it carries out its duties to enforce the Code and Ethics Standards. A major goal of these Enforcement Procedures is to ensure objectivity and fundamental fairness to all individuals who may be parties in an ethics complaint.

The Enforcement Procedures are used to help ensure compliance with the Code and Ethics Standards, which represent the values and principles that members of the profession have identified as important. Acceptance of AOTA membership commits individuals to adherence to the Code and Ethics Standards and cooperation with its Enforcement Procedures. These are established and maintained by the EC: The EC and AOTA's Ethics Office make the Enforcement Procedures public and available to members of the profession, state regulatory boards, consumers, and others for their use.

The EC urges particular attention to the following issues:

1.1. Professional Responsibility, Other Processes—All occupational therapy personnel have an obligation to maintain the Code and Ethics Standards of their profession and to promote and support these Standards among their colleagues. Each AOTA member must be alert to practices that undermine these Standards and is obligated to take action that is appropriate in the circumstances. At the same time, members must carefully weigh their judgments as to potentially unethical practice to ensure that they are based on objective evaluation and not on personal bias or prejudice, inadequate information, or simply differences of professional viewpoint. It is recognized that individual occupational therapy personnel may not have the authority or ability to address or correct all situations of concern. Whenever feasible and appropriate, members should first pursue other corrective steps within the relevant institution or setting and discuss ethical concerns directly with the potential Respondent before resorting to AOTA's ethics complaint process.

1.2. Jurisdiction—The Code and Ethics Standards apply to persons who are or were AOTA members at the time of the conduct in question. Later nonrenewal or relinquishment of membership does not affect Association jurisdiction. The Enforcement Procedures that shall be utilized in any complaint shall be those in effect at the time the complaint is initiated.

1.3. Disciplinary Actions/Sanctions (Pursuing a Complaint)—If the EC determines that unethical conduct has occurred, it may impose sanctions, including reprimand, censure, probation (with terms), suspension, or permanent revocation of AOTA membership. In all cases, except those involving only reprimand, the Association will report the conclusions and sanctions in its official publications and also will communicate to any appropriate persons or entities. The potential sanctions are defined as follows:

1.3.1. Reprimand—A formal expression of disapproval of conduct communicated privately by letter from the EC Chairperson that is nondisclosable and noncommunicative to other bodies (e.g., state regulatory boards [SRBs], National Board for Certification in Occupational Therapy® [NBCOT®]).

1.3.2. Censure—A formal expression of disapproval that is public.

1.3.3. Probation of Membership Subject to Terms—Failure to meet terms will subject an AOTA member to any of the disciplinary actions or sanctions.

1.3.4. Suspension—Removal of AOTA membership for a specified period of time.

1.3.5. Revocation—Permanent denial of AOTA membership.

1.3.5.1. If an individual is on either the Roster of Fellows (ROF) or the Roster of Honor (ROH), the EC Chairperson (via the EC Staff Liaison) shall notify the Recognitions Committee Chairperson (and AOTA Executive Director) of their membership revocation. That individual shall have their name removed from either the ROF or the ROH and no longer has the right to use the designated credential of FAOTA or ROH.

1.4. Educative Letters—If the EC determines that the alleged conduct may or may not be a true breach of the Code and Ethics Standards but in any event does not warrant any of the sanctions set forth in Section 1.3 or is not completely in keeping with the aspirational nature of the Code and Ethics Standards or within the prevailing standards of practice or good professionalism, the EC may send a letter to educate the Respondent about relevant standards of practice and/or appropriate professional behavior. In addition, a different educative letter, if appropriate, may be sent to the Complainant.

1.5. Advisory Opinions—The EC may issue general advisory opinions on ethical issues to inform and educate the AOTA membership. These opinions shall be publicized to the membership and are available in the *Reference Guide to the Occupational Therapy Code of Ethics and Ethics Standards* as well as in other locations.

1.6. Rules of Evidence—The EC proceedings shall be conducted in accordance with fundamental fairness. However, formal rules of evidence that are used in legal proceedings do not apply to these Enforcement Procedures. The Disciplinary Council (see Section 5) and the Appeal Panel (see Section 6) can consider any evidence that they deem appropriate and pertinent.

1.7. Confidentiality and Disclosure—The EC develops and adheres to strict rules of confidentiality in every aspect of its work. This requires that participants in the process refrain from any communication relating to the existence and subject matter of the complaint other than with those directly involved in the enforcement process. Maintaining confidentiality throughout the investigation and enforcement process of a formal ethics complaint is essential in order to ensure fairness to all parties involved. These rules of confidentiality pertain not only to the EC but also apply to others involved in the complaint process. Beginning with the EC Staff Liaison and support staff, strict rules of confidentiality are followed. These same rules of confidentiality apply to Complainants, Respondents and their attorneys, and witnesses involved with the EC's investigatory process. Due diligence must be exercised by everyone involved in the investigation to avoid compromising the confidential nature of the process. Any AOTA member who breaches these rules of confidentiality may become subject to an ethics complaint/investigatory process himself or herself. Non–AOTA members may lodge an ethics complaint against an Association member, and these individuals are still expected to adhere to the Association's confidentiality rules. The Association reserves the right to take appropriate action against non–AOTA members who violate confidentiality rules, including notification of their appropriate licensure boards.

1.7.1. Disclosure—When the EC investigates a complaint, it may request information from a variety of sources. The process of obtaining additional information is carefully executed in order to maintain confidentiality. The EC may request information from a variety of sources, including state licensing agencies, academic councils, courts, employers, and other persons and entities. It is within the EC's purview to determine what disclosures are appropriate for particular parties in order to effectively implement its investigatory obligations. Public sanctions by the EC, Disciplinary Council, or Appeal Panel will be publicized as provided in these Enforcement Procedures. Normally, the EC does not disclose information or documentation reviewed in the course of an investigation unless the EC determines that disclosure is necessary to obtain additional, relevant evidence or to administer the ethics process or is legally required.

Individuals who file a complaint (i.e., *Complainant*) and those who are the subject of one (i.e., *Respondent*) must not disclose to anyone outside of those involved in the complaint process their role in an ethics complaint. Disclosing this information in and of itself may jeopardize the ethics process and violate the rules of fundamental fairness by which all parties are protected. Disclosure of information related to any case under investigation by the EC is prohibited and, if done, will lead to repercussions as outlined in these Enforcement Procedures (see Section 2.2.3).

2. COMPLAINTS

2.1. Interested Party Complaints

2.1.1. Complaints stating an alleged violation of the Code and Ethics Standards may originate from any individual, group, or entity within or outside AOTA. All complaints must be in writing, signed by the Complainant(s), and submitted to the EC Chairperson at the address of the AOTA Headquarters. Complainants must complete the Formal Statement of Complaint Form at the end of this document. All complaints shall identify the person against whom the complaint is directed (the Respondent), the ethical principles that the Complainant believes have been violated, and the key facts and date(s) of the alleged ethical violations. If lawfully available, supporting documentation should be attached.

2.1.2. Within 90 days of receipt of a complaint, the EC shall make a preliminary assessment of the complaint and decide whether it presents sufficient questions as to a potential ethics violation that an investigation is warranted in accordance with Section 3. Commencing an investigation does not imply a conclusion that an ethical violation has in fact occurred or any judgment as to the ultimate sanction, if any, that may be appropriate. In the event the EC determines at the completion of an investigation that the complaint does rise to the level of an ethical violation, the EC may initiate a charge as set forth in Section 4 below. In the event the EC determines that the complaint does not rise to the level of an ethical violation, the EC may direct the parties to utilize *Roberts Rules* and/or other conflict resolution resources via an educative letter. This applies to all complaints including those involving AOTA elected/volunteer leadership related to their official roles.

2.2. Complaints Initiated by the EC

2.2.1. The EC itself may initiate a complaint (a *sua sponte complaint*) when it receives information from a governmental body, certification or similar body, public media, or other source indicating that a person subject to its jurisdiction may have committed acts that violate the Code and Ethics Standards. The Association will ordinarily act promptly after learning of the basis of a sua sponte complaint, but there is no specified time limit.

If the EC passes a motion to initiate a sua sponte complaint, the AOTA Staff Liaison to the EC will complete the Formal Statement of Complaint Form (at the end of this document) and will describe the nature of the factual allegations that led to the complaint and the manner in which the EC learned of the matter. The Complaint Form will be signed by the EC Chairperson on behalf of the EC. The form will be filed with the case material in the Association's Ethics Office.

2.2.2. De Jure Complaints—Where the source of a sua sponte complaint is the findings and conclusions of another official body, the EC classifies such sua sponte complaints as *de jure*. The procedure in such cases is addressed in Section 4.2.

2.2.3. The EC shall have the jurisdiction to investigate, charge, or sanction any matter or person for violations based on information learned in the course of investigating a complaint under Section 2.2.2.

2.3. Continuation of Complaint Process—If an AOTA member relinquishes membership, fails to

renew membership, or fails to cooperate with the ethics investigation, the EC shall nevertheless continue to process the complaint, noting in its report the circumstances of the Respondent's action. Such actions shall not deprive the EC of jurisdiction. All correspondence related to the EC complaint process is in writing and sent by certified mail, return receipt requested. In the event that any written correspondence does not have delivery confirmation, the AOTA Ethics Office will make an attempt to search for an alternate address or make a second attempt to send to the original address. If Respondent does not claim correspondence after two attempts to deliver, delivery cannot be confirmed, or correspondence is returned to the Association as undeliverable, the EC shall consider that it has made good-faith effort and shall proceed with the ethics enforcement process.

3. EC REVIEW AND INVESTIGATIONS

3.1. Initial Action—The purpose of the preliminary review is to decide whether or not the information submitted with the complaint warrants opening the case. If in its preliminary review of the complaint the EC determines that an investigation is not warranted, the Complainant will be so notified.

3.2. Dismissal of Complaints—The EC may at any time dismiss a complaint for any of the following reasons:

3.2.1. Lack of Jurisdiction—The EC determines that it has no jurisdiction over the Respondent (e.g., a complaint against a person who is or was not an AOTA member at the time of the alleged incident or who has never been a member).

3.2.2. Absolute Time Limit/Not Timely Filed—The EC determines that the violation of the Code and Ethics Standards is alleged to have occurred more than 7 years prior to the filing of the complaint.

3.2.3. Subject to Jurisdiction of Another Authority—The EC determines that the complaint is based on matters that are within the authority of and are more properly dealt with by another governmental or nongovernmental body, such as an SRB, NBCOT, an Association component other than the EC, an employer, or a court (e.g., accusing a superior of sexual harassment at work, accusing someone of anticompetitive practices subject to the antitrust laws).

3.2.4. No Ethics Violation—The EC finds that the complaint, even if proven, does not state a basis for action under the Code and Ethics Standards (e.g., simply accusing someone of being unpleasant or rude on an occasion).

3.2.5. Insufficient Evidence—The EC determines that there clearly would not be sufficient factual evidence to support a finding of an ethics violation.

3.2.6. Corrected Violation—The EC determines that any violation it might find already has been or is being corrected and that this is an adequate result in the given case.

3.2.7. Other Good Cause.

3.3. Investigator (Avoidance of Conflict of Interest)—The investigator chosen shall not have a conflict of interest (i.e., shall never have had a substantial professional, personal, financial, business, or volunteer relationship with either the Complainant or the Respondent). In the event that the EC Staff Liaison has such a conflict, the EC Chairperson shall appoint an alternate investigator who has no conflict of interest.

3.4. Investigation—If an investigation is deemed warranted, the EC Chairperson shall do the following within thirty (30) days: Appoint the EC Staff Liaison at the AOTA Headquarters to investigate the complaint and notify the Respondent (by certified, return-receipt mail) that a complaint has been received and an investigation is being conducted. A copy of the complaint and supporting documentation shall be enclosed with this notification. The Complainant also will receive notification by certified, return-receipt mail that the complaint is being investigated.

3.4.1. Ordinarily, the Investigator will send questions formulated by the EC to be answered by the Complainant and/or the Respondent.

3.4.2. The Complainant shall be given thirty (30) days from receipt of the questions to respond in writing to the investigator.

3.4.3. The Respondent shall be given thirty (30) days from receipt of the questions to respond in writing to the Investigator.

3.4.4. The EC ordinarily will notify the Complainant of any substantive new evidence adverse to the Complainant's initial complaint that is discovered in the course of the ethics investigation and allow the Complainant to respond to such adverse evidence. In such cases, the Complainant will be given a copy of such evidence and will have fourteen (14) days in which to submit a written response. If the new evidence clearly shows that there has been no ethics violation, the EC may terminate the proceeding. In addition, if the investigation includes questions for both the Respondent and the Complainant, the evidence submitted by each party in response to the investigatory questions shall be provided to the Respondent and available to the Complainant on request. The EC may request reasonable payment for copying expenses depending on the volume of material to be sent.

3.4.5. The Investigator, in consultation with the EC, may obtain evidence directly from third parties without permission from the Complainant or Respondent.

3.5. Investigation Timeline—The investigation will be completed within ninety (90) days after receipt of notification by the Respondent or his or her designee that an investigation is being conducted, unless the EC determines that special circumstances warrant additional time for the investigation. All timelines noted here can be extended for good cause at the discretion of the EC, including the EC's schedule and additional requests of the Respondent. The Respondent and the Complainant shall be notified in writing if a delay occurs or if the investigational process requires more time.

3.6. Case Files—The investigative files shall include the complaint and any documentation on which the EC relied in initiating the investigation.

3.7. Cooperation by Member—Every AOTA member has a duty to cooperate reasonably with enforcement processes for the Code and Ethics Standards. Failure of the Respondent to participate and/or cooperate with the investigative process of the EC shall not prevent continuation of the ethics process, and this behavior itself may constitute a violation of the Code and Ethics Standards.

3.8. Referral of Complaint—The EC may at any time refer a matter to NBCOT, the SRB, or other recognized authorities for appropriate action. Despite such referral to an appropriate authority, the EC shall retain jurisdiction. EC action may be stayed for a reasonable period pending notification of a decision by that authority, at the discretion of the EC (and such delays will extend the time periods under these Procedures). A stay in conducting an investigation shall not constitute a waiver by the EC of jurisdiction over the matters. The EC shall provide written notice by mail (requiring signature and proof of date of receipt) to the Respondent and the Complainant of any such stay of action.

4. EC REVIEW AND DECISION

4.1. Regular Complaint Process

4.1.1. Charges—The EC shall review the relevant materials resulting from the investigation and shall render a decision on whether a charge by the EC is warranted within 90 days of receipt. The EC may, in the conduct of its review, take whatever further investigatory actions it deems necessary. If the EC determines that an ethics complaint warrants a charge, the EC shall proceed with a disciplinary proceeding by promptly sending a notice of the charge(s) to the Respondent and Complainant by mail with signature and proof of date received. The notice of the charge(s) shall describe the alleged conduct that, if proven in accordance with these Enforcement Procedures, would constitute a violation of the Code and Ethics Standards. The notice of charge(s) shall describe the conduct in sufficient detail to inform the Respondent of the nature of the unethical be-

havior that is alleged. The EC may indicate in the notice its preliminary view (absent contrary facts or mitigating circumstances) as to what sanction would be warranted if the violation is proven in accordance with these Enforcement Procedures.

4.1.2. Respondent's Response—Within 30 days of notification of the EC's decision to charge, and proposed sanction, if any, the Respondent shall

> **4.1.2.1.** Advise the EC Chairperson in writing that he or she accepts the EC's charge of an ethics violation and the proposed sanction and waives any right to a Disciplinary Council hearing, or

> **4.1.2.2.** Advise the EC Chairperson in writing that he or she accepts the EC's charge of an ethics violation but believes the sanction is not justified or should be reduced with a rationale to support a reduced sanction.

> **4.1.2.3.** Advise the EC Chairperson in writing that he or she contests the EC's charge and the proposed sanction and requests a hearing before the Disciplinary Council.

Failure of the Respondent to take one of these actions within the time specified will be deemed to constitute acceptance of the charge and proposed sanction. If the Respondent requests a Disciplinary Council hearing, it will be scheduled. If the Respondent does not request a Disciplinary Council hearing but accepts the decision, the EC will notify all relevant parties and implement the sanction.

4.2. De Jure Complaint Process

4.2.1. The EC Staff Liaison will present to the EC any findings from external sources (as described above) that come to his or her attention and that may warrant sua sponte complaints pertaining to individuals who are or were AOTA members at the time of the alleged incident.

4.2.2. Because de jure complaints are based on the findings of fact or conclusions of another official body, the EC will decide whether or not to act based on such findings or conclusions and will not ordinarily initiate another investigation, absent clear and convincing evidence that such findings and conclusions were erroneous or not supported by substantial evidence. Based on the information presented by the EC Staff Liaison, the EC will determine whether the findings of the public body also are sufficient to demonstrate an egregious violation of the Code and Ethics Standards and therefore warrant an ethics charge.

4.2.3. If the EC decides that a formal charge is warranted, the EC Chairperson will notify the Respondent in writing of the formal charge and the proposed education and/or disciplinary action. In response to the de jure sua sponte charge by the EC, the Respondent may

> **4.2.3.1.** Accept the decision of the EC (as to both the ethics violation and the sanction) based solely on the findings of fact and conclusions of the EC or the public body, or
>
> **4.2.3.2.** Accept the charge that the Respondent committed unethical conduct but within thirty (30) days submit to the EC a statement setting forth the reasons why any sanction should not be imposed or reasons why the sanction should be mitigated or reduced.
>
> **4.2.3.3.** Within thirty (30) days, present information showing the findings of fact of the official body relied on by the EC to initiate the charge are clearly erroneous and request reconsideration by the EC. The EC may have the option of opening an investigation or modifying the sanction in the event they find clear and convincing evidence that the findings and the conclusions of the other body are erroneous.

4.2.4. In cases of de jure complaints, a Disciplinary Council hearing can later be requested (pursuant to Section 5 below) only if the Respondent has first exercised Options 4.2.3.2 or 4.2.3.3.

4.2.5. Respondents in an ethics case may utilize Options 4.2.3.2 or 4.2.3.3 (reconsideration) once in responding to the EC. Following one review of the additional information submitted by the Respondent, if the EC reaffirms its original sanction, the Respondent has the option of accepting the violation and proposed sanction or requesting a Disciplinary Council hearing. Repeated requests for reconsideration will not be accepted by the EC.

5. DISCIPLINARY COUNCIL

5.1. Purpose—The purpose of the Disciplinary Council (hereinafter to be known as *the Council*) hearing is to provide the Respondent an opportunity to present evidence and witnesses to answer and refute the charge and/or the proposed sanction and to permit the EC Chairperson or designee to present evidence and witnesses in support of his or her charge. The Council shall consider the matters alleged in the complaint; the matters raised in defense as well as other relevant facts, ethical principles, and federal or state law, if applicable. The Council may question the parties concerned and determine ethical issues arising from the factual matters in the case even if those specific ethical issues were not raised by the Complainant. The Council also may choose to apply Principles or other language from the AOTA Code and Ethics Standards not originally identified by the EC. The Council may affirm the decision of the EC or reverse or modify it if it finds that the decision was clearly erroneous or a material departure from its written procedure.

5.2. Parties—The parties to a Council Hearing are the Respondent and the EC Chairperson.

5.3. Criteria and Process for Selection of Council Chairperson

> **5.3.1. Criteria**
>
> > **5.3.1.1.** Must have experience in analyzing/reviewing cases.
> >
> > **5.3.1.2.** May be selected from the pool of candidates for the Council or a former EC member who has been off the EC for at least three (3) years.

5.3.1.3. The EC Chairperson shall not serve as the Council Chairperson.

5.3.2. Process

5.3.2.1. The Representative Assembly (RA) Speaker (in consultation with EC Staff Liaison) will select the Council Chairperson.

5.3.2.2. If the RA Speaker needs to be recused from this duty, the RA Vice Speaker will select the Council Chairperson.

5.4. Criteria and Process for Selection of Council Members

5.4.1. Criteria

5.4.1.1. AOTA Administrative SOP guidelines in Policy 2.6 shall be considered in the selection of qualified potential candidates for the Council, which shall be composed of qualified individuals and AOTA members drawn from a pool of candidates who meet the criteria outlined below. In the interest of financial prudence and efficiency, every effort will be made to assemble Council members who meet the criteria below but also who are within geographic proximity to the AOTA Headquarters.

5.4.1.2. Members ideally will have some knowledge or experience in the areas of activity that are at issue in the case. They also will have experience in disciplinary hearings and/or general knowledge about ethics as demonstrated by education, presentations, and/or publications.

5.4.1.3. No conflict of interest may exist with either the Complainant or the Respondent (refer to Association Policy 1.22—Conflict of Interest for guidance).

5.4.1.4. No individual may serve on the Council who is currently a member of the EC or the AOTA Board of Directors.

5.4.1.5. No individual may serve on the Council who has previously been the subject of an ethics complaint that resulted in a specific EC disciplinary action.

5.4.1.6. The public member on the Council shall have knowledge of the profession and ethical issues.

5.4.1.7. The public member shall not be an occupational therapy practitioner, educator, or researcher.

5.4.2. Process

5.4.2.1. Potential candidates for the Council pool will be recruited through public postings in AOTA publications and via the electronic forums. Association leadership will be encouraged to recruit qualified candidates. Potential members of the Council shall be interviewed to ascertain the following:

> a. Willingness to serve on the Council and availability for a period of three (3) years and
>
> b. Qualifications per criteria outlined in Section 5.3.1.

5.4.2.2. The AOTA President and EC Staff Liaison will maintain a pool of no less than six (6) and no more than twelve (12) qualified individuals.

5.4.2.3. The President, with input from the EC Staff Liaison, will select from the pool the members of each Council within thirty (30) days of notification by a Respondent that a Council is being requested.

5.4.2.4. Each Council shall be composed of three (3) AOTA members in good standing and a public member.

5.4.2.5. The EC Staff Liaison will remove anyone with a potential conflict of interest in a particular case from the potential Council pool.

5.5. Notification of Parties (EC Chairperson, Complainant, Respondent, Council Members)

5.5.1. The EC Staff Liaison shall schedule a hearing date in coordination with the Council Chairperson.

5.5.2. The Council (via the EC Staff Liaison) shall notify all parties at least forty-five

(45) days prior to the hearing of the date, time, and place.

5.5.3. Case material will be sent to all parties and the Council members by national delivery service or mail with signature required and proof of date received with return receipt.

5.6. Hearing Witnesses, Materials, and Evidence

5.6.1. Within thirty (30) days of notification of the hearing, the Respondent shall submit to the Council a written response to the charges, including a detailed statement as to the reasons that he or she is appealing the decision and a list of potential witnesses (if any) with a statement indicating the subject matter they will be addressing.

5.6.2. The Complainant before the Council also will submit a list of potential witnesses (if any) to the Council with a statement indicating the subject matter they will be addressing. Only under limited circumstances may the Council consider additional material evidence from the Respondent or the Complainant not presented or available prior to the issuance of their proposed sanction. Such new or additional evidence may be considered by the Council if the Council is satisfied that the Respondent or the Complainant has demonstrated the new evidence was previously unavailable and provided it is submitted to all parties in writing no later than fifteen (15) days prior to the hearing.

5.6.3. The Council Chairperson may permit testimony by conference call (at no expense to the participant), limit participation of witnesses in order to curtail repetitive testimony, or prescribe other reasonable arrangements or limitations. The Respondent may elect to appear (at Respondent's own expense) and present testimony. If alternative technology options are available for the hearing, the Respondent, Council members, and EC Chairperson shall be so informed when the hearing arrangements are sent.

5.7. Counsel—The Respondent may be represented by legal counsel at his or her own expense. AOTA's Legal Counsel shall advise and represent the Association at the hearing. AOTA's Legal Counsel also may advise the Council regarding procedural matters to ensure fairness to all parties. All parties and the AOTA Legal Counsel (at the request of the EC or the Council) shall have the opportunity to question witnesses.

5.8. Hearing

5.8.1. The Council hearing shall be recorded by a professional transcription service or telephone recording transcribed for Council members and shall be limited to two (2) hours.

5.8.2. The Council Chairperson will conduct the hearing and does not vote except in the case of a tie.

5.8.3. Each person present shall be identified for the record, and the Council Chairperson will describe the procedures for the Council hearing. An oral affirmation of truthfulness will be requested from each participant who gives factual testimony in the Council hearing.

5.8.4. The Council Chairperson shall allow for questions.

5.8.5. The EC Chairperson shall present the ethics charge, a summary of the evidence resulting from the investigation, and the EC proposed disciplinary action against the Respondent.

5.8.6. The Respondent may present a defense to the charge(s) after the EC presents its case.

5.8.7. Each party and/or his or her legal representative shall have the opportunity to call witnesses to present testimony and to question any witnesses including the EC Chairperson or his or her designee. The Council Chairperson shall be entitled to provide reasonable limits on the extent of any witnesses' testimony or any questioning.

5.8.8. The Council Chairperson may recess the hearing at any time.

5.8.9. The Council Chairperson shall call for final statements from each party before concluding the hearing.

5.8.10. Decisions of the Council will be by majority vote.

5.9. Disciplinary Council Decision

5.9.1. An official copy of the transcript shall be sent to each Council member, the EC Chairperson, the AOTA Legal Counsel, the EC Staff Liaison, and the Respondent and his or her counsel as soon as it is available from the transcription company.

5.9.2. The Council Chairperson shall work with the EC Staff Liaison and the AOTA Legal Counsel in preparing the text of the final decision.

5.9.3. The Council shall issue a decision in writing to the AOTA Executive Director within thirty (30) days of receiving the written transcription of the hearing (unless special circumstances warrant additional time). The Council decision shall be based on the record and evidence presented and may affirm, modify, or reverse the decision of the EC, including increasing or decreasing the level of sanction or determining that no disciplinary action is warranted.

5.10. Action, Notification, and Timeline Adjustments

5.10.1. A copy of the Council's official decision and appeal process (Section 6) is sent to the Respondent, the EC Chairperson, and other appropriate parties within fifteen (15) business days via mail (with signature and proof of date received) after notification of the AOTA Executive Director.

5.10.2. The time limits specified in the *Enforcement Procedures for the Occupational Therapy Code of Ethics and Ethics Standards* may be extended by mutual consent of the Respondent, Complainant, and Council Chairperson for good cause by the Chairperson.

5.10.3. Other features of the preceding Enforcement Procedures may be adjusted in particular cases in light of extraordinary circumstances, consistent with fundamental fairness.

5.11. Appeal—Within thirty (30) days after notification of the Council's decision, a Respondent upon whom a sanction was imposed may appeal the decision as provided in Section 6. Within thirty (30) days after notification of the Council's decision, the EC also may appeal the decision as provided in Section 6. If no appeal is filed within that time, the AOTA Executive Director or EC Staff Liaison shall publish the decision in accordance with these procedures and make any other notifications deemed necessary.

6. APPEAL PROCESS

6.1. Appeals—Either the EC or the Respondent may appeal. Appeals shall be written, signed by the appealing party, and sent by certified mail to the AOTA Executive Director in care of the AOTA Ethics Office. The grounds for the appeal shall be fully explained in this document. When an appeal is requested, the other party will be notified.

6.2. Grounds for Appeal—Appeals shall generally address only the issues, procedures, or sanctions that are part of the record before the Council. However, in the interest of fairness, the Appeal Panel may consider newly available evidence relating to the original charge only under extraordinary circumstances.

6.3. Composition and Leadership of Appeal Panel—The AOTA Vice President, Secretary, and Treasurer shall constitute the Appeal Panel. In the event of vacancies in these positions or the existence of a conflict of interest, the Vice President shall appoint replacements drawn from among the other AOTA Board of Directors members. If the entire Board has a conflict of interest (e.g., the Complainant or Respondent is or was recently a member of the Board), the Board Appeal process shall be followed. The President shall not serve on the Appeal Panel. No individual may serve on the Council who has previously been the subject of an ethics complaint that resulted in a specific EC disciplinary action.

The Appeal Panel Chairperson will be selected by its members from among themselves.

6.4. Appeal Process—The AOTA Executive Director shall forward any letter of appeal to the Appeal Panel within fifteen (15) business days of receipt. Within thirty (30) days after the Appeal Panel receives the appeal, the Panel shall determine whether a hearing is warranted. If the Panel decides that a hearing is warranted, timely notice for such hearing shall be given to the parties. Participants at the hearing shall be limited to the Respondent and legal counsel (if so desired), the EC Chairperson, the Council Chairperson, the AOTA Legal Counsel, or others approved in advance by the Appeal Panel as necessary to the proceedings.

6.5. Decision

    6.5.1. The Appeal Panel shall have the power to (a) affirm the decision; or (b) modify the decision; or (c) reverse or remand to the EC, but only if there were procedural errors materially prejudicial to the outcome of the proceeding or if the Council decision was against the clear weight of the evidence.

    6.5.2. Within thirty (30) days after receipt of the appeal if no hearing was granted, or within thirty (30) days after receipt of the transcript if a hearing was held, the Appeal Panel shall notify the AOTA Executive Director of its decision. The AOTA Executive Director shall promptly notify the Respondent, the original Complainant, appropriate Association bodies, and any other parties deemed appropriate (e.g., SRB, NBCOT). For Association purposes, the decision of the Appeal Panel shall be final.

7. NOTIFICATIONS

All notifications referred to in these Enforcement Procedures shall be in writing and shall be delivered by national delivery service or mail with signature and proof of date of receipt required.

8. RECORDS AND REPORTS

At the completion of the enforcement process, the written records and reports that state the initial basis for the complaint, material evidence, and the disposition of the complaint shall be retained in the AOTA Ethics Office for a period of five (5) years.

9. PUBLICATION

Final decisions will be publicized only after any Appeal Panel process has been completed.

10. MODIFICATION

AOTA reserves the right to (a) modify the time periods, procedures, or application of these Enforcement Procedures for good cause consistent with fundamental fairness in a given case and (b) modify its Code and Ethics Standards and/or these Enforcement Procedures, with such modifications to be applied only prospectively.

Adopted by the Representative Assembly 2009CONov146 as Attachment A of the Standard Operating Procedures (SOP) of the Ethics Commission.

Reviewed by BPPC 1/04, 1/05, 9/06, 1/07, 9/09
Adopted by RA 4/96, 5/04, 5/05, 11/06, 4/07, 11/09
Revised by SEC 4/98, 4/00, 1/02, 1/04, 12/04, 9/06
Revised by EC 12/06, 2/07, 8/09

Note. The Commission on Standards and Ethics (SEC) changed to Ethics Commission (EC) in September 2005 as per Association Bylaws.

Citation. American Occupational Therapy Association. (2010). Enforcement procedures for the *Occupational Therapy Code of Ethics and Ethics Standards. American Journal of Occupational Therapy, 64*(6,Suppl.), S4–S16. doi: 10.5014/ajot.2010.64S4

AMERICAN OCCUPATIONAL THERAPY ASSOCIATION
ETHICS COMMISSION

Formal Complaint of Alleged Violation of the *Occupational Therapy Code of Ethics and Ethics Standards*

If an investigation is deemed necessary, a copy of this form will be provided to the individual against whom the complaint is filed.

Date

Complainant: (Information regarding individual filing the complaint)

Name

Phone

Address

Email

City   State   Zip Code

Respondent: (Information regarding individual against whom the complaint is directed)

Name

Phone

Address

Email

City   State   Zip Code

1. **Summarize** in a written attachment the **facts and circumstances, including dates and events**, which support a violation of the *Code of Ethics and Ethics Standards* and this complaint. Include steps, if any, that have been taken to resolve this complaint before filing.
2. **Please sign and date all documents you have written and are submitting**. *Do not include confidential documents such as patient or employment records.*
3. **If you have filed a complaint about this same matter with any other agency (e.g., NBCOT; SRB; academic institution; any federal, state, or local official), indicate to whom it was submitted, the approximate date(s), and resolution if known.**

I certify that the statements/information within this complaint are correct and truthful to the best of my knowledge and are submitted in good faith, not for resolution of private business, legal, or other disputes for which other appropriate forums exist.

_____

Signature

Send completed form, with accompanying documentation, **IN AN ENVELOPE MARKED *CONFIDENTIAL*** to:

Ethics Commission
American Occupational Therapy Association, Inc.
Attn: Staff Liaison to the EC/Ethics Office
4720 Montgomery Lane, PO Box 31220
Bethesda, MD 20824-1220

Office Use Only:

Membership Dates:_____

Verified by:_____

Appendix C
Scope of Practice

STATEMENT OF PURPOSE

The purpose of this document is to

A. Define the scope of practice in occupational therapy by

1. Delineating the domain of occupational therapy practice that directs the focus and actions of services provided by occupational therapists and occupational therapy assistants;
2. Delineating the dynamic process of occupational therapy evaluation and intervention services used to achieve outcomes that support the participation of clients in their everyday life activities (occupations);
3. Describing the education and certification requirements needed to practice as an occupational therapist and occupational therapy assistant;

B. Inform consumers, health care providers, educators, the community, funding agencies, payers, referral sources, and policymakers regarding the scope of occupational therapy.

INTRODUCTION

The occupational therapy scope of practice is based on the American Occupational Therapy Association (AOTA) document *Occupational Therapy Practice Framework: Domain and Process* (AOTA, 2008, 2nd ed.) and on the *Philosophical Base of Occupational Therapy,* which states that "the understanding and use of occupations shall be at the central core of occupational therapy practice, education, and research" (AOTA, 2006b, Policy 1.11). Occupational therapy is a dynamic and evolving profession that is responsive to consumer needs and to emerging knowledge and research.

This scope of practice document is designed to support and be used in conjunction with the *Definition of Occupational Therapy Practice for the Model Practice Act* (AOTA, 2004b). While this scope of practice document helps support state laws and regulations that govern the practice of occupational therapy, it does not supersede those existing laws and other regulatory requirements. Occupational therapists and occupational therapy assistants are required to abide by statutes and regulations when providing occupational therapy services. State laws and other regulatory requirements typically include statements about educational requirements to practice occupational therapy, procedures to practice occupational therapy legally within the defined area of jurisdiction, the definition and scope of occupational therapy practice, and supervision requirements.

It is the position of AOTA that a referral is not required for the provision of occupational therapy services and that "an occupational therapist accepts and responds to referrals in compliance with state laws or other regulatory requirements" (AOTA 2005a, Standard II.1, p. 664). State laws and other regulatory requirements should be viewed as minimum criteria to practice occupational therapy. Ethical guidelines that ensure safe and effective delivery of occupational therapy services to clients always influence occupational therapy practice (AOTA, 2005b). Policies of payers such as insurance companies also must be followed.

Occupational therapy services may be provided by two levels of practitioners—the occupational therapist and the occupational therapy assistant. Occupational therapists function as autonomous practitioners and are responsible for all aspects of occupational therapy service delivery and are accountable for the safety and effectiveness of the occupational therapy service delivery process.

The occupational therapy assistant delivers occupational therapy services under the supervision of and in partnership with the occupational therapist (AOTA, 2009). When the term *occupational therapy practitioner* is used in this document, it refers to both occupational therapists and occupational therapy assistants (AOTA, 2006a).

DEFINITION OF OCCUPATIONAL THERAPY

AOTA's *Definition of Occupational Therapy for the Model Practice Act* defines occupational therapy as

The therapeutic use of everyday life activities (occupations) with individuals or groups for the purpose of participation in roles and situations in home, school, workplace, community, and other settings. Occupational therapy services are provided for the purpose of promoting health and wellness and to those who have or are at risk for developing an illness, injury, disease, disorder, condition, impairment, disability, activity limitation, or participation restriction. Occupational

therapy addresses the physical, cognitive, psychosocial, sensory, and other aspects of performance in a variety of contexts to support engagement in everyday life activities that affect health, well-being, and quality of life. (AOTA, 2004b)

OCCUPATIONAL THERAPY PRACTICE

Occupational therapists and occupational therapy assistants are experts at analyzing the performance skills and patterns necessary for people to engage in their everyday activities in the contexts and environments in which those activities and occupations occur. The practice of occupational therapy includes

A. Methods or strategies selected to direct the process of interventions, such as

1. Establishment, remediation, or restoration of a skill or ability that has not yet developed or is impaired.
2. Compensation, modification, or adaptation of activity or environment to enhance performance.
3. Maintenance and enhancement of capabilities without which performance in everyday life activities would decline.
4. Health promotion and wellness to enable or enhance performance in everyday life activities.
5. Prevention of barriers to performance, including disability prevention.

B. Evaluation of factors affecting activities of daily living (ADLs), instrumental activities of daily living (IADLs), education, work, play, leisure, and social participation, including

1. Client factors, including body functions (e.g., neuromuscular, sensory, visual, perceptual, cognitive) and body structures (e.g., cardiovascular, digestive, integumentary, genitourinary systems).
2. Habits, routines, roles, and behavior patterns.
3. Cultural, physical, environmental, social, and spiritual contexts and activity demands that affect performance.

4. Performance skills, including motor, process, and communication/interaction skills.

C. Interventions and procedures to promote or enhance safety and performance in activities of daily living (ADLs), instrumental activities of daily living (IADLs), education, work, play, leisure, and social participation, including

1. Therapeutic use of occupations, exercises, and activities.
2. Training in self-care, self-management, home management, and community/work reintegration.
3. Development, remediation, or compensation of physical, cognitive, neuromuscular, sensory functions, and behavioral skills.
4. Therapeutic use of self, including one's personality, insights, perceptions, and judgments, as part of the therapeutic process.
5. Education and training of individuals, including family members, caregivers, and others.
6. Care coordination, case management, and transition services.
7. Consultative services to groups, programs, organizations, or communities.
8. Modification of environments (e.g., home, work, school, community) and adaptation of processes, including the application of ergonomic principles.
9. Assessment, design, fabrication, application, fitting, and training in assistive technology, adaptive devices, and orthotic devices, and training in the use of prosthetic devices.
10. Assessment, recommendation, and training in techniques to enhance functional mobility, including wheelchair management.
11. Driver rehabilitation and community mobility.
12. Management of feeding, eating, and swallowing to enable eating and feeding performance.
13. Application of physical agent modalities and use of a range of specific therapeutic procedures (e.g., wound care management; techniques to enhance sensory, perceptual, and cognitive processing; manual therapy techniques) to enhance performance skills (AOTA, 2004b).

SCOPE OF PRACTICE: DOMAIN AND PROCESS

The scope of practice includes the domain (see Figure 1) and process (see Figure 2) of occupational therapy services. These two concepts are intertwined, with the *domain* defining the focus of occupational therapy and the *process* defining the delivery of occupational therapy (see Figure 3). The domain of occupational therapy is the everyday life activities (occupations) that people find meaningful and purposeful. Within this domain, occupational therapy services enable clients to engage (participate) in their everyday life activities in their desired roles, contexts and environments, and life situations. Clients may be individuals or persons, organizations or populations. The occupations in which clients engage occur throughout the life span and include

- ADLs (self-care activities);
- Education (activities to participate in as a learner in a learning environment);
- IADLs (multistep activities to care for self and others, such as household management, financial management, and child care);
- Rest and sleep (activities relating to obtaining rest and sleep, including identifying need for rest and sleep, preparing for sleep, and participating in rest and sleep);
- Leisure (nonobligatory, discretionary, and intrinsically rewarding activities);
- Play (spontaneous and organized activities that promote pleasure, amusement, and diversion);
- Social participation (activities expected of individuals or individuals interacting with others); and
- Work (employment-related and volunteer activities).

Within their domain of practice, occupational therapists and occupational therapy assistants consider the repertoire of occupations in which the client engages, the performance skills and patterns the client uses, the contexts and environments influencing engagement, the features and demands of the activity, and the client's body functions and structures. Occupational therapists and occupational therapy assistants use their

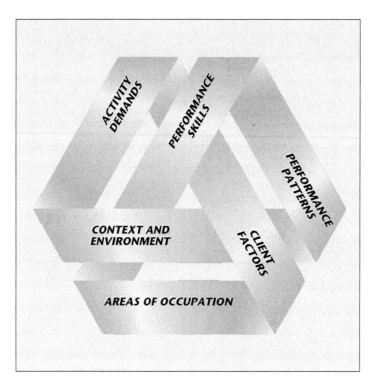

FIGURE 1

Occupational therapy's domain.
Supporting health and participation in life through engagement in occupation (AOTA, 2008).
Note. Mobius originally designed by Mark Dow. Used with permission.

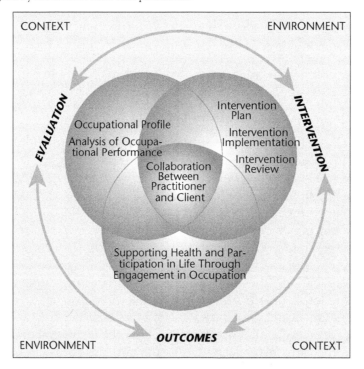

FIGURE 2

Occupational therapy's process.
Collaboration between the practitioner and the client is central to the interactive nature of service delivery (AOTA, 2008).

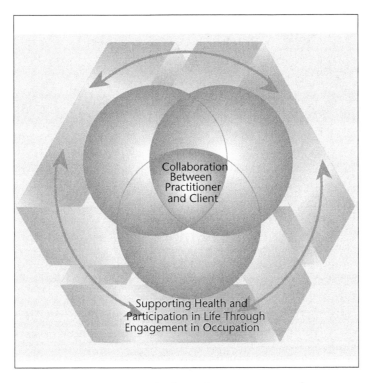

FIGURE 3

Occupational therapy.
The domain and process are inextricably linked (AOTA, 2008).
Note. Mobius originally designed by Mark Dow. Used with permission.

knowledge and skills to help clients attain and resume daily life activities that support function and health throughout the life span. Participation in activities and occupations that are meaningful to the client involves emotional, psychosocial, cognitive, and physical aspects of performance. Participation in meaningful activities and occupations enhances health, well-being, and life satisfaction.

The domain of occupational therapy practice complements the World Health Organization's (WHO) conceptualization of participation and health articulated in the *International Classification of Functioning, Disability and Health* (*ICF;* WHO, 2001). Occupational therapy incorporates the basic constructs of ICF, including environment, participation, activities, and body structures and functions, when addressing the complexity and richness of occupations and occupational engagement.

The process of occupational therapy refers to the delivery of services and includes evaluating, intervening, and targeting outcomes. Occupation

remains central to the occupational therapy process. It is client-centered, involving collaboration with the client throughout each aspect of service delivery. During the evaluation, the therapist develops an occupational profile; analyzes the client's ability to carry out everyday life activities; and determines the client's occupational needs, problems, and priorities for intervention.

Evaluation and intervention may address one or more aspects of the domain (see Figure 4) that influence occupational performance. Intervention includes planning and implementing occupational therapy services and involves therapeutic use of self, activities, and occupations, as well as consultation, education, and advocacy. The occupational therapist and occupational therapy assistant utilize occupation-based theories, frames of reference, evidence, and clinical reasoning to guide the intervention (AOTA, 2008).

The outcome of occupational therapy intervention is directed toward "supporting health and participation in life through engagement in

AREAS OF OCCUPATION	CLIENT FACTORS	PERFORMANCE SKILLS	PERFORMANCE PATTERNS	CONTEXT AND ENVIRONMENT	ACTIVITY DEMANDS
Activities of Daily Living (ADL)*	Values, Beliefs, and Spirituality	Sensory Perceptual Skills	Habits	Cultural	Objects Used and Their Properties
Instrumental Activities of Daily Living (IADL)	Body Functions	Motor and Praxis Skills	Routines	Personal	Space Demands
Rest and Sleep	Body Structures	Emotional Regulation Skills	Roles	Physical	Social Demands
Education		Cognitive Skills	Rituals	Social	Sequencing and Timing
Work		Communication and Social Skills		Temporal	Required Actions
Play				Virtual	Required Body Functions
Leisure					Required Body Structures
Social Participation					

*Also referred to as basic activities of *daily living* (BADL) or personal activities of daily living (PADL).

FIGURE 4

Aspects of occupational therapy's domain.
All aspects of the domain transact to support engagement, participation, and health. This figure does not imply a hierarchy (AOTA, 2008).

occupations" (AOTA, 2008, p. 660). Outcomes of the intervention determine future actions with the client. Outcomes include the client's occupational performance, adaptation, health and wellness, participation, prevention, quality of life, role competence, self-advocacy, and occupational justice initiatives (AOTA, 2008, pp. 662–663).

SITES OF INTERVENTION AND AREAS OF FOCUS

Occupational therapy services are provided to persons, organizations, and populations. People served come from all age groups. Practitioners work with individuals one to one, in organizations, or at the population level to address occupational needs and issues in mental health, work and industry, rehabilitation, disability and participation, productive aging, and health and wellness.

Along the continuum of service, occupational therapy services may be provided to clients throughout the life span in a variety of settings. The settings may include, but are not limited to, the following:

- Institutional settings (inpatient) (e.g., acute rehabilitation, psychiatric hospital, community and specialty-focused hospitals, nursing facilities, prisons)
- Outpatient settings (e.g., hospitals, clinics, medical and therapy offices)

- Home and community settings (e.g., home care, group homes, assisted living, schools, early intervention centers, day care centers, industry and business, hospice, sheltered workshops, transitional-living facilities, wellness and fitness centers, community mental health facilities)
- Research facilities.

EDUCATION AND CERTIFICATION REQUIREMENTS

To practice as an occupational therapist, an individual

- Must have graduated from an occupational therapy program accredited by the Accreditation Council for Occupational Therapy Education (ACOTE®) or predecessor organizations,[1] and
- Must have successfully completed a period of supervised fieldwork experience required by the recognized educational institution where the applicant met the academic requirements of an educational program for occupational

[1]Foreign-educated graduates of occupational therapy programs approved by the World Federation of Occupational Therapy also may be eligible for certification/licensure as an occupational therapist provided that additional requirements are met.

therapists that is accredited by ACOTE® or predecessor organization.
- Must have successfully passed the national certification examination for occupational therapists and/or met state requirements for licensure/registration.

To practice as an occupational therapy assistant, an individual
- Must have graduated from an occupational therapy assistant program accredited by ACOTE® or predecessor organizations,
- Must have successfully completed a period of supervised fieldwork experience required by the recognized educational institution where the applicant met the academic requirements of an educational program for occupational therapy assistants that is accredited by ACOTE® or predecessor organizations.
- Must have successfully passed the national certification examination for occupational therapy assistants and/or met state requirements for licensure/registration.[2]

AOTA supports licensure of qualified occupational therapists and occupational therapy assistants (AOTA, 2004a, Policy 5.3). State and other legislative or regulatory agencies may impose additional requirements to practice as occupational therapists and occupational therapy assistants in their area of jurisdiction.

REFERENCES

Accreditation Council for Occupational Therapy Education. (2007a). Accreditation standards for a doctoral-degree-level educational program for the occupational therapist. *American Journal of Occupational Therapy, 61,* 641–651.

---

[2]The majority of this information is taken from the *Accreditation Standards for a Doctoral-Degree-Level Educational Program for the Occupational Therapist* (ACOTE, 2007a), *Accreditation Standards for a Master's-Degree-Level Educational Program for the Occupational Therapist* (ACOTE, 2007b), and *Accreditation Standards for an Educational Program for the Occupational Therapy Assistant* (ACOTE, 2007c).

Accreditation Council for Occupational Therapy Education. (2007b). Accreditation standards for a master's-degree-level educational program for the occupational therapist. *American Journal of Occupational Therapy, 61,* 652–661.
Accreditation Council for Occupational Therapy Education. (2007c). Accreditation standards for an educational program for the occupational therapy assistant. *American Journal of Occupational Therapy, 61,* 662–671.
American Occupational Therapy Association. (2004a). Policy 5.3: Licensure. *Policy manual* (2008 ed., p. 64). Bethesda, MD: Author.
American Occupational Therapy Association. (2004b). Definition of occupational therapy practice for the AOTA Model Practice Act. (Available from the State Affairs Group, American Occupational Therapy Association, PO Box 31220, Bethesda, MD 20824-1220. E-mail: stpd@aota.org)
American Occupational Therapy Association. (2005a). Standards of practice for occupational therapy. *American Journal of Occupational Therapy, 59,* 663–665.
American Occupational Therapy Association. (2005b). Occupational therapy code of ethics (2005). *American Journal of Occupational Therapy, 54,* 614–616.
American Occupational Therapy Association. (2006a). Policy 1.44: Categories of occupational therapy personnel. In *Policy manual* (2008 ed., p. 10). Bethesda, MD: Author.
American Occupational Therapy Association. (2006b). Policy 1.11: The philosophical base of occupational therapy. In *Policy manual* (2008 ed., pp. 33–34). Bethesda, MD: Author.
American Occupational Therapy Association. (2008). Occupational therapy practice framework: Domain and process (2nd ed.). *American Journal of Occupational Therapy, 62,* 625–688.
American Occupational Therapy Association. (2009). Guidelines for supervision, roles, and responsibilities during the delivery of occupational therapy services. *American Journal of Occupational Therapy, 63,* 797–803.
World Health Organization. (2001). *International classification of functioning, disability, and health (ICF).* Geneva, Switzerland: Author.

ADDITIONAL READING

Moyers, P., & Dale, L. (Eds.). (2007). *The guide to occupational therapy practice* (2nd ed.). Bethesda, MD: AOTA Press.

AUTHORS

The Commission on Practice:
  Sara Jane Brayman, PhD, OTR/L, FAOTA,
    Chairperson, 2002–2005
  Gloria Frolek Clark, MS, OTR/L, FAOTA
  Janet V. DeLany, DEd, OTR/L
  Eileen R. Garza, PhD, OTR, ATP
  Mary V. Radomski, MA, OTR/L, FAOTA
  Ruth Ramsey, MS, OTR/L
  Carol Siebert, MS, OTR/L
  Kristi Voelkerding, BS, COTA/L
  Patricia D. LaVesser, PhD, OTR/L, *SIS Liaison*
  Lenna Aird, *ASD Liaison*
  Deborah Lieberman, MHSA, OTR/L, FAOTA,
    AOTA Headquarters Liaison

for

The Commission on Practice
  Sara Jane Brayman, PhD, OTR/L FAOTA,
    Chairperson

Adopted by the Representative Assembly 2004C23
Edited by the Commission on Practice 2005
Edited by the Commission on Practice 2009

Note: This replaces the 2004 document Scope of Practice (previously published and copyrighted in 2004 by the *American Journal of Occupational Therapy, 58,* 673–677).

Copyright © 2010 by the American Occupational Therapy Association.

Citation. American Occupational Therapy Association. (2010). Scope of practice. *American Journal of Occupational Therapy, 64*(6,Suppl.), S70–S77. doi: 10.5014/ajot.2010.64S70

Appendix D
NBCOT® Candidate/Certificant Code of Conduct

PREAMBLE

The National Board for Certification in Occupational Therapy, Inc. ("NBCOT," formerly known as "AOTCB") is a professional organization that supports and promotes occupational therapy practitioner certification. This Candidate/Certificant Code of Conduct enables NBCOT to define and clarify the professional responsibilities for present and future NBCOT certificants, i.e., OCCUPATIONAL THERAPIST REGISTERED OTR® (OTR) henceforth OTR, and CERTIFIED OCCUPATIONAL THERAPY ASSISTANT COTA® (COTA) henceforth COTA.

It is vital that NBCOT certificants conduct their work in an appropriate and professional manner to earn and maintain the confidence and respect of recipients of occupational therapy, colleagues, employers, students, and the public.

As certified professionals in the field of occupational therapy, NBCOT certificants will at all times act with integrity and adhere to high standards for personal and professional conduct, accept responsibility for their actions, both personally and professionally, continually seek to enhance their professional capabilities, practice with fairness and honesty, abide by all federal, state, and local laws and regulations, and encourage others to act in a professional manner consistent with the certification standards and responsibilities set forth below.

Where the term "certificant" is used, the term "applicant or candidate" is included in its scope.

PRINCIPLE 1

Certificants shall provide accurate and truthful representations to NBCOT concerning all information related to aspects of the Certification Program, including, but not limited to, the submission of information:

- On the examination and certification renewal applications, and renewal audit form;
- Requested by NBCOT for a disciplinary action situation or
- Requested by NBCOT concerning allegations related to:
  - test security violations and/or disclosure of confidential examination material content to unauthorized parties;
  - misrepresentations by a certificant regarding his/her credential(s) and/or education;
  - the unauthorized use of NBCOT's intellectual property, certification marks, and other copyrighted materials.

PRINCIPLE 2

Certificants who are the subject of a complaint shall cooperate with NBCOT concerning investigations of violations of the Candidate/Certificant Code of Conduct, including the collection of relevant information.

PRINCIPLE 3

Certificants shall be accurate, truthful, and complete in any and all communications relating to their education, professional work, research, and contributions to the field of occupational therapy.

PRINCIPLE 4

Certificants shall comply with laws, regulations, and statutes governing the practice of occupational therapy.

PRINCIPLE 5

Certificants shall not have been convicted of a crime, the circumstances of which substantially relate to the practice of occupational therapy or indicate an inability to engage in the practice of occupational therapy safely, and/or competently.

PRINCIPLE 6

Certificants shall not engage in behavior or conduct, lawful or otherwise that causes them to be, or reasonably perceived to be, a threat or potential threat to the health, well-being, or safety of recipients or potential recipients of occupational therapy services.

PRINCIPLE 7

Certificants shall not engage in the practice of occupational therapy while one's ability to practice is impaired due to chemical (i.e., legal and/or illegal) drug or alcohol abuse.

Appendix E
Procedures for the Enforcement of the *NBCOT® Candidate/ Certificant Code of Conduct*

SECTION A. PREAMBLE

In exercising its responsibility for promoting and maintaining standards of professional conduct in the practice of occupational therapy and in order to protect the public from those practitioners whose behavior falls short of these standards, the National Board for Certification in Occupational Therapy, Inc. ("NBCOT®," formerly known as "AOTCB") has adopted a Candidate/Certificant Code of Conduct. The NBCOT has adopted these procedures for resolving issues arising under the Candidate/Certificant Code of Conduct with respect to persons who have been certified by the NBCOT or who have applied for such certification. These procedures are intended to enable the NBCOT, through its Qualifications and Compliance Review Committee ("QCRC"), to act fairly in the performance of its responsibilities to the public as a certifying agency, and to ensure that the rights of candidates and certificants are protected.

SECTION B. BASIS FOR SANCTION

A violation of the Candidate/Certificant Code of Conduct provides basis for action and sanction under these Procedures.

SECTION C. SANCTIONS

1. Violations of the Candidate/Certificant Code of Conduct may result in one or more of the following sanctions:

   a. Ineligibility for certification, which means that an individual is barred from becoming certified by the NBCOT, either indefinitely or for a certain duration.
   b. Reprimand, which means a formal expression of disapproval, which shall be retained in the certificant's file, but shall not be publicly announced.
   c. Censure, which means a formal expression of disapproval which is publicly announced.
   d. Probation, which means continued certification is subject to fulfillment of specified conditions, e.g., monitoring, education, supervision, and/or counseling.
   e. Suspension, which means the loss of certification for a certain duration, after which the individual may be required to apply for reinstatement.
   f. Revocation, which means permanent loss of certification.

2. All sanctions other than reprimand shall be announced publicly, in accordance with

Section D.7. All sanctions other than reprimand shall be disclosed in response to inquiries in accordance with Section D.7.

SECTION D. QUALIFICATIONS AND COMPLIANCE REVIEW PROCEDURES

1. Jurisdiction

The NBCOT has jurisdiction over all individuals who have been certified as an OCCUPATIONAL THERAPIST REGISTERED OTR (OTR®) henceforth OTR, or CERTIFIED OCCUPATIONAL THERAPY ASSISTANT COTA (COTA®) henceforth COTA, or who are planning to apply for or have applied for certification, or have applied for Occupational Therapy Eligibility Determination (OTED) to take the NBCOT Certification Examination for OTR. In addition, NBCOT has jurisdiction over all individuals who have applied for an Early Determination Review to determine eligibility to take the Certification Examination for OTR or COTA; Jurisdiction, in this case, is for the limited purpose of acting upon a request for an Early Determination.

2. Initiation of the Process

The QCRC Staff ("Staff") shall initiate the process upon receipt by the QCRC of information indicating that an individual subject to QCRC's jurisdiction may have violated the Candidate/Certificant Code of Conduct. Receipt of such information shall be considered a complaint for the purposes of these procedures, regardless of the source.

3. Staff Investigation and Action

a. Staff shall review all complaints and investigate these complaints, as it deems appropriate.
b. Staff may review any evidence, which it deems appropriate and relevant.

   i. If Staff determines that the evidence does not support the allegation(s), no file shall be opened and the complainant shall be notified of the Staff's decision.
   ii. If Staff determines that the evidence does support the allegation(s) and decides to investigate, the subject of the complaint as well as the complainant shall be notified. This notification shall be in writing and shall include a description of the complaint and the identity of the complainant. The subject of the complaint shall have thirty (30) days from the date notification is sent to respond in writing to the complaint. The Staff may extend this period up to an additional thirty (30) days upon request, provided sufficient justification for the extension is given.
   iii. The subject of a complaint may request voluntary forfeiture of his/her certification. This request must be submitted in writing and can be made while the complaint is either under active investigation or when disciplinary action has been taken by the QCRC but the terms of the sanction remain incomplete.

   If the subject applies to regain certification, to restore back to a current status, after voluntary forfeiture, the subject must meet all of the following requirements:

   a. submit request to regain certification in writing
   b. satisfy current certification examination eligibility requirements (including academic and fieldwork requirements) and
   c. re-take and pass the national certification examination

   Further, any pending investigation will be resumed upon request to regain certification.
   If the subject's certification is voluntarily forfeited, public notice may be given in accordance with Section D. 7 of these procedures.

   iv. If the subject does not respond to investigative inquiries, subject's certification will be placed on Noncompliant-Inactive status. This means that the subject CANNOT a) identify themselves to the public as an OCCUPATIONAL THER-

APIST REGISTERED (OTR) or CER-TIFIED OCCUPATIONAL THERAPY ASSISTANT (COTA) or b) use the OTR or COTA credential after their name.

If the subject applies to renew certification, to restore back to a current status, after being placed on Non Compliant–Inactive status, the subject must meet all of the following requirements:

a. submit request to regain certification in writing
b. satisfy current certification renewal requirements, and
c. cooperate with and provide written response and supporting documentation to the NBCOT investigative inquiry

c. Upon the completion of its investigation, Staff shall either:

i. Dismiss the case due to insufficient evidence, the matter being insufficiently serious, or other reasons as may be warranted. The qualifications and compliance review shall be considered closed at the time such decision is made; or
ii. Propose a settlement agreement.

4. QCRC Review and Decision

Staff shall prepare a case summary of its investigation along with the proposed settlement for the QCRC to consider. The report shall include the basis for Staff's findings, as well as any written responses, or other materials submitted in relation to the investigation of the complaint. Upon review of Staff's investigation, findings, and recommendation, the QCRC may either:

a. Approve the proposed settlement agreement. Upon the subject's acceptance of the settlement, the qualifications and compliance process shall be considered closed. The public notification standards of Section D.7 are applicable if the settlement contains a sanction that warrants such announcement be made; or
b. Reject the proposed settlement. Should the QCRC reject the settlement, it may either

instruct Staff with modifications or revisions to the proposed settlement or it may dismiss the case altogether.

Upon notification of the proposed settlement, the subject of the complaint may either:

a. Agree to the proposed settlement and thereby waive his/her right to a hearing; or
b. Not agree to the proposed settlement and request a hearing before the QCRC.

i. The subject of the complaint may be represented at the hearing by his/her legal counsel, or any other individual of his/her choosing.
ii. The subject of the complaint shall be solely responsible for all of his/her own expenses related to the hearing. Hearings can be conducted via teleconference call or in person at the sole discretion of the QCRC. Should the subject cancel the hearing, he/she must notify the QCRC of the cancellation no less than five (5) days prior to the hearing date. Should the subject cancel the hearing within five (5) days of the hearing date or not appear at the scheduled hearing, all costs associated with the preparation of the hearing shall be paid by the subject (e.g. court reporting fees, teleconference fees, hearing manual preparation fees).
iii. The subject of the complaint shall provide the QCRC with any and all materials he/she may wish to include for the hearing no less than ten (10) days prior to the hearing date.

Following the hearing, Staff shall notify (in writing) the complainant and the subject of the complaint of the QCRC's decision within thirty (30) days of the decision. The decision shall take effect immediately unless otherwise provided by the QCRC.

5. Appeals Process

Within thirty (30) days after the notification of the QCRC's decision, any individual(s) sanctioned by the QCRC at the hearing may appeal the hearing decision to the NBCOT Directors. A notice of appeal, which must be in writing and signed by the appealing party, shall be sent by the appealing party to the NBCOT Chairperson in care of the President/Chief Executive Officer. The basis for the appeal shall be fully explained in this notice.

The Chairperson shall form an Appeals Panel within thirty (30) days after receipt of the notice of appeal. The Appeals Panel shall be comprised of three (3) NBCOT Directors and shall include at least one (1) OTR or one (1) COTA and one (1) public member. Members of the QCRC who participated in any aspect of the proceedings related to the complaint shall not serve on the Appeals Panel.

An appeal must relate to evidence, issues and procedures that are part of the record of the QCRC hearing and decision. The appeal may also address the substance of the disciplinary action. However, the Panel may in its discretion consider additional evidence.

Within fifteen (15) days after the notice of appeal is received by the Appeals Panel, the Panel shall either decide the appeal or schedule a hearing.

The Appeals Panel may either:

a. Affirm the QCRC's decision;
b. Deny the QCRC's decision;
c. Refer the case back to the QCRC for further investigation and resolution with full right of appeal; or
d. Modify the decision, but not in a manner that would be more adverse to the subject.

If a hearing is scheduled the appealing party shall be given at least thirty (30) days notice of the hearing. The appealing party may be represented at the hearing by legal counsel or any other individual of his/her choosing. The appealing party shall be solely responsible for all of his/her own expenses related to the hearing. Within fifteen (15) days after the appeals hearing, the Panel shall notify the Chairperson of its decision.

The Chairperson shall promptly notify the appealing party of the Appeals Panel's decision. The decision of the Appeals Panel shall be final.

6. Cooperation with NBCOT Enforcement Procedures

Failure to respond to any aspect of the Enforcement Procedures, will be considered a violation of the Candidate/Certificant Code of Conduct,

Principle 2, and is sufficient grounds for the imposition of sanction by the QCRC.

7. Noncompliant–Inactive

Individuals who do not satisfy the NBCOT certification renewal requirements by their scheduled renewal date, or who are non-responsive to NBCOT investigative inquiries are "Noncompliant–Inactive" and CANNOT a) identify themselves to the public as an OCCUPATIONAL THERAPIST REGISTERED (OTR) or CERTIFIED OCCUPATIONAL THERAPY ASSISTANT (COTA) or b) use the OTR or COTA credential after their name.

8. Announcement of Sanction

If an individual's certification status is voluntarily forfeited, suspended or revoked, or he/she is censured or placed on probation, occupational therapy state regulatory bodies shall be notified and an announcement included in one or more publications of general circulation to persons engaged or otherwise interested in the profession of occupational therapy. The NBCOT may also disclose its final decision, including ineligibility for certification, to others as it deems appropriate, including, but not limited to, persons inquiring about the status of an individual's certification, employers, third party payers and the general public.

9. Notification

All notifications referred to in these procedures shall be in writing and shall be by confirmation of signature, return receipt mail, unless otherwise indicated. Subjects of complaints who live outside of the U.S. may be given additional time to respond to any notifications they are sent, as determined by the Staff in its discretion.

10. Records and Reports

At the completion of this procedure, all records and reports shall be returned to the Staff. The complete files in the qualifications and compliance review proceedings shall be maintained.

11. Expedited Action

The QCRC Chair may expedite a matter by shortening any notice or response period provided for under these procedures if the responsible party determines in its sole discretion that shortening the period is appropriate in order to protect against the possibility of harm to recipients of occupational therapy services.

In matters where the severity of the allegations and evidence provided warrant such action in order to protect the public, the QCRC may authorize immediate suspension/revocation of certification. The subject will be duly notified of the action and given fifteen (15) days to contest the suspension or revocation.

12. Standard of Proof

The NBCOT's QCRC and Appeals Panel shall take disciplinary action against an individual only where there is clear and convincing evidence of a violation of the Candidate/Certificant Code of Conduct.

13. Special Accommodations

The NBCOT recognizes the definition of disability as defined by the Americans with Disabilities Act (ADA) and acknowledges the provisions and protections of the Act. The NBCOT shall offer hearings related to qualifications and compliance review or the appeals process in a site and manner, which is architecturally accessible to persons with disabilities or offer alternative arrangements for such individuals.

An individual with a documented disability may request special accommodations for a hearing by providing reasonable advance notice to the NBCOT of his or her disability and of the modifications or aids needed at the hearing at his or her own expense.

14. Amendment to Procedures

These procedures may be amended at any time by the NBCOT Directors.

Revised: February 6, 2010

© Copyright 2010 NBCOT, Inc. Reprinted with permission.

Appendix F
Occupational Therapy Profession— Continuing Competence Requirements

STATE	STATUS	REQUIREMENTS
Alabama	Mandatory	**OT:** 3.0 CEUs (or 30 contact hours) biennially **OTA:** 2.0 CEUs (or 20 contact hours) biennially
Alaska	Mandatory	**OT:** 12 months or more of the concluding licensing period must have completed 24. Less than 12 months of the concluding licensing period must have completed 12 contact hours of continuing education during that licensing period. **OTA:** 12 months or more of the concluding licensing period must have completed 12 contact hours. Less than 12 months of the concluding licensing period must have completed 6 contact hours.
Arizona	Mandatory	**OT:** 20 hours for renewal of a 2-year license period **OTA:** 12 hours for renewal of a 2-year license period
Arkansas	Mandatory	**OT:** 10 hours of continuing education each year **OTA:** 10 hours of continuing education each year
California	Mandatory	**OT:** 24 PDUs for each biennial renewal period **OTA:** 24 PDUs for each biennial renewal period 1 PDU = 60 minutes
Colorado	No requirements	**OT:** No requirements **OTA:** No requirements
Connecticut	Mandatory	**OT:** 12 units of qualifying continuing competency during the preceding 2-year period for which the license is being renewed; will increase to 24 contact hours for licenses being renewed after 1/1/2011 **OTA:** 9 units of qualifying continuing competency during the preceding 2-year period for which the license is being renewed; will increase to 18 contact hours for licenses being renewed after 1/1/2011

STATE	STATUS	REQUIREMENTS
Delaware	Mandatory	**OT:** 20 hours CEUs for each license renewed biennially; new licensees prorated **OTA:** 20 hours CEUs for each license renewed biennially; new licensees prorated
District of Columbia	Mandatory	**OT:** 24 hours of approved continuing education credit biennially **OTA:** 12 hours of approved continuing education credit biennially
Florida[i]	Mandatory	**OT:** 22 hours continuing education + 2 hours of Florida OT Laws & Rules + 2 hours of Prevention of Medical Errors = total 26 hours biennially **OTA:** 22 hours continuing education + 2 hours of Florida OT Laws & Rules + 2 hours of Prevention of Medical Errors = total 26 hours biennially
Georgia	Mandatory	**OT:** 24 hours of continuing education biennially; 16 hours must be related to direct "hands on" patient care **OTA:** 24 hours of continuing education biennially; 16 hours must be related to direct "hands on" patient care
Hawaii	No requirements	**OT:** No requirements **OTA:** No requirements
Idaho	Mandatory	**OT:** At least 2 CE units and 10 hours of professional development units biennially **OTA:** At least 2 CE units and 10 hours of professional development units biennially (Requirements go into effect for the biennium following the 2010 license renewal)
Illinois	Mandatory	**OT:** 24 contact hours of CE relevant to the practice of occupational therapy the 24 months preceding December 31 in the year of the renewal. **OTA:** 24 contact hours of CE relevant to the practice of occupational therapy during the 24 months preceding December 31 in the year of the renewal.
Indiana	Mandatory[ii]	**OT:** 18 hours biennially, prorated if less than 24 months since license was issued. **OTA:** 18 hours biennially, prorated if less than 24 months since license was issued.
Iowa	Mandatory	**OT:** 30 hours of continuing education each biennium (by birth month); minimum of 15 hours shall be clinical in nature. **OTA:** 15 hours of continuing education each biennium (by birth month); minimum of 8 hours shall be clinical in nature.
Kansas	Mandatory	**OT:** 40 hours of continuing education (CEU) for the preceding 2-year period, reported during the odd-numbered years. No evidence of CEU is required during even-numbered years. **OTA:** 40 hours of continuing education (CEU) for the preceding 2-year period, reported during the odd-numbered years. No evidence of CEU is required during even-numbered years.

STATE	STATUS	REQUIREMENTS
Kentucky	Mandatory	**OT:** (12) CCUs of qualified activities for maintaining continuing competence during the preceding annual renewal period (prorated if licensed less than 1-year) **OTA:** (12) CCUs of qualified activities for maintaining continuing competence during the preceding annual renewal period (prorated if licensed less than 1-year)
Louisiana	Mandatory	**OT:** 15 hours or 1.5 CEUs annually; one CEU constitutes 10 hours of participation in an organized continuing professional education program approved by the board **OTA:** 15 hours or 1.5 CEUs annually; one CEU constitutes 10 hours of participation in an organized continuing professional education program approved by the board
Maine	Mandatory	**OT:** 36 hours of study equivalent to 3.6 CEUs which shall be completed for every biennial license renewal **OTA:** 36 hours of study equivalent to 3.6 CEUs which shall be completed for every biennial license renewal
Maryland	Mandatory	**OT:** 12 contact hours consisting of a minimum of 8 contact hours related to occupational therapy principles and procedures and a maximum of 4 contact hours through occupational therapy role-related activities **OTA:** 12 contact hours consisting of a minimum of 8 contact hours related to occupational therapy principles and procedures and a maximum of 4 contact hours through occupational therapy role-related activities
Massachusetts	No requirements	**OT:** No requirements **OTA:** No requirements
Michigan	No requirements[iii]	**OT:** No requirements **OTA:** No requirements
Minnesota	Mandatory	**OT:** 24 contact hours of continuing education in the 2-year licensure period; licensees who are issued licenses for a period of less than 2 years shall obtain a prorated number of contact hours required for licensure renewal based on the number of months licensed during the 2-year licensure period. **OTA:** 18 contact hours of continuing education in the 2-year licensure period; licensees who are issued licenses for a period of less than 2 years shall obtain a prorated number of contact hours required for licensure renewal based on the number of months licensed during the 2-year licensure period.
Mississippi	Mandatory	**OT:** 20 contact hours (CH) or 2 CEUs to be accrued during the licensure period. At least 6 CH or .6 CEU must be directly related to the clinical practice of occupational therapy. **OTA:** 20 contact hours (CH) or 2 CEUs to be accrued during the licensure period. At least 6 CH or .6 CEU must be directly related to the clinical practice of occupational therapy.

STATE	STATUS	REQUIREMENTS
Missouri	Mandatory	**OT:** 24 continuing competence credits (CCCs) for the 2-year license period. At least 50% of the CCCs must be directly related to the delivery of occupational therapy services, and the remaining CCCs must be related to one's practice area or setting. **OTA:** 24 continuing competence credits (CCCs) for the 2-year license period. At least 50% of the CCCs must be directly related to the delivery of occupational therapy services, and the remaining CCCs must be related to one's practice area or setting. 1 CEU = 10 CCCs; 1 contact hour = 1 CCC
Montana	Mandatory	**OT:** 10 hours of continuing education annually **OTA:** 10 hours of continuing education annually
Nebraska	Mandatory	**OT:** 20 hours of continuing education for biennial license renewal beginning August 1 each even-numbered year through August 1 the following even-numbered year. **OTA:** 15 hours of continuing education for biennial license renewal beginning August 1 each even-numbered year through August 1 the following even-numbered year.
Nevada	Mandatory	**OT:** 10 hours of continuing education at annual renewal **OTA:** 10 hours of continuing education at annual renewal
New Hampshire	Mandatory	**OT:** 12 hours of continuing professional education annually, 6 of those hours need to be clinical application; 24 hours of continuing professional education biennially, 12 of those hours need to be clinical application. **OTA:** 12 hours of continuing professional education annually, 6 of those hours need to be clinical application; 24 hours of continuing professional education biennially, 12 of those hours need to be clinical application.
New Jersey	No requirements	**OT:** No requirements **OTA:** No requirements
New Mexico	Mandatory	**OT:** 20 continuing education contact hours annually **OTA:** 20 continuing education contact hours annually
New York	No requirements	**OT:** No requirements **OTA:** No requirements
North Carolina	Mandatory	**OT:** 15 hours each (annual) renewal year, every 2 years all licensees shall document completion of at least 1 contact hour (one point) of an ethics course **OTA:** 15 hours each (annual) renewal year, every 2 years all licensees shall document completion of at least 1 contact hour (one point) of an ethics course
North Dakota	Mandatory	**OT:** 20 contact hours (2.0 CEUs) within the 24 months prior to the date the completed application for renewal of licensure is received **OTA:** 20 contact hours (2.0 CEUs) within the 24 months prior to the date the completed application for renewal of licensure is received
Ohio	Mandatory	**OT:** 20 contact hours of continuing education activities within a 2-year renewal cycle, at least 1 contact hour of an ethics course **OTA:** 20 contact hours of continuing education activities within a 2-year renewal cycle, at least 1 contact hour of an ethics course

STATE	STATUS	REQUIREMENTS
Oklahoma	Mandatory	**OT:** 20 hours every 2 years **OTA:** 20 hours every 2 years
Oregon	Mandatory[iv]	**OT:** 30 points of CE for the 2 years preceding the date of the 2-year license renewal **OTA:** 30 points of CE for the 2 years preceding the date of the 2-year license renewal Unless stated otherwise, 1 point equals 1 contact hour
Pennsylvania	No requirements	**OT:** No requirements **OTA:** No requirements
Rhode Island	Mandatory	**OT:** 20 hours biennially **OTA:** 20 hours biennially
South Carolina	Mandatory	**OT:** 16 hours of continuing education credit per biennium year, 8 must be related to direct patient care **OTA:** 16 hours of continuing education credit per biennium year, 8 must be related to direct patient care One contact hour is 50 minutes of instruction or organized learning.
South Dakota	Mandatory	**OT:** 12 continuing competency points in 1-year period in professional education activities **OTA:** 12 continuing competency points in 1-year period in professional education activities
Tennessee	Mandatory[v]	**OT:** 24 continued competency credits for the 2 years preceding the date of the 2-year license renewal **OTA:** 24 continued competency credits for the 2 years preceding the date of the 2-year license renewal
Texas	Mandatory	**OT:** 30 hours of continuing education every 2 years; a minimum of 15 hours of continuing education must be in skills specific to occupational therapy practice **OTA:** 30 hours of continuing education every 2 years; a minimum of 15 hours of continuing education must be in skills specific to occupational therapy practice
Utah	No requirements	**OT:** No requirements **OTA:** No requirements
Vermont	Mandatory	**OT:** 20 hours of continuing education during the preceding 2-year licensure period, 50% of continuing competency hours must be directly related to the delivery of occupational therapy services **OTA:** 20 hours of continuing education during the preceding 2-year licensure period, 50% of continuing competency hours must be directly related to the delivery of occupational therapy services
Virginia	Mandatory[vi]	**OT:** 20 contact hours of continuing education activities every 2 years **OTA:** 20 contact hours of continuing education activities every 2 years
Washington	Mandatory	**OT:** 30 hours of continuing education every 2 years, a minimum of 20 hours must be directly related to the practice of occupational therapy **OTA:** 30 hours of continuing education every 2 years, a minimum of 20 hours must be directly related to the practice of occupational therapy

STATE	STATUS	REQUIREMENTS
West Virginia	Mandatory	**OT:** 24 hours of continuing education activities obtained within 2-year period **OTA:** 24 hours of continuing education activities obtained within 2-year period
Wisconsin	Mandatory	**OT:** 24 points of acceptable continuing education in a 2-year period; at least 12 of the points shall be accumulated through professional development activities related to occupational therapy **OTA:** 24 points of acceptable continuing education in a 2-year period; at least 12 of the points shall be accumulated through professional development activities related to occupational therapy
Wyoming	Mandatory	**OT:** 16 hours of continuing education per year **OTA:** 16 hours of continuing education per year

[i]**Florida**—1 hour of HIV/AIDS training is required for the first renewal period only.

[ii]**Indiana**—The committee will require 1/2 of the required continuing education (CE) to be completed for the December 31, 2010, renewal. That means that you will be required to complete 9 hours (at least 1/2 of which must be CAT 1) of CE for this renewal cycle. If a license or certificate is valid for less than 12 months, no continuing competency is required for renewal. If the license or certificate is valid for 12 to 24 months, 9 hours of continuing competency is required for renewal.

[iii]**Michigan**—Legislation enacted in 2009 (SB 921) requires the Board to establish continuing competence requirements beginning with the license renewal cycle after the effective date of the rules. Rules to implement the new requirement are in development.

[iv]**Oregon**—Effective January 2008, a one-time requirement of 7 points of CE on pain management must be completed as part of the 30 points of continuing education currently required.

[v]**Tennessee**—Beginning January 1, 2008, all applicants for licensure, renewal of licensure, reactivation of licensure, or reinstatement of licensure must attest to having completed continued competence requirements for the 2 calendar years (January 1–December 31) that precede the licensure renewal, reactivation, or reinstatement year.

[vi]**Virginia**—10 contact hours shall be Type 1 continuing learning activities as documented by a sponsor or organization recognized by the profession of occupational therapy to designate learning activities for credit or other value. An additional 10 contact hours shall be Type 2 continuing learning activities, which may or may not be approved for credit by a sponsor or organization recognized by the profession to designate learning activities for credit or other value. Occupational therapists shall document their own participation in Type 2 learning activities.

Note. CCU = continuing competency unit; CE = continuing education; CEU = continuing education unit; OT = occupational therapist; OTA = occupational therapy assistant; PDU = professional development unit.

Appendix G
Ethics Resources

PRINT RESOURCES

American Occupational Therapy Association. (2010). Occupational therapy code of ethics and ethics standards (2010). *American Journal of Occupational Therapy,* 64(6 Suppl.), S17–S26. doi: 10.5014/ajot.2010.64S17

American Occupational Therapy Association. (2010). Standards for continuing competence. *American Journal of Occupational Therapy,* 64(6 Suppl.), S103–S105. doi: 10.5014/ajot.2010.64S103

Barker, P. (Ed.). (2011). *Mental health ethics: The human context.* New York: Routledge.

Beauchamp, T. L., & Childress, J. F. (2009). *Principles of biomedical ethics.* New York: Oxford University Press.

College of Occupational Therapists. (2005). College of Occupational Therapists: Code of ethics and professional conduct. *British Journal of Occupational Therapy,* 68, 527–532.

Corey, G., Schneider-Corey, M., & Callanan, P. (1998). *Issues and ethics in the helping professions.* Pacific Grove, CA: Brooks/Cole.

Kornblau, B. L., & Burkhardt, A. (2012). *Ethics in rehabilitation: A clinical perspective* (2nd ed.). Thorofare, NJ: Slack.

Kyler, P. (2010). Ethical issues in evaluation. In J. Hinojosa, P. Kramer, & P. Crist (Eds.), *Occupational therapy evaluation: Obtaining and interpreting data* (3rd ed., pp. 295–319). Bethesda, MD: AOTA Press.

Lerner, K. L., & Lerner, B. W. (2006). *Medicine health and bioethics: Essential primary sources.* Detroit: Thomson/Gale.

National Bioethics Advisory Commission. (2001). *Research involving human biological materials: Ethical issues and policy guidance.* Rockville, MD: Author.

Purtilo, R., & Doherty, R. F. (2011). *Ethical dimensions in the health professions* (5th ed.). St. Louis, MO: Elsevier.

Purtilo, R., Royeen, C., & Jensen, G. (Eds.). (2005). *Educating for moral action: A sourcebook in health and rehabilitation ethics.* Philadelphia: F. A. Davis.

Romano, J. L. (2011). *Legal rights of the seriously ill and injured: A family guide.* Pittsburgh: Author.

Slater, D. Y. (Ed.). (2011). *Reference guide to the Occupational Therapy Code of Ethics and Ethics Standards* (2010 ed.). Bethesda, MD: AOTA Press.

U.S. Department of Health and Human Services. (2003). *Institutional review boards and the HIPAA privacy rules* (NIH Publication No. 03-5428). Washington, DC: Author. Retrieved from http://privacyruleandresearch.nih.gov/pdf/IRB_Factsheet.pdf

World Federation of Occupational Therapists. (2005). *Code of ethics.* Forrestfield, Western Australia: Author. Retrieved from http://www.wfot.org/ResourceCentre.aspx

WEB SITES

- American Medical Association Ethics Resource Center
  http://www.ama-assn.org/ama/pub/physician-resources/medical-ethics/about-ethics-group/ethics-resource-center.page
- American Occupational Therapy Association (AOTA) ethics resources
  http://www.aota.org/Consumers/Ethics.aspx
- AOTA evidence-based practice and research resources
  http://www.aota.org/ebp
- AOTA Professional Development Tool
  http://www.aota.org/Practitioners/ProfDev/PDT.aspx
- Applied Ethics Resources on WWW
  http://www.ethicsweb.ca/resources/
- Clinical Ethics Resource
  http://clinicalethics.info/
- Globethics.net
  http://www.globethics.net/

- Hastings Center
  http://www.thehastingscenter.org/
- Institutional Review Boards
  http://www.hhs.gov/ohrp/assurances/irb/index.html
- International Center for Academic Integrity
  http://www.academicintegrity.org/icai/home.php
- Kennedy Institute of Ethics
  http://kennedyinstitute.georgetown.edu
- National Board for Certification in Occupational Therapy (NBCOT) *Certification Examination Handbook*
  http://www.nbcot.org/pdf/Cert-Exam-Handbook.pdf
- NBCOT certification renewal
  http://www.nbcot.org/index.php?option=com_content&view=article&id=48&Itemid=9
- NBCOT Professional Development Log
  http://www.nbcot.org/index.php?option=com_content&view=article&id=62&Itemid=2
- National Center for Ethics in Health Care
  http://www.ethics.va.gov/
- World Federation of Occupational Therapists (WFOT)
  http://www.wfot.org/SearchResults.aspx?Search=ethics

Index

Note: Pages numbers in italics indicate figures, tables, and boxes.

academic dishonesty
  case studies, 209–212
  understanding, 207–209
  see also higher education
academic settings
  Fidelity, 99–100
  health promotion and wellness, 162
  Nonmaleficence, 48–50, 52–53
  Procedural Justice, 83–84
accreditation, definition, xix
Accreditation Council for Occupational Therapy
    Education (ACOTE)
  accreditation standards, 206–207
  standards for addressing ethical conflicts, *207*
  standards related to health promotion and
      community-based practice, *163*
  see also health promotion and wellness
accreditation for institutions, 243–244
acute care hospitals, Beneficence, 41–42
aging in place, 140–143
  see also productive aging
aging-in-place clients, productive aging, 141–142
altruism, xix
  see also Core Values and Attitudes of Occupa-
      tional Therapy Practice
American Counseling Association (ACA), 66, 80,
    182
  see also disability
American Journal of Occupational Therapy (AJOT),
    217, 218
American Nurses Association, *80*
American Physical Therapy Association, 66, 80
American Psychological Association, 67, 80

American Speech–Language–Hearing Association,
    67, 80
Americans With Disabilities Act (ADA), 182
  see also disability
ancient world, ethics in, 6–8
AOTA
  disciplinary actions, 23, 24–25
  oversight of ethical practice, 22, 23, 24–25, 26
Asian immigrants, Social Justice, 72–73
assessments, appropriate use of, 41
  see also evidence-based practice
assistive technology, Autonomy and Confidentiality, 61
asylum reform, 10–12
attribution
  definition, xix
  and Veracity, 93–95
autism, 152–153
Autonomy and Confidentiality
  excerpt from Code and Ethics Standards, 55–56
  case studies, 57–58, 60–61, 182–183, 185–186
  children and youth, 151, 154–155
  and collaboration, 62
  and communication, 58–61
  consent, 61–62
  definition of Autonomy, xix
  definition of Confidentiality, 56, xx
  health promotion and wellness, 164
  institutions, 252–253
  private practice, 199
  vignettes, 57, 61, 62

Basic Principles of Occupational Therapy (1919), 15
Belmont Report, 222

Beneficence
    excerpt from Code and Ethics Standards, 37–38
    case studies, 40, 41–42
    children and youth, 150–153, *150*
    definition, xix
    health promotion and wellness, 161–162
    institutions, 251–252
    private practice, 198
    through competence, 38–40
    through evidence-based practice, 40–42
    vignettes, 39
bioethics, definition, xix
Board of Certification for the Athletic Trainer, *80*
boundaries (professional), definition, xix
bullying, 233–236
business ethics, 245–246, 252

care ethics, definition, xix
Centennial Vision, 165, 216
cerebrovascular accident patients
    Autonomy and Confidentiality, 182–183
    ethical dilemmas, 113–114
    productive aging, 142–143
certification, xix–xx, 23–25, 26, 285–286
children and youth
    and autism, 152–153
    Autonomy and Confidentiality, 61, *151*, 154–155
    Beneficence, 150–153, *150*
    and Down syndrome, 153–154
    Fidelity, *152*, 158
    legal compliance, 244–245
    Nonmaleficence, *151*
    outpatient facilities, 156–157
    Procedural Justice, 84–85, *152*, 156–157
    and seizure disorders, 154–155
    Social Justice, *151*, 155
    Veracity, *152*, 157–158
    vignettes, 152–158
clinical trials, 225
clubhouse model, 130–131
    see also mental health practice
Code and Ethics Standards
    full text, 255–263
    comparison to past codes, *17–19*
    development of, 19–21
    enforcement procedures, 265–276
    revisions, 16–19, *17–19*
    Social Justice in, 69
    vignettes describing breaches, *150–151*
code of ethics, xx
collaboration, and Autonomy and Confidentiality, 62
colleague, xx
Commission on Practice (COP), role of, 20

Commission on Standards and Ethics (SEC), role of, 20
communication
    and Autonomy and Confidentiality, 58–61
    with the public, 88–91
    see also Veracity
community centers, Autonomy and Confidentiality, 60–61
community fall prevention programs, health promotion and wellness, 166
community settings
    ethics in, 131
    Fidelity, 101–102
    productive aging, 140, 141–142
    Social Justice, 69, 72–73
community-based practice
    Autonomy and Confidentiality, 61
    Beneficence, 39
    see also mental health practice
compensatory justice, xxi
competence
    Beneficence through, 38–40
    definition, xx
    ensuring, 116
    in mental health practice, 124–125
conflict of commitment, xx
conflict of interest, xx
conflicts
    case studies, 183–184
    duality of interest, 248–250
    prevention of, 101–102
    see also Fidelity
consent
    Autonomy and Confidentiality, 61–62
    definition, xx
    see also Autonomy and Confidentiality
consumer-run nonprofit settings, ethics in, 133
continuing competence requirements, 293–298
Core Values and Attitudes of Occupational Therapy Practice (AOTA)
    description of, *21*
    development of, 20–21, *21*
    structure of, 21–22
county hospitals, 232–233
credentials
    definition, xx
    and Procedural Justice, 79–81, *82*
cultural competence, xx

decision making
    models for, 109–112, *110*, *111*
    process, 112–116
    in work and industry, 172–175
deontology, xx

dignity, xx
  see also Core Values and Attitudes of Occupational Therapy Practice
disability
  case studies, 182–186
  definitions, 178–181
  disability model, 179
  empowerment model, 179
  ethical dilemmas, 180
  medical model, 178
  moral model, 178
  occupational therapy model, 179
  policies, 181–182
  rehabilitation model, 178–179
  rights model, 179–180
  social model, 179
  tragedy/charity models, 178
  see also participation; rehabilitation
disaster survivors, Social Justice, 73
discharge planning, 144–145
  see also productive aging
disciplinary actions
  AOTA enforcement procedures, 22, *23*, *24–25*, *26*, 265–276
  jurisdiction, 27, *29*
  National Board for Certification in Occupational Therapy (NBCOT), *26*
  reporting on, 28–30
  state regulatory boards (SRBs), *26*, *27*
discrimination, 233
  see also institutions
distance teaching, Nonmaleficence, 52
distributive justice
  definition, xxi
  see also Social Justice
documentation, and Veracity, 91–93
Down syndrome, 153–154
duplicate data publications, 226
  see also research
duty, xx

early intervention settings
  children and youth, 152–154
  external relationships, 244–245
EBM (evidence-based medicine), 217–221, *219*, *220*
  see also research
EC (Ethics Commission), 22, 265–276
education requirements, 285–286
education system issues, 243
  see also institutions
employee, xx
employee relationships, Nonmaleficence, 47–48
empowerment model, 179
  see also disability

end-of-life care, 145–146
  see also productive aging
The Enlightenment, 9–12
equality, xx
  see also Core Values and Attitudes of Occupational Therapy Practice
ethical decision making
  private practice, 200–202
  in work and industry, 172–175
ethical dilemmas
  case studies, 113–116
  definition, 109, xx
  disability, 180
  prevention of, 202
  private practice, 197–200
  in productive aging, 140–146
  three-step model for evaluating, 109–112, *110*, *111*
ethics
  business ethics, 252
  definition, 5, xx
  historical context, 6–12, *6*
  in mental health practice, 124–133
  in private practice, 190–196
  and research, 222–225
  resources, 299–300
Ethics Commission (EC), 22, 265–276
evidence-based medicine (EBM), 217–221, *219*, *220*
  see also research
evidence-based practice
  Beneficence through, 40–42
  definition, xx
exploitation, avoidance of, 46–48
  see also Nonmaleficence

facility settings
  Fidelity, 100
  Procedural Justice, 83
families, professional morality, 191–192
Fidelity
  excerpt from Code and Ethics Standards, 97–98
  case studies, 100–102
  children and youth, *152*, 158
  definition, xx
  health promotion and wellness, 166–167
  prevention and analysis of potential ethical breaches, 100–101
  prevention of conflicts, 101–102
  private practice, 200
  and respect, 99–100
  stewardship of resources, 102–104
  vignettes, 99–100, 102–104
fiduciary
  definition, 98, xxi
  historical context, 98–99

fieldwork students
  and ethics, 211–212
  Procedural Justice, 84–85
fraud, xxi
freedom, xxi
  see also Core Values and Attitudes of Occupational Therapy Practice

gifts, 250
golden rule, 6–7
government agencies, 246–248
  see also institutions
groupthink, 231
guidelines, xxi

hand therapy clients, professional morality, 193
harm
  avoidance of, 50–52, 153–154
  prevention of, 48
  see also Nonmaleficence
health care system issues, 242–243
  see also institutions
health promotion and wellness
  Autonomy and Confidentiality, 164
  Beneficence, 161–162
  case studies, 162, 164–165
  definition, 161
  Fidelity, 166–167
  Nonmaleficence, 162–163
  Procedural Justice, 165–166, *165, 166*
  Social Justice, 165
  Veracity, 166
  vignettes, 166–167
higher education
  academic dishonesty, 207–209
  accreditation standards, *207*
  case studies, 209–212
  cheating in, 205–206
  ethics in, 209–211, 212
higher education settings, health promotion and
    wellness, 166–167
Hippocratic Oath, 7, 8
Hispanic clients, Autonomy and Confidentiality, 60–61
home care settings
  Beneficence, 40
  children and youth, 158
  productive aging, 142–143
hospice, 145–146
  see also productive aging
hospital settings
  ethical dilemmas, 113–115
  ethics in, 128–129

Fidelity, 102–104
  gifts, 250–251
  health promotion and wellness, 164–165
  internal relationships, 232–233
  mobbing in, 236–238
  Nonmaleficence, 47–48
  Procedural Justice, 81–83
  productive aging, 144–145
  and research, 225

individuals with developmental disabilities, Procedural Justice, 83
infants and toddlers. *See* children and youth
injured workers, 169–172
inpatient services, 70, 128
  see also mental health practice
institutional care, 143–144
  see also productive aging
Institutional Review Board (IRB), 229–230
institutions
  accreditation for, 243–244
  Autonomy and Confidentiality, 252–253
  Beneficence, 251–252
  bullying, 233–236
  case studies, 233, 235–238, 244–248, 249–252
  discrimination, 233
  duality of interest, 248–250
  education system issues, 243
  external relationships, 241–253
  government agencies, 246–248
  health care system issues, 242–243
  internal relationships, 231–238
  legal compliance, 244–245
  Nonmaleficence, 251–252
  sabotaging and mobbing, 236–238
  use of term, 231
  vignettes, 232–233, 252
International Center for Clubhouse Development
    (ICCD), 130–131

jurisdiction, xxi, 27, 29, xxi, 265–276
jurisprudence, xxi
jurisprudence exam, xxi
justice, xxi
  see also Core Values and Attitudes of Occupational Therapy Practice

lack of inclusion, 233
  see also institutions
large outpatient clinics, bullying, 235–236
law, definition, xxi
leisure settings, Social Justice, 69

Level II fieldwork students, productive aging, 144–145
liability, xxi
licensure, xxi
long-term care settings, Veracity, 89–90

manufacturing companies, 185–186
medical model, 178
  see also disability
medieval guilds, 9, *10*
mental health practice
  case studies, 128–129, 132–133
  community-based practice, 130–131
  competence in, 124–125
  consumer-run organizations, 133
  current settings, 123–124
  ethics in, 124–133
  inpatient services, 128
  partial hospitalization programs, 129
  private practice, 132–133
  and reimbursement, 125–126
  scope of practice, 126–127
  service delivery models, 127–128
  supervision in, 124–125
  and therapeutic relationships, 127
  vignettes, 129–130, 131, 133
mental health settings, ethics in, 131
mindfulness, to avoid harm, 50–52
moral courage, 89–90, xxi
  see also Veracity
moral distress, xxi
moral model, 178
  see also disability
moral treatment, 10–12, xxi
morality, 190–191, xxi
  see also ethics
MyPlate, *166*
  see also health promotion and wellness
MyPyramid, *165*
  see also health promotion and wellness

National Association of Social Workers, 67, *81*
National Board for Certification in Occupational Therapy (NBCOT)
  code of conduct, 285–286
  disciplinary actions, *26*
  formation of, 26
Nonmaleficence
  excerpt from Code and Ethics Standards, 45–46
  avoidance of exploitation, 46–48
  avoidance of harm, 153–154
  case studies, 47–48, 51

children and youth, *151*, 153–154
definition, xxi
health promotion and wellness, 162–163
institutions, 251–252
prevention of harm, 48
private practice, 198–199
self-care, 52–53
vignettes, 48–53
  see also harm
not-for-profit teaching hospitals, Veracity, 92–93
Nuremberg trials, 222, 229
Nurses' Ethical Reasoning Skills (NERS) model, 111

occupational potential, definition, 98
occupational therapy assistant supervision, Procedural Justice, 81–83
occupational therapy assistants, 114–115, 252–253
Occupational Therapy Code of Ethics and Ethics Standards (2010). *See* Code and Ethics Standards
occupational therapy model, 179
  see also disability
occupational therapy practice
  definition, ix, 285–286
  use of term, ix–x
occupational therapy profession, continuing competence requirements, 293–298
occupational therapy students
  academic dishonesty, 209–212
  Procedural Justice, 83–84
older adults
  Autonomy and Confidentiality, 61
  Fidelity, 100–101
  Nonmaleficence, 50
  Procedural Justice, 79–81
  and productive aging, 140–146
  Social Justice, 70–72
  see also productive aging
organizational morality, 194–196
  see also private practice
outpatient facilities
  Beneficence, 251–252
  children and youth, 156–157
  ethical dilemmas, 116
  Nonmaleficence, 251–252
  service delivery, 184–185
  Social Justice, 70–72
  Veracity, 90–91
oversight, definition, xxi
oversight of ethical practice, 22–30, 27–28, *29*
  AOTA, 22, *23*, 24–25, *26*
  AOTA enforcement procedures, *24–25*
  state regulatory boards (SRBs), 25–27, *26*, *27*

parent programs, health promotion and wellness,
164–165
partial hospitalization programs (PHPs), 128–129
see also mental health practice
participation
case studies, 182–186
definition, 177–178
see also disability; rehabilitation
paternalism, xxi
pediatric inpatient rehabilitation settings, Veracity, 91
personal morality, 191–192, *192*
see also private practice
plagiarism, 226, xxii
see also research
privacy, right to, 113–114
private practice
Autonomy and Confidentiality, 199
Beneficence, 39, 198
case studies, 193, 195
ethical decision making, 200–202
ethical dilemmas, 197–200
ethics in, 190–196
Fidelity, 200
legal and regulatory issues, 196–197, *197*
mental health, 132–133
Nonmaleficence, 198–199
Procedural Justice, 199–200
Social Justice, 199
Veracity, 89–90, 200
vignettes, 191–192
see also mental health practice
private practice settings
children and youth, 155
ethics in, 132–133
external relationships, 247–248
personal morality, 191–192
Procedural Justice, 84–85
professional morality, 191–192
Procedural Justice
excerpt from Code and Ethics Standards, 77–78
case studies, 79–81
children and youth, *152*, 156–157
credentials, 79–81, *82*
current knowledge of regulations, 81–83
definition, xxi, xxii
financial and business relationships, 84–85
health promotion and wellness, 165–166, *165*, *166*
policies and procedures to ensure ethical practice,
83–84
private practice, 199–200
vignettes, 81–85

productive aging
case studies, 141–143
demographic trends, 139–140
discharge planning, 144–145
end-of-life care, 145–146
ethical dilemmas in service delivery, 140–146
hospice, 145–146
institutional care, 143–144
role of OT, 137–139
use of term, 137
vignettes, 140, 144–146
see also older adults
Professional and Technical Role Analysis (PATRA),
20
professional associations
decision-making models, 109–112, *110*, *111*
Nonmaleficence, 51–52
policies relevant to Procedural Justice, *80–81*
professional boundaries, protecting, 114–115
professional conferences
Nonmaleficence, 52
Veracity, 95
professional morality, 192–194, *194*
see also private practice
professional relationships, use of term, 98
prudence, xxii
see also Core Values and Attitudes of Occupational Therapy Practice
public
communication with, 88–91
definition, xxii
Public Hospital for Persons of Insane and Disordered
Minds, *11*
public restaurants, Autonomy and Confidentiality,
57–58
publication of research, 225–227

randomized controlled trials (RCTs), 217–221
see also research
regulation, xxii
rehabilitation
case studies, 182–186
definition, 181
see also disability; participation
rehabilitation facilities, 211–212, 249–250
rehabilitation model, 178–179
see also disability
reimbursement, 125–126
relationships among professionals, bullying, 235–236
religion, 6–8
Representative Assembly, role of, 20

research
  American Journal of Occupational Therapy (AJOT), 217, *218*
  design and conduct of, 221–225
  and ethics, 222–223
  importance to profession, 216–221, *218, 219, 220*
  and publishing, 225–227
  randomized controlled trials (RCTs), 217–221
  vignettes, 225
  see also evidence-based medicine (EBM)
research participants, xxii
resources, stewardship of, 102–104
  see also Fidelity
respect
  definition, xxii
  and Fidelity, 99–100
return to work
  Procedural Justice, 79–81
  Social Justice, 69
rheumatoid arthritis patients, 184–185
rights, definition, xxii
rights model, 179–180
  see also disability

school settings, 245–246
school-based practice, 154–155, 157–158
scope of practice
  full text, 277–284
  definition, xxii
  domain and practice, 277–284, *280, 281, 282*
  mental health practice, 126–127
seizure disorders, 154–155
self-care, 52–53
  see also Nonmaleficence
self-determination principle. *See* Autonomy and Confidentiality
self-reflection, to avoid harm, 50–52
self-regulation, 192
  see also professional morality
service delivery, and productive aging, 140–146
service delivery models, 127–128
  see also mental health practice
skilled nursing facilities
  conflicts, 183–184
  Fidelity, 100–101
  Nonmaleficence, 50, 51
  productive aging, 144
Slagle, Eleanor Clarke, 15
Social Justice
  excerpt from Code and Ethics Standards, 65–66

case studies, 70–72, 185–186
children and youth, *151, 155*
in the Code and Ethics Standards, 69
definition, xxii
health promotion and wellness, 165
historical links, 68
private practice, 199
in professional associations, *66–67*
securing, 69–73
vignettes, 69, 70, 72–73
social model, 179
  see also disability
Society for Public Health Education, *67, 81*
Socrates, 7, *9*
spinal cord injury patients
  conflicts, 183–184
  gifts, 250–251
  Veracity, 91
stakeholders, xxii
standards, xxii
state regulatory boards (SRBs)
  definition, xxii
  disciplinary actions, *26, 27*
  oversight of ethical practice, 25–27
stewardship, xxii
strong paternalism, xxi
students
  definition, xxii
  and ethics, 209–211
  Fidelity, 100
  Nonmaleficence, 50
subacute care facilities
  Autonomy and Confidentiality, 182–183
  Veracity, 89–90
supervision, in mental health practice, 124–125
supervisory duties, and Procedural Justice, 79–81, *82*

Taoism, 7, *7*
therapeutic relationships, 127
  see also mental health practice
trademark, definition, xxii
tragedy/charity models, 178
  see also disability
traumatic head injury patients
  Confidentiality and Social Justice, 185–186
  duality of interest, 249–250
  Veracity, 91
truth, xxii
  see also Core Values and Attitudes of Occupational Therapy Practice

Veracity
    excerpt from Code and Ethics Standards, 87–88
    and attribution, 93–95
    case studies, 89–93
    children and youth, *152*, 157–158
    communication with the public, 88–91
    definition, xxii
    and documentation, 91–93
    health promotion and wellness, 166
    private practice, 200
    vignettes, 91, 95

weak paternalism, xxi
work and industry
    case studies, 169–172
    ethical decision making in, 172–175
work rehabilitation
    Autonomy and Confidentiality, 57
    injury prevention programs, 169–172

youth. *See* children and youth